Music and Soulmaking

Toward a New Theory of Music Therapy

Barbara J. Crowe

THE SCARECROW PRESS, INC.
Lanham, Maryland • Toronto • Oxford
2004

SCARECROW PRESS, INC.

Published in the United States of America
by Scarecrow Press, Inc.
A wholly owned subsidary of
The Rowman & Littlefield Publishing Group, Inc.
4501 Forbes Boulevard, Suite 200, Lanham, Maryland 20706
www.scarecrowpress.com

PO Box 317
Oxford
OX2 9RU, UK

British Library Cataloguing in Publication Information Available

Library of Congress Cataloging-in-Publication Data

Crowe, Barbara J.
  Music and soulmaking : toward a new theory of music therapy / Barbara J.
Crowe.
    p. cm.
  Includes bibliographical references (p.   ) and index.
  ISBN 0-8108-5143-1 (hardcover : alk. paper)
  1. Music therapy. 2. Music—Psychological aspects. I. Title.
ML3920.C898 2004
615.8'5154—dc22

                                                                  2004010790

∞™ The paper used in this publication meets the minimum requirements of
American National Standard for Information Sciences—Permanence of Paper for
Printed Library Materials, ANSI/NISO Z39.48-1992.
Manufactured in the United States of America.

This book is dedicated to my mother, Jean Menefee Crowe,
and especially to my late father, James A. O. Crowe,
who made me the musician and writer I am today.

And to my beloved husband, Ross Whiteaker, whose unwavering support
and encouragement made this book possible.

~

Contents

~

Acknowledgments

This book constitutes my life's work in music therapy. It is the culmination of my experiences as a musician, a clinician in music therapy, a music therapy educator, a client experiencing music therapy interventions, an academic researcher, and a seeker after spirit and deep personal truth. All the people who contributed to this book are too numerous to mention. I will acknowledge as many as I can.

I first want to thank the people who shaped my love of music and whatever talent I may have. I first must acknowledge my late father, who rocked me to sleep to the glorious contrapuntal complexity of Bach fugues and who took me to my first symphony when I was three years old and my first ballet when I was four. My deep connection to and unabashed love of music comes from him. I am profoundly grateful to my early music teachers—Mrs. Frank, my piano teacher, and Miss Heaton, my first violin teacher—whose strong but caring teaching style has been a model for me throughout my teaching career. And to the conductors I have played under, the peers who challenged me for my chair in the second violin section, my friends whom I played guitar with and sang meaningful songs as an adolescent, I offer my thanks for inspiring me, encouraging me, and pushing me forward in my musical career. I also must acknowledge other, diverse musical influences—Judy Collins, whose deeply felt songs healed me during the dark times of adolescence; The Beatles, for teaching me there was more to music than symphonies and violin concerti; Stevie Wonder, who showed me that "popular" music could also be intricate and complex; Joni Mitchell, who taught me that the message in the lyrics can be intensified by the right music; and so many others.

I have been fortunate to have many mentors and influences in music therapy. I first want to acknowledge the late Robert Unkefer, my first music therapy teacher, for his knowledge, insight, humor, and, most important, loving care. I also want to acknowledge Dr. Charles Eagle for the brilliance of his thinking and the ideas that are the foundation of this book, and Dr. Kenneth Bruscia, Music Therapist–Board Certified (MT-BC), who has taught me more than I can ever express. He is a true mentor. I also want to thank the work and ideas of Dr. Carolyn Kenny, MT-BC, Dr. Even Ruud, Barbara Hesser, MT, Dr. Barbara Wheeler, MT-BC, Francis Goldberg, MT-BC, and Dr. Helen Bonny, MT-BC. From personal conversations to your published ideas, you have all had a profound impact on me. And I particularly want to acknowledge my friend and colleague Barry Bernstein, MT-BC, for broadening my concepts of music therapy and teaching me to drum. Perhaps the greatest influence on me as a practicing music therapist are my clients. To them all, I give my thanks and deepest respect.

I want to thank my colleagues and administrators at Arizona State University (ASU) for their ongoing support in the completion of this book—Dr. Robert Wills, fine arts dean; the School of Music directors during the time I wrote the book, Dr. George Umberson, Dr. Toni-Marie Montgomery, and Dr. Wayne Bailey; and the Arizona State librarians, especially Brian Doherty. My music therapy colleagues have been particularly helpful and supportive—Robin Rio, MT-BC, Jane Price, MT-BC, Sally Niles, MT-BC, and Dalena Watson, MT-BC. I have bounced ideas off them and asked them to take on added responsibility to free me to write, and they have broadened my ideas about our profession. And, in particular, I want to thank my students past and present. My knowledge of music therapy has broadened and deepened during the time I prepared to teach you.

I also want to thank several colleagues from other departments at ASU. My deepest thanks go to Dr. Stephen Helms Tillery, neuroscientist in the ASU Department of Bioengineering, for his invaluable input and assistance with neurophysiology, and to Dr. Ching-Leng Lai, Department of Mathematics, for the computer-generated fractal illustrations. I also want to thank my friend Bill Brauckman, ASU Master of Fine Art, for his wonderful illustrations.

As this book is about complexity and the influence of music on all areas of human functioning, including spirit, I want to thank Dr. Michael Harner and Sandra Ingerman for introducing me to the ancient wisdom tradition of shamanism and the first use of music as a healing tool. I also want to thank a special group of friends for their unique support and contributions to this book—Linda Parsons, Pat Dolan, Ramona Johnson, Debra Chesnut, Paula Klempay, Hib Sabin, Joseph Williams, Steven Farmer, Sara Sifers, Anne Scholder, Marsalee Forrester, Netanya Selman, Dixie Pearson, Kim Erickson, Anne Pym McDonald, and Dean Vusikas.

A number of people read the manuscript at various points in the writing process. Their feedback and input proved to be invaluable—Sarah Sifers, Anne Parker, Stanley Jordan, Robin Rio, Barbara Reuer, Laura Wilkinson, and Andrea Farbman. I especially want to thank my dear friend Karen Stromberg for her professional editing, insightful comments, and important input, and especially my "soul friend" and colleague Tomas Winn, MT-BC, for the long talks, challenges, and fearless criticism of the book in all stages of its development.

I am grateful to my editor Bruce Phillips and the staff at Scarecrow Press for their time and invaluable input. As a first-time author, I could not have completed this project without them. I particularly want to thank Bruce Phillips for the willingness and courage to publish a book that didn't fit neatly into any publishing category.

During the entire process of writing this book, I wrote to a soundtrack of the rich, complex classical music of Romantic and twentieth-century composers. I want to acknowledge these composers whose music provided a fertile envelope for my creative process—Beethoven, Schumann, Brahms, Dvorak, Wagner, Vaughn Williams, Faure, Ravel, Bruch, Holst, Mendelssohn, Tchaikovsky, Barber, Massenet, Mahler, Respighi, Rachmaninov, Schubert, and Hovhaness. Thanks for the music.

~

Introduction

The air was full of music. So full it seemed there was room for nothing else. And each particle of air seemed to have its own music, so that as Richard moved his head he heard a new and different music, though the new and different music fitted quite perfectly with the music that lay beside it in the air. . . . He knew he had been listening to the music of life itself. The music of light dancing on water that rippled with the wind and the tides, of the life that moved through the water, of the life that moved on the land, warmed by the light. . . . "Such music," he said. "I'm not religious, but if I were I would say it was like a glimpse into the mind of God."

—Douglas Adams, *Dirk Gently's Holistic Detective Agency*

Music is humankind's greatest joy and biggest mystery. This book is about music's ability to touch people in deep, profound ways. It is about using music for healing and particularly the planned intervention of therapy. It is also about music's impact on the four levels of human functioning—mind, emotion, body, and spirit. Using music to affect human functioning is not a simple process. It is, in fact, very complicated. This book, then, is really about complexity—of sound and music, of human functioning, and of disease and health. The book, too, will be complex, touching on many subjects to make two basic points: first that music is a powerful tool for healing and, second, that it is a source of human knowledge and understanding. In exploring the complex interaction of music and human functioning and acknowledging the limits of the current, empirical scientific model, especially in health care, the book explores the new scientific breakthrough of complexity science. It challenges our assumptions of how our world works and how healing occurs. The book examines how music affects all aspects of human functioning—mind, body, emotion, and spirit. Based on this total involvement, a new theory for music healing—"music and soulmaking"—is developed. The book makes a case for how this new theory can lead into a new paradigm of health and healing based on understanding the natural world's complexity and essential wholeness.

I am a *music therapist* by profession and training. I hold degrees and credentials in *music therapy*, an established health care profession using music as the basis of the therapeutic interaction. Music therapy is the systematic use of music by a trained professional to achieve individual therapeutic goals for a wide variety of clients. When I talk about music therapy or the effects of music therapy throughout this book, I am referring to the impact of both the music itself and the trained music therapist. Music therapy emerges from the unique situation of a specially trained individual using music, particularly live music making, to positively impact client functioning. In my thirty years as a practicing music therapist, I have seen music affect people in amazing ways. I have worked with clients of all ages and disabilities—eighty-year-old clients with Alzheimer's disease, adolescents who are depressed and suicidal, year-old children with Down syndrome, patients in oncology units of hospitals, adults with traumatic brain injury, and schoolchildren at risk for gang involvement. The systematic uses of music therapy interventions have positively affected them all. I would call these responses miracles if I did not understand some of the mechanisms involved. But I do know why an agitated, confused patient with Alzheimer's disease can focus his or her attention and smile when singing a familiar song. I understand how a child with cognitive delay can learn to count by playing a musical game. I know the neurological processes involved when a stroke victim relearns to walk faster and better with rhythmic music.

Since the formal establishment of the profession of music therapy in 1950, four questions are routinely asked: Is music an effective therapy? How does music affect functioning? Why does music help achieve such a diverse body of goals for so many different types of clients? What explains the effectiveness of music for therapy? This book is an attempt to answer these questions and formulate a philosophy of music therapy. A philosophy tries to form a correct representation of the world—in this case, the world of music therapy. The book endeavors to explain the music therapy "world" by exploring the impact of music on all aspects of human functioning. But as Abram (1996) notes, "To explain is not to present a set of finished reasons, but to tell a story" (p. 265). In telling the story of music as therapy, information and in-sights from many disciplines—physics, biology, chemistry, neuroscience, psy-chology, sociology, musicology, acoustics, psychoacoustics, cognitive sci-ences, education, wisdom and spiritual traditions, and the new sciences of quantum physics and especially *complexity science*, the new physics science of the macro-world—are utilized. Theories from all these disciplines are needed to deal with the immense complexity of human functioning. Any one theory may be necessary yet insufficient to explain a phenomenon (Edelman, 1992).

The place to begin an explanation of music therapy's impact on human functioning is with the information gathered from the methods and proce-dures of current, empirical scientific research. The profession of music ther-apy has done this since its inception. Much information has been gained from the quantitative and qualitative research that has been conducted over the fifty-year history of the music therapy profession, which is summarized throughout the book. However, I am increasingly frustrated with the ability of current science alone to satisfactorily explain the results I see from music therapy interventions. As a practicing music therapist, I see the affect of a music therapy intervention on a client. It is clear to me that the music ther-apy interventions make a positive, beneficial difference to the client and the client's functioning. In an effort to "prove" that music therapy "works," I em-barked on a research project. As required by scientific method, I set a hy-pothesis and designed the research protocols controlling all variables except the music or aspect of music I thought was "causing" the positive therapeu-tic change. Yet time and again, I got "no significant results" as determined by inferential statistics. The research actually "proves" that what I observed, had known deeply and absolutely through my experience of the effects of the music therapy, was wrong. Can my experience be that inaccurate? Am I de-luding myself? What about the agitated client with Alzheimer's disease who talked and smiled during a rhythm-based music therapy activity? What about the child with severe disabilities who showed her first and only response to the environment through music? How could these results and countless oth-ers not really exist?

It became clear to me that the tool for researching the complex, intricate processes involved in music therapy, the empirical, scientific method, was neither appropriate nor adequate. An empirical approach does not take into account the interaction of the various facets of human functioning. As Den-nis Fry (1971) observes,

> In the case of music there is also continuously interaction between the physical
> character of the musical stimulus and its physiological and psychological effects

so that a more thorough study of music would demand at least the combining of a physical, physiological and psychological approach. Modern science has relatively little information about the links between physics, physiology and psychology and is certainly not in a position to specify how the effects are related in music, but most scientists would recognize here a gap in scientific knowledge and would not want to deny the fact of a connection. (quoted in Aldridge, 1996, p. 23)

Even utilizing the current approach, there are clearly gaps and deficiencies that prevent these methods from substantiating the impact of music therapy interventions. But the empirical method also leaves out a large body of human experience, particularly subjective experiences. "Human beings are complex organisms. We are not merely objects that can be reduced to one or two dimensions and be explained in deterministic terms. What makes us unique as a species is our subjectivity—and the ability to experience ourselves as subjects. The challenge of the human condition, then, is to fully grasp the complexity of subjective experience" (Bruscia, 1995, p. 196). Empirical science does not do this for us.

There is nothing wrong with the empirical approach. It brings us a wealth of knowledge. It just is not the complete picture. As Wilber (1996) writes, ". . . I in no way deny the general importance of empirical representation. It's just not the whole story; its not even the most interesting part of the story" (p. 107). In exploring the processes and effects of music therapy, I found that the empirical method is definitely not the whole story. So I began a search for a scientific paradigm that "fit better" with what I experienced and observed in music therapy. I found that paradigm in *complexity science*, the science of complex systems in motion.

Complexity science, with its emphasis on chaos theory, is a newly developed scientific paradigm related to systems theory. It is the science of the global nature of *dynamical systems*—systems in motion. Complexity science recognizes basic underlying interrelatedness and interdependency of the various parts of a whole system (deQuincey, 2002). It focuses on hidden patterns, nuances, and the extreme sensitivity of real things. Complexity science asserts that *everything* in nature is complex—from weather systems to economic trends, to population growth, to the formation of mountains and rivers, to the functioning of the human body, to health and disease. This complexity also includes the functioning of the human mind and its products, like consciousness and music, and, as I assert, the interaction of music and human functioning seen in music therapy. Nature, then, is recognized as a highly complex, interlocking network of nested, dynamical systems. Dynamical systems are nonlinear in nature—the whole is greater than the sum of the parts. Things do not necessarily add up, and small things can and do have a huge impact. Because dynamical systems are systems in motion, complexity science is the science of the real, practical, messy world. "Relationships between 'parts' are dynamic, ever-changing, because they involve complex networks of feedback and feedforward loops. It becomes difficult, if not meaningless, to identify or isolate individual causes. . . . Such nonlinear evolution means it is impossible to accurately predict the behavior of complex systems . . ." (deQuincey, 2002, pp. 30–31). Dynamical systems are simultaneously stable and ever changing. They are in a constant state of renewal and change. Complexity science establishes the "rules" or constants for how the seemingly unpredictable leads to the new (Briggs & Peat, 1999). Dynamical systems must be considered in their wholeness. They cannot be cut up and reduced to constituent parts. To do so is to destroy the system.

In complexity science, I found a scientific paradigm that fits what I observe in music therapy. Music as therapy, like music itself, is more than the sum of its parts. We can gain some understanding, some reasons how and why music can be therapeutic, but reducing this process to only small, measurable effects does not explain what is really happening. Music therapy must be looked at as a whole process in all its frustrating, beautiful complexity.

As I explored complexity science and applied its principles to the processes inherent in music therapy, I formed a theory of music therapy I call "music and soulmaking." Throughout the book, I move through the steps that brought me to this theory. Music and soulmaking looks at human functioning in its wholeness. For the purposes of this theory, soul is what is most genuine and unique in each of us. It is our unique experience of being in its totality. Soul includes the full range and depth of the human being. Soul ". . . is the experiencer and the site of experience. It not only experiences and feels itself, but it is also responsive and alive. . . . The soul is you that is living, experiencing, thinking, feeling, responding. . . . It is a unified, total wholeness that is alive and energetic, that feels and acts as a unit" (Almaas quoted in Davis, 1999, p. 54). Soul is our experience of ourselves, and, as such, it is dynamic, malleable, and ever growing and changing. The soul learns and grows through the experiences of our lives. It is manifested through body, mind, emotion, and spirit.

Soulmaking as therapy provides experiences in all areas of human functioning to foster a more complete way of being in the world. As Davis (1999) notes, soulmaking is living ". . . more fully in our bodies, becoming more available and honest in our relationships, healing unresolved traumas, removing the barriers to fulfillment in our work lives, engaging our life transitions with confidence and openness, as well as meditation, contemplation and inquiry [as] important aspects of awakening the soul to its possibilities" (p. 49). This is the process of becoming whole, the true definition of health, and the ultimate goal of any therapeutic intervention. The theory of music and soulmaking is based on the contention that music is a fundamental, holistic experience that impacts functioning in all areas—body, mind, emotion, and spirit. As such, it provides the opportunity for soulmaking.

In chapter 1, "Music in Therapy and Healing," the journey to understand how music affects health begins by looking at the history of music in human cultures. Human civilizations have used music as a source of knowledge, in the worship of the Divine, and as a form of healing. Then the modern profession of music therapy is introduced. Current music therapy practice is a well-established professional discipline serving a wide variety of clients—children with autism, patients with Alzheimer's disease, persons experiencing depression, and more. It was developed as a behavioral science, and a fifty-year history of research literature and clinical practice has established the effectiveness of music therapy interventions. Music therapy is defined, and an overview of the various interventions used with clients is presented.

In chapter 2, "Complexity Science: A New Scientific Paradigm," the scientific paradigm of complexity science is introduced. Complexity science is the science of the real world and challenges the assumptions of current empirical scientific method. Of particular importance are the principles of complexity science in living systems. Factors of complexity science like nonlinearity, fractal structures and fractal time, and self-organization are all observed in living systems, including human anatomy and physiology. All biological life is a special kind of self-organization known as complex adaptive systems. Such systems are adaptive because they are in a constant state of flux and change to maintain optimum vigor. This process is known as autopoiesis. Additionally, complex adaptive systems are recursively organized—they have systems embedded within systems. Each level of the system is a prerequisite for the formation of the next level, and each is enfolded into the next level. Every level is important in its own right. Input or change on any level of organization changes the whole system. The influence can move from the bottom up (change in DNA changes molecules) or from the top down (consciousness changes DNA). This makes the potential influence of music therapy great, as music can affect human functioning on all levels of this recursive organization.

Chapter 3, "Of Sound and Music," explores the complexity of music itself and its impact on human functioning. To understand music, sound—the perception of physical vibration—must first be understood. Sound vibration is a complex mechanical energy involving frequency, amplitude, resonance, and duration. Human perception of sound is also a complex process. The human ear collects and changes vibrational energy into electrochemical impulses. Chapter 3 continues with a discussion of music. Music is the organization of sound and silence for human expression. Put in another way, music is sound meeting human consciousness (Hughes, 1948). Defining music is approached by asking four questions: What is the experience of music? What are the origins of music? What purpose does music serve? And what behaviors constitute music?

The experience of music is an acoustical event combining the building blocks of music—rhythm, melody, harmony, timbre, and form. The origins of music are theorized as a biological adaptation, an aspect of human consciousness, and a cultural device. Many authors have speculated about the purposes of music. They include pleasure, aesthetic response, support to humanity, touching the Divine, communication, effect on activity level, and support for human culture.

The last question, on the behaviors that constitute music, is important since music therapy practice involves much more than listening to music. It also involves musical performance, improvisation, and composition. When music is used for therapy, the client actually makes music or responds in some physical way. This adds a layer of complexity, since even simple musical performance is a skilled motor behavior (Wilson, 1986). This motor behavior uses many fine motor skills and activates more of the brain than any other single activity. Music is itself a complex, dynamical system. It meets the criteria for a dynamical system, including sensitivity to initial conditions, use of iterative feedback, action of attractors, emergent properties, wholeness, and nonlinearity. Music can be defined as a self-organizing stream of energetic information. Human interaction with music just may be the most complex dynamical system known.

In chapter 4, "Music Therapy and Problems of Brain and Mind," the various aspects of the mind beginning with a review of brain anatomy are explored. Because of their importance to an understanding of music therapy practice and its impact on clients, a review of the brain and nervous system structures involved in perception of sound and in motor coordination is undertaken. As with any complex system, however, examining the parts does not provide a true sense of how the brain functions. The vast connections and recursive organization of the brain are "sculpted" by our experience with the world around us. Our experiences of sound and music are an important part of brain development, since a fetus in utero can perceive sound by age five and a half months. Our experience of sound, especially music, is an important sensory experience with the world around us. Research has shown that brain functioning, especially higher brain functioning, is musical in nature (Leng & Shaw, 1991). It is also nonlinear in its processing, making the brain a dynamical system. Brain processes show fractal time variations, like the 1/f spectrum. This fractal time is the spectrum most commonly seen in nature. Music has 1/f spectrum time intervals in many aspects, making musical input a potentially useful tool in influencing neurological function and the products of that functioning—aspects of mind. The chapter concludes with an overview of the impact of music on aspects of mind—sensation, perception, discrimination, concept development, cognition and higher brain function, behavior, motivation and drives, learning and memory, intelligence, creativity and imagery, speech and language, and consciousness. Music therapy practice in work with problems in all these areas of mind are also reviewed.

Our discovery journey continues in chapter 5, "Music Therapy and Problems of the Body," by studying music's impact on the physical body. The *content* of medical interventions—some agent or action that alleviates or remediates dysfunction—is first addressed. The content of healing provided by traditional Western medicine addresses the physical body primarily from a chemistry perspective. Chemical and, to some extent, structural interventions have been the focus of content of treatment for the body. These interventions include surgery, chemotherapy, medication, and now gene therapy. First, medical music therapy is explored by overviewing the use of music in the content of healing—impact on physical aspects, interface with the essential rhythm of physical functioning, and vibrotactile stimulation. However, there are other processes occurring in the body that have been recognized by non-Western medicine for centuries and are now increasingly recognized by Western medical practice. These include energetic systems in the body and the use of energy medicine, the mind–body connection and the link of emotion and immune system functioning, and the nonlinear, edge-of-chaos dynamics of typical optimum vigor. The *context* of healing—the external and internal environment conducive to recovery and health—is then addressed.

In chapter 6, "Music Therapy and Problems of Emotion and Feeling," our journey into the complexity of music therapy process continues by exploring the close relationship of music and emotion and feeling. Expression of emotion through sound is a primal, biological function that humans share with all primates (Wallin, 1991). Controlled by the limbic system of the midbrain, we perceive and express emotional states through sound tone and timbre. Music is an emotional art directly touching and communicating emotions and feelings (emotions with memory) that cannot be expressed in words. This chapter addresses the issues of human psychology—the study of human nature. Psychology deals with the mental structure of a person, especially as a motivating force. This study goes beyond the properties and faculties of mind into the human psyche's relationship, not only to biology and the environment but to the particularly human interactions of culture and society. It also addresses the problems that can arise in this area—mental illness. This chapter addresses psychological growth, consciousness development, and the problems of feeling, mood, and temperament and how music therapy practice can have an effect in these areas. It also looks at psychiatric music therapy and the various ways it can help in the treatment of mental illness.

Chapter 7, "Music Therapy and Problems of Spirit," looks at issues of human spirit as another factor in health and healing. Music and spirit have always been closely linked. The human spirit needs vitality, playfulness, and belonging. Music embodies this spirit, inspiring us to sing, dance, play, laugh, and cry for joy. Music is socially acceptable play for children and adults alike. However, human spirit is best expressed and enhanced through relationships with other people. Music is a natural social event. It gives us a reason for being together and makes it easier to interact with others (Gaston, 1968a). Music's strong rhythmic element creates an actual physical entrainment among people—a synchronization of brain waves and movement patterns. It helps us feel that we belong. Spirit also means moving past our own egos and personal dramas to experience wholeness and unity with the life force. Music has been used for millennia to evoke these transpersonal and transformative experiences. Music touches the Divine. In our culture, we often experience this in aesthetic reaction or "peak experience" when listening to music. We get goose bumps and are completely captivated by the experience. Music Therapy practice relating to spirit involves relationships to others and the need for affiliation, play, quality of life, ritual, deeply transformative experiences through altered states of consciousness and integrative consciousness, and relation to the Divine source.

The book concludes in chapter 8, "Toward a New Theory of Music and Healing," with the new model for music and healing—music and soulmaking. For the purpose of this theory, soul is defined as a quality of human functioning: the essence of being that makes each of us unique. It reflects our true nature, separate from individual self. Soul and music are related because they are one and the same process. Music and soulmaking, then, is an ongoing process of health in mind, emotion, body, and spirit, with music as a fundamental force in maintaining a harmonious relationship among all these elements of functioning. It is a dynamic process of right relationship of all aspects of functioning. Health, like all functioning in living systems, is a dynamical system in motion. It is all aspects of functioning poised at the edge of chaos—the place of optimum vigor and adaptability. Music therapy interventions infuse the human system with complexity, information, that keeps it at the edge of chaos and in the right balance of all aspects of functioning. This perspective changes how music therapists work and do research.

Investigating music as complexity will expand all human knowledge including health and healing methods. Throughout history, the study of music has served to expand our knowledge. Science as we know it grew from an intense study of music by the Greek mathematician Pythagoras (Levenson, 1994). As we push into the new science of complexity and chaos, a close study of music will reveal much. Music will again lead us to new understanding, knowledge, and wisdom.

Music and Soulmaking is about music in all its forms—from popular songs to opera, from bluegrass fiddle tunes to classical symphonies, from rock and roll to lullabies, from country ballads to Indian ragas. A music therapist uses any and all music that motivates client participation and meets the therapeutic needs. The book focuses on the music itself. The lyrics of songs are not considered, though they add another wonderful layer of complexity to music. This book does not make judgments about what music is "good" for us or "inappropriate." When the complexity of human participation in music is understood, there will be no claims for absolutes in music therapy and healing. There are no special tones or timbres, no scales or tuning systems, and no instruments or sound devices that intrinsically heal. The process is too complex to make predictions and simplified prescriptions of music.

I have loved music since I was a small child and believe fervently in its power to effect change, to "heal." I have spent most of my adult life discovering how and why it is an effective tool for therapy. I hope this book will excite interest in the potential of music to heal, to positively affect our lives, and to expand our knowledge. I hope it will generate a new appreciation for music and how it can benefit everyone in wide-ranging ways.

~

CHAPTER ONE

Music in Therapy and Healing

Becky's mother arrives at the Arizona State University Music Therapy Clinic with her three-year-old severely handicapped daughter in her arms. Becky has athetoid cerebral palsy and is cortically blind, probably deaf, and nonverbal. In fact, Becky doesn't have much going for her. She is very small and frail. A pair of thick, black-framed glasses overwhelms her tiny, pale face. The athetoid cerebral palsy makes her muscles limp and weak. Like a rag doll, she can't sit up, can't reach for an object, can't make her needs known, can't move around. She doesn't look around, doesn't respond to sounds or objects, doesn't seem aware of the world around her at all. She cries some but not much more.

Because music therapy techniques are based on the client participating in or reacting to the music activity presented, developing a music therapy program for her is a challenge. Becky can't join in, can't respond. I begin exposing her to sound vibrations. I place her back against a stereo speaker or roll her on a large drum and play it rhythmically. I use music boxes and musical toys to grab her attention. I sew bells on her socks to encourage her to move her feet and stand her on a cassette tape recorder playing many different kinds of music. Nothing very dramatic happens at first, but I do notice some response. Her facial expression changes when she feels and hears the music. She particularly likes Ravel's Boléro. She makes an attempt to follow the movement of a music box, but her body just won't cooperate. She has such limited muscle control that she just flops over. But I notice she does one movement spontaneously—she kneads the fingers of her right hand, flexes them on her own.

Flexibility and the ability to meet clients on their level of functioning are basic principles of music therapy. How can I use this small reflexive finger movement in

1

an active music experience? How can I be flexible with music in this case? Her arms are so weak she can't lift them to use the movement she has. I put her in a bouncing chair hung over the doorframe. This frees her arms a little. She now can use her arms and fingers slightly. I take an electronic keyboard and push it up under her hand. As she begins to knead her fingers, she activates the keys and a sound is produced. A small thing really—a note sounds and a basic rhythm track plays.

But an amazing thing happens. She startles at the sound. She reacts—the first reaction I've observed. She can hear, is aware of things going on around her. Her startle movements cause her to swing in the hanging chair and her hand slips off the keyboard. The note and the rhythm stop. Then something truly miraculous happens. On her own, she pushes off the floor with her foot, swings herself around, and lands her hand back on the keyboard. This child whom everyone thought was totally unaware of herself or her environment knows she can make the sound, knows how to get herself in the right position to do it. I have much more to work with than I realized.

From this point, Becky's therapy progresses rapidly. I find other ways for her to affect and control her environment—electronic switches to turn on the tape recorder, special chairs to improve her mobility, rhythm instruments suspended on strings for her to grab and play. She responds more, attempts more movement, laughs a little, and cries less. Becky is still a child with severe disabilities, but she now can interact a little with the world around her, and whatever potential she has can now be developed.

The case study above is just one example of the use of music as a therapeutic agent. Music for healing and therapy is one way in which humans use music. Most people have some relationship with music. You turn on a radio in the morning to "get yourself going" or use a favorite tape to make your daily walk less boring. A large percentage of people report music is their first choice as a stress reducer. What new mother has not learned very quickly that gentle singing and rocking soothes her baby? Music is chosen for entertainment at a party and to express the deep sadness of a funeral. Music is an important part of our social and religious ceremonies. Hymns are sung in church and bands play at Saturday afternoon football games. Everyone knows that music can deeply touch emotions. There are special songs to make us cry, and we attend concerts to experience deep thrills and physical chills. Everyone has experienced music's effects on the body, the mind, the emotion, and the spirit. These reactions are clearly beneficial and useful. However, alone they do not make the lasting changes in behavior and functioning defined as therapy. A *music therapist* is trained to use music as the basis of a systematic, planned course of treatment that creates the lasting changes of therapy (Bruscia, 1998a). To begin the exploration of the complex processes involved in music therapy, the history of the use of music for healing and therapy is examined and then current music therapy practice is defined and explored.

History of Music and Healing

Music is pervasive in human cultures. Based on the best anthropological knowledge, all human cultures—primitive and developed—had some form of music (Merriam, 1964). The specific forms that constitute "music" are as varied as the cultures of the world. These all have one thing in common—they involve the organization of sound and silence for the purpose of human expression (Hughes, 1948). Music involves the conscious human act of choosing and combining pitches and placing them in a rhythmic pattern over time. Composer Igor Stravinsky (1947) writes, "I conclude that tonal elements become music only by virtue of their being organized, and that such organization presupposes a conscious human act" (pp. 23–24). To date, research has shown that music is a uniquely and exclusively human behavior and a defining element of a culture linked with worship, ritual, acquisition of knowledge, and, often, healing.

Why has music been such a common element in human cultures from the earliest times? Most human behavior persists because it has survival benefit, yet there is no obvious survival benefit to music. It doesn't help us gather food or protect us from the elements. There is no obvious evolutionary advantage to this human behavior we call music (Pinker, 1997). Expression and communication, clearly important elements of music, do have survival benefits. Music, as chant, likely preceded speech as human communication. "There is anthropological evidence that music came before speech. . . . Early human skeletal remains reveal signs that the use of the voice to produce speech goes back only eighty thousand years, while also suggesting that chanting [early forms of music] began perhaps half a million years earlier" (Menuhin & Davis, 1979, p. 7). But music is much more than chant's basic vocal tone quality variations. Why did we put certain sound combinations together and then remember them for future use? Why did we begin to beat on hollow logs and stretched animal hides in repetitive rhythmic patterns? Why did we make holes in a bamboo stalk to make a flute? Why music? Humans from the beginning of history have asked this simple question. Music's various roles in past cultures give us some idea of how they answered the question.

The Role of Music in Ancient Cultures

Music had a variety of uses in early human civilization. The three roles that most relate to the history of music and healing include music as the key to knowledge of universal law; as a way to worship, interact with, placate, and engage the Divine; and as a direct healing tool and support for general well-being.

Music as a Source of Knowledge

Our ancestors believed music existed as an expression of divinely bestowed natural law. In most cultures, music revealed God's will and the deepest secrets of creation. In the ancient worldview (belief system), numbers, mathematics, and sound were interrelated, divine manifestations of natural laws and were the mystical vehicles to the knowledge of those truths. Mysticism is an immediate intuition of spiritual truths through direct union with the Divine. The ancients believed mathematics and sound combinations provided this direct understanding of divinely established natural law. "Because of the mixture of the esoteric and the practical, the otherworldly and the temporal, the universal and the particular, music and mathematics have held almost a mystical power since ancient times" (Rothstein, 1995, p. 14). Number mysticism was an important concept in ancient knowledge, and this number mysticism included music.

Many in ancient cultures developed a philosophy of number mysticism, including the great Greek philosopher and mathematician Pythagoras. Since the Greek ideas so greatly influenced the development of Western thought, a summary will help illustrate this important concept. For the Greeks, the study of numbers and their relationships (mathematics) was a direct path leading to the mind of the Divine. Mathematics was accompanied by " number mysticism, with each integer having a metaphysical significance. . . . This went along with a mysticism about music, which was itself linked to number and to the character of emotional and intellectual life" (Rothstein, 1995, p. 20). The Greeks sought the gods' perfect order in the measurement of nature. It is important to note, however, that the Greeks did not think of "measurement" as we do today—a comparison of an object with an external standard.

To the Greeks, measurement was "right measure," an important aspect of number mysticism. As physicist David Bohm (1980) wrote, right measure was an inner measure,

> . . . which played an essential role in everything. When something went beyond its proper measure, this meant not merely that it was not conforming to some external standard of what was right but, much more, that it was inwardly out of harmony, so that it was bound to lose its integrity and break up into fragments. (p. 20)

Right measure was expressed through proportion and ratio. The term *ratio* implies comparing two objects in the universe using a number relationship.

A ratio requires comparison between one object and another, a measurement of their relationship, and an assessment of their differences and similarities.

To lead a healthy, happy, productive life, one must achieve the perfect proportion, the perfect balance experienced through the right measurement of ratio. This is the Greek belief in harmony. Since the Divine's perfect order was inherent in the ratio relationships that expressed right measure, such a state of harmony was inevitable and the basis of health. This emphasis on ratios over numerical qualities is an acoustical calculation.

The connection between number and music may seem tenuous, but they have been intimately linked from the earliest human history. Our most basic sound perception involves constant processing of numbers. This is explored in detail in chapter 3. The human ear is bombarded with number relationships over time. Pitch perception is the ear evaluating how many sound waves occur in a second. Tone quality is the numerical relation of pitches in the overtone series. And rhythm is all about cutting up time mathematically. The connection of sound and number ". . . is not arbitrary. It is not a metaphor; if we interpret the words properly, sound is simply heard number; number is latent sound" (Rothstein, 1995, p. 23). Many ancient civilizations, including Babylon, Egypt, and China, explored the connection between number and music. However, the concept of right measure and the use of mathematics and music as keys to fundamental knowledge culminated in the work of the Greek mathematician Pythagoras.

Pythagoras lived in the sixth century B.C.E. and traveled extensively, studying for twenty-one years in Egypt and later studying with priests in Babylon. He was known to be an initiate of several mystical orders including the Cretean Rites (Abraham, 1994), where he learned the mystical and secret information concerning number and music. History sees Pythagoras as the inventor of Western mathematics, science, and music theory. His writings and those of his students profoundly shaped Western culture. Pythagoras searched for the Divine order in numbers. He saw the earthly manifestation of that order in the movement of heavenly bodies, the laws of music, and the physical and mental worlds of human beings. Pythagoras calculated the ratios of musical intervals and created a system of musical scales based on mathematics and this number mysticism. He calculated planetary movement in the same way. He developed a mathematical model based on the musical scale (Levenson, 1994). For Pythagoras, there was no difference between music and the study of how our world works. The study of music was a primary source of knowledge. This idea informed Western thinking through the European Renaissance, where an educated man was musically trained (Boxberger, 1962).

Music in Worship of the Divine

To many ancient people, music and number revealed the divinely inspired natural laws of the universe. Music was also connected to the Divine in other ways. Historically, music was typically associated with ancient worship rituals and temple ceremonies. The link of music and religious worship is still strong today. We sing hymns in the Protestant Christian church, have full musical masses in the Catholic cathedral, are called to prayer through chant in Islam, and listen to a cantor sing prayers in the Jewish temple. We know, touch, praise, and worship the Divine through music. Music gives us a direct experience of God. The Shaker hymn "Amazing Grace" tells us how we can experience God by beginning, "Amazing Grace, how sweet the *sound. . . .*" According to this lovely hymn, the grace of God is a sweet sound.

The relationship of music with the Divine is so strong that sound is considered by many cultures to be the force of creation itself. This force is not just vibration but the limited and specific vibrations constituting sound. "From the standpoint of physics, there are billions of different possible vibrations. But the cosmos—the universe—chooses from these billions of possibilities with overwhelming preference for those few thousand vibrations that make harmonic sense . . ." (Berendt, 1983, p. 90). For many cultures, this limited choice of vibrations cannot be by chance. A Divine intelligence is implied. For the ancient Egyptians, the world began when the singing sun sang light into existence. Hindu texts express that through the sound of the Vedas, the supreme divinity made all things (Daniélou, 1995). Australian Aborigines tell stories of the Dreamtime when the world was sung into being. The Gospel of John declares, "In the beginning was the Word, and the Word was with God, and the Word was God." And what is a word but a particular combination of sounds? Or as expressed by Tibetan Buddhists, in the beginning was the OM. In the Hindu religion, the concept of Nada Brahma—God is sound, sound is God—is a central tenet. Brahma is the All-Creator. Nada Brahma is the primal sound of being. "The world is sound. It sounds in pulsars and planetary orbits, in the spin of electrons, in the quanta of atoms and the structure of molecules, in the microcosm and in the macrocosm" (Berendt, 1983, p. 76). The creation story in the *Rgveda*, an ancient Hindu text, credits singers with creating the whole universe with their minds (McClain, 1976).

In the Middle East, sound is also recognized for its creative potential. As modern Sufi philosopher Hazrat Inayat Khan writes, "The creative source in its first step towards manifestation was audible, and in its next step visible. . . . It also shows that all we see in this objective world, every form, has been constructed by sound and is the phenomenon of sound" (Godwin, 1987, p.

261). In the northern hemisphere, the Keres people believe the world began with the song of Spider Woman, while the Athabascan people report life began when Asintmah wove songs into the Great Blanket of Earth (Hale, 1995, p. 45). For the early Anasazi people of the Southwest, Kokopelli, the cricket, is much more than a fertility figure. He represents the force of creation—the high-pitched sound of the cricket. He is later represented as the hunchbacked flute player, but the idea is the same. The sound of the flute, like the cricket call, is the creative force.

These early creation myths reveal our ancestors' intuition—sound is the Divine creative force. Scientific research has begun to support this belief. The early work of Ernst Chladni demonstrated how sound vibration moved and organized sand grains into symmetrical patterns. Sand is placed on a glass plate. When a violin bow is drawn across the edge of the plate, the particles jump, move, and create a form (Berendt, 1983). In the early twentieth century, the Swiss scientist Hans Jenny elaborated on this idea. Taking a steel plate, he vibrated a variety of materials like water, sand, iron filings, and thick fluids with different frequencies (pitches). What he found was astonishing. Each frequency at a particular loudness created specific, recognizable forms—spirals, leaf patterns, shells, the iris of the human eye. And even more astonishing, these forms were repeated at the given frequency in the same material. Through ten years of research, Jenny demonstrated the power of sound to create form (Goldman, 1992). Perhaps the creation myths of the past express an understanding of sound's power that we are only now able to verify scientifically.

Music for Healing and Therapy

For the earliest humans, worship of the Divine, magic, ritual, healing, and music were all part of the same activity. Though "healing" may have been defined differently in different cultures, music was frequently linked with these rituals—from shamanic practices to the healing temples of Greece and Rome. The use of music/sound as a healing agent is a very, very old idea. Music's connection to the Divine and the belief in sound as the creative force led naturally to music for healing. Throughout history, two basic ideas have existed about music healing: (1) music is a direct curative agent and is a form of content of healing, and (2) music is a support to natural balance, harmony, and wellness and is part of the context of health. Some cultures held one belief over the other, while, at times, both ideas were present in a culture's approach to music and healing.

The first idea about music and healing involves music as a direct curative agent, where music or certain sounds have an impact on some aspect of anatomy or physiology. The sound combinations influence functioning and create a change that leads to the cure for the physical problem. This is a form of content of healing—the methods or procedures used to "fix" the physical problem. Today we would think of surgery procedures or specific medications as the primary forms of healing content. But the direct application of sound and music is historically one of the first forms of healing content.

Shamanic practices of early hunter/gatherer cultures developed healing or medicine songs. These songs, often revealed to the shaman in altered states of consciousness or dreams, are believed to cure specific illnesses or conditions. The Navaho Blessing Way tradition includes such songs (Hale, 1995), while the Tohono O'Odham people of southern Arizona have a rich tradition of songs for power and healing (Underhill, 1938). A medicine song tradition can be found in healing practices in India, South America, Mexico, and Africa (Cook, 1997). Medicine songs from all world cultures have similar musical characteristics. They have irregular melodic accent, hypnotic rhythm, slow tempo with unexpected interruptions, and limited melodic range (McClellan, 1988). The sound combinations are the direct means to positively affect the patient and help cure the illness.

The developed cultures of the ancient Eastern world also used music in their healing practices. Chinese medicine as early as the second century B.C.E. indicated the use of music for healing. In this system, specific scale patterns or modes are assigned to each human emotion. The Hindu civilization of India developed a highly specific system of pitch organization known as ragas. Each raga promotes a distinct mood or psychological temperament (Hamel, 1976) and is used to positively influence physical and mental health. One highly developed medical system with a long history, Ayurvedic medicine, incorporates specific tones and music as part of comprehensive medical treatment (Chopra, 1990). Modern sound healing techniques reflect this approach (Leeds, 2001).

The second idea about music for healing involves the use of music to support balance, harmony, and general wellness. This is the idea of music in the context of healing. Context of healing is the internal and external environment of the patient that is conducive to overall health and recovery from illness. A patient's internal environment includes his or her emotional state, belief in the effectiveness of treatments used, and a general sense of hope. The external environment includes the physical surroundings and the community's attitudes toward the patient. Sound and music have also been used as part of the context of healing since ancient times.

Returning to the Greek idea of right measure, health involves proper attunement of the body and soul to the universe. Melody and rhythm can assist in restoring the soul to order and harmony, thus supporting the body's return to health. This state of harmony constitutes the context for health. David Bohm (1980) illustrates this point by tracing the early meanings of key English words related to health and healing:

> Thus, the Latin "mederi" meaning "to cure" (the root of the modern "medicine") is based on a root meaning "to measure." This reflects the view that physical health is to be regarded as the outcome of a state of right inward measure in all parts and processes of the body. Similarly, the word "moderation," which describes one of the prime ancient notions of virtue, is based on the same root, and this shows that such virtue was regarded as the outcome of a right inner measure underlying man's social action and behaviour. Again, the word "meditation," which is based on the same root, implies a kind of weighing, pondering, or measuring of the whole process of thought, which could bring the inner activities of the mind to a state of harmonious measure. So, physically, socially and mentally, awareness of the inner measure of things was seen as the essential key to a healthy, happy, harmonious life. (p. 20)

Ancient references to the effects of music on emotional states, including the biblical account of David curing Saul's melancholy with his harp playing, speak to the use of music as part of the overall context of healing.

Modern Music Therapy

The history of modern music therapy begins in the mid-1700s. Many physicians of the time were also trained as musicians and wrote about the use of music in medicine. In 1748, Louis Roger wrote A Treatise on the Effects of Music on the Human Body, establishing basic principles of acoustics (the science of sound), human sound perception, and the psychology of music. He also speculated on the vibrational effects of music on the human body as the basis of medical intervention (McClellan, 1988). Other works on music and medicine included a 1729 publication by Richard Brown entitled Medicina Musica (Musical Medicine). In 1790, an article was published in the London Journal of Medicine, "An Account of the Singular Effects of Music on a Patient," as was the 1806 book entitled On the Effects of Music in Curing and Palliating Disease. Writings also emphasized the psychological effects of music. The 1621 book The Anatomy of Melancholy included an entire chapter on music (Peters, 1987).

By the mid-1800s, scientific medicine was the norm, and the curative claims of music were being closely examined and largely rejected. Reports on medical uses of music did still exist, however. In 1875, the French writer Chomet wrote The Influence of Music on Health and Life, and in 1918,

Pothey's *The Power of Music and the Healing Art* was published. Though medical uses of music declined, it continued to be used as a treatment for the mentally ill and became a therapeutic activity in institutions and special education programs for individuals who were blind, deaf, and mentally retarded (Solomon, 1981). In the early twentieth century, interest in the use of music as therapy was revitalized when the phonograph was invented. Many types of music became available in hospitals, clinics, surgery theaters, and rehabilitation programs. In a 1914 letter to the American Medical Association, Dr. Evan O'Neil reported on his use of a phonograph in the operating room to ". . . mitigate the dread of operations . . ." (Boxberger, 1962, p. 139).

During the early twentieth century, research increased on music's physical and psychological effects and its use for various clinical situations (Taylor, 1981). What emerged was the concept of music as therapy. The word *therapy* is based on the Greek word *therapia* meaning "to attend, help, or serve" (Bruscia, 1998a). In modern usage, therapy means the treatment of disease by some remedial or curative process. It also refers to the rehabilitation of emotional and social problems. Perhaps the first instance of modern *music therapy* came in 1903 when music therapy pioneer Eva Vescelius founded the National Therapeutic Society of New York City. She published her article "Music and Health" in 1918. Based on many of the classic ideas about music for healing, Vescelius believed music cured diseases "based upon the law of harmonious rhythmic vibration" (1918, p. 379). She stressed the importance of correct musical selection for desired results. During this time period, others established organizations to promote music therapy, including the National Association for Music in Hospitals (1926) and, in the 1930s, the National Foundation for Music Therapy. None of these organizations sustained any general interest in music therapy or established a professional field of study (Boxberger, 1963).

In the period between the two world wars, a shift occurred in the treatment of patients with mental illness that greatly influenced the development of modern music therapy. During this period of reform, more humane treatment was introduced, including activity therapy. The idea was to involve patients in planned, productive activities during the day rather than restrain them in chairs, lock them in cells, or have them sit staring into space. Arts and crafts activities were introduced first and became the basis of occupational therapy. Soon, other activities including music were instituted. Musicians and music teachers were brought into hospitals to perform and later teach music skills to the patients. According to Unkefer (1961), the development of music therapy as a profession is more closely related to the development of the activity therapy movement than to the historical precedents for music's healing effects.

During and after World War II, veterans' hospitals in the United States employed many musicians to work in their activity therapy departments. By the late 1940s, a new therapeutic discipline had emerged. Soon, early practi-tioners recognized the need for formal education and research in the use of music as a therapy. The first university degree program was established in 1944 at what is now Michigan State University, followed in 1945 by a pro-gram at the University of Kansas. In 1950, the National Association for Mu-sic Therapy (NAMT) was formed from a special interest group of the Music Educators National Conference to support "the progressive development of the therapeutic use of music in hospital, educational, and community set-tings and the advancement of education, training, and research in music therapy" (1994, p. xix). As Boxberger (1963) reports, "It was the need to make music applicable to the scientific aspects of medicine in the twentieth century that initiated the drive toward an organization based on common goals and purposes" (p. 133). NAMT pursued a vigorous research program and, since 1968, has published a research journal, *The Journal of Music Ther-apy*. In 1971, a second national organization, the American Association for Music Therapy, was formed with similar goals. By 1981, the need for inde-pendent credentialing for professional music therapists was recognized, and the Certification Board for Music Therapists was formed. In January 1998, the National Association and the American Association merged to form the American Music Therapy Association. There are currently over 5,000 cre-dentialed music therapists in this country.

During this same time, music therapy practice developed in other countries. The largest and most well-established profession exists in England, where the British Society for Music Therapy was formed in 1958 by Juliette Alvin. Mu-sic therapy exists in other European countries including France, Germany, Denmark, Austria, Switzerland, and Belgium. The Canadian Association for Music Therapy was formed in 1974, and the Australian Music Therapy Asso-ciation, in 1975. Professional music therapy is currently developing in Japan, Brazil, Korea, Israel, Turkey, South Africa, and other countries.

Defining Music Therapy

As a music therapist, I am asked one question over and over again: "So what is music therapy anyway?" This is not an easy question to answer. Music ther-apy can be very hard to define. It is a process-based intervention combining the art of music and the interpersonal interaction of therapy verified by sci-ence. Unlike a profession like speech therapy, which is defined by the clients served (people with speech and communication problems), music therapy is broadly defined by the process involved—engaging people in experiencing and making music to accomplish nonmusical goals in various areas of functioning. Music therapy is a very diverse treatment modality. It is used successfully for the very old and the very young, for people with physical challenges and cognitive delay, for violent teenagers and depressed adults, for children with autism and patients paralyzed by stroke, and much more. The specific definition of music therapy is different for all these applications. What music therapy is for a child with autism is not the same as that for an adult with depression. And it is different again when working to rehabilitate a patient recovering from a stroke (Bruscia, 1998a). Music therapy is indeed hard to define.

In 1960, NAMT defined music therapy as ". . . the scientific application of the art of music to accomplish therapeutic aims. It is the use of music and of the therapist's self to influence changes in behavior." By 1983, NAMT published another definition: "Music therapy is the specialized use of music in the service of persons with needs in mental health, physical health, habilitation, rehabilitation, or special education. . . . [T]he purpose is to help individuals attain and maintain their maximum levels of functioning" (1983, p. 2). Dr. Kenneth Bruscia (1987) defines music therapy as ". . . a goal-directed process in which the therapist helps the client to improve, maintain, or restore a state of well-being, using musical experiences and the relationships that develop through them as dynamic forces of change" (p. 5). The Canadian Association for Music Therapy (n.d.) states in one of its brochures that music therapy

> . . . is the use of music to aid the physical, psychological and emotional integration of the individual, and in the treatment of illness or disability. It can be applied to all age groups, in a variety of treatment settings. . . . The nature of music therapy emphasizes a creative approach in work with handicapped individuals. Music therapy provides a viable and humanistic approach that recognizes and develops the often untapped inner resources of the client. Music therapists wish to help the individual to move towards an improved self-concept, and in the broadest sense, to develop each human being to their own greatest potential.

Author Jacqueline Peters (1987) defines music therapy as ". . . the prescribed, structured use of music or music activities under the direction of specially trained personnel (i.e., music therapists) to influence changes in maladaptive conditions or behavior patterns, thereby helping clients achieve therapeutic goals" (p. 5). All these definitions provide a general overview of this therapeutic discipline.

Music therapy uses the inherent therapeutic potential found in the basic components of sound and in music as a complex art form (Sekeles, 1996). However, therapy cannot be defined merely by client outcomes. It requires an ongoing process of intervention planned and carried out by a trained professional music therapist. "In order for *therapy* to take place, the process of intervention must be carried out by a person who, by qualification and intent, acts in the capacity of a 'therapist' . . ." (Bruscia, 1998a, p. 38).

Music therapy is now a well-established professional discipline, which developed within and as part of the scientific, biomedical model. As a professional discipline, it is considered a behavioral science. This implies that the trained music therapist uses a general procedure for work with clients. First, assessment of client needs and functioning is undertaken. Based on this information, goals are set and a treatment plan is created. With the nonmusical goals in mind, the music therapist creates music activity interventions and implements them in the therapy session. Evaluation of results helps to ensure effectiveness of treatment. Music therapists are trained both as performing musicians and as therapists. University curricula in music therapy are music degrees with a specialization in music therapy. Many music therapy interventions involve the client in active music making. The therapy derives from the music therapist and the client making music together. The client actively participates in music performance. Extensive experimental research, much of which will be reviewed in subsequent chapters, has verified the effectiveness of music therapy interventions. The complexity of the music therapy process comes, in part, from the vast variety of music activities used as therapeutic interventions. Because these are referred to throughout the book, they are briefly overviewed here.

Music Therapy Activity Interventions

When modern music therapy was developed in the United States in the middle of the twentieth century, it was primarily an activity-based therapeutic intervention (Unkefer, 1961). An intervention implies something that comes between or addresses some aspect of client functioning that is affecting his or her health (Bruscia, 1998a). An activity intervention in music therapy is a musical experience or event that is planned and implemented by a trained, professional music therapist. The idea is that the music therapy intervention can assist the client in achieving the therapeutic goals by engaging him or her in a music experience or event.

There are a number of reasons why the activity of music is particularly well suited for engaging clients in the therapeutic interaction. First, music is a basic human behavior. All humans make music and have, in fact, always made music. As explored in chapter 3, we are "hardwired" for music. Second, music provides flexibility of response. In music therapy, the music can be as simple or as complex as needed to meet the clients at their level of functioning. This can be hard to understand if we think music skill is only available to naturally talented people after many years of hard study. And there are many examples of this type of highly developed, complex musical skill— performers like Elton John or Isaac Stern, composers like Leonard Bernstein or Ludwig von Beethoven, and modern songwriters like Carol King or Billy Joel. But a musical response can also be a vocalization, clapping to the beat, playing a rhythm instrument on cue, or, for someone like Becky, pushing the keys. I have yet to find a client, no matter how impaired, that I can't engage in a music therapy intervention. Music is that flexible. A well-structured music activity intervention matches the client's physical, musical, cognitive, and social/emotional functioning. This means the music activity can be a successful and enjoyable experience for anyone.

A third reason why music is a good basis for a therapeutic interaction is the fact the music is a social event. Music is made by people to communicate with other people. A music experience becomes the reason for being together. Music provides a means for nonthreatening familiarity. It makes it safe to interact with another person. And as a social event, music has the ability to form groups and provide opportunities for socialization. Playing music together gives us a sense of belonging, of being part of something. A group music activity fosters teamwork and cooperation just as well as any team sport. Finally, music is a rewarding activity. People are motivated to participate in music and receive rewards for using musical skill. In order for a therapeutic intervention to work, the client must be willing to participate. People are usually eager to become involved in a musical event (Gaston, 1968a).

Product-Oriented Music Therapy Interventions
The vast range of music therapy interventions can be roughly categorized in two groups: product-oriented interventions and process-oriented interventions (Unkefer, 1990). In product-oriented music therapy interventions, the goals are achieved primarily through the client's active music making or direct response to the musical stimuli. This promotes participation and the practice or rehearsal of healthy behavior and response (Unkefer, 1990). Goals are achieved as the client actively makes music or responds to music in some fashion. The actual activity in music used in the session will vary based on the client's age; cognitive, physical, emotional, and social functioning; musical background and skill; and musical preferences. Product-

oriented music therapy interventions include music performance/skill building, music activity therapy, composing music and songs, movement to music/dance, music combined with other arts, and social/recreational music.

Music Performance/Skill Building

The earliest music therapy interventions were performance and skill-building experiences. The original music therapy theoretical principles, "Experiences in Structure" (Sears, 1968), were predicated on the assumption that the client would be involved in complex, skilled music making. Learning a musical skill such as playing an instrument (guitar, piano, drums) or performing a particular style of music (rock, blues, Tejano) is common in music therapy practice. The music therapist provides individual or group learning experiences. This often leads to individual and group performances. The music therapist often creates special and adaptive means for the performance to occur. When I worked in a school for students with special needs, we had a performing handbell choir and a jazz combo. Both groups were given special support to allow the performance to occur. The handbell choir could not read music, but they knew when to play the complicated arrangements through a system of hand signals. Special tuning systems for guitar (Krout, 1995) constitute another example of this. Music therapists will often create special designs for musical instruments and adaptive devices to make music performance more accessible to a wide range of clients. In a collaborative project with the Arizona State University Department of Industrial Design, instruments were created with slanting heads, special mallet grips, and alternative means of playing bells to ensure performance opportunities for all clients.

A newer performance approach is rhythm-based music therapy (Reuer & Crowe, 1995). Developed and researched by music therapists (Clair & Bernstein, 1990b; Clair, Bernstein, & Johnson, 1995), these activities involve learning ethnic drumming forms such as modified African drumming and playing in groups. I developed a program for disadvantaged youth in an inner-city school that used this drum circle performance approach as the basis of a gang prevention program. The involvement in these performance activities fostered personal self-esteem, positive peer identification, a sense of belonging, learning conflict resolution strategies, and emotional awareness and expression.

Performance-based music therapy interventions can also utilize client's existing musical skill, training, and talent. Senior band programs are an example. In these performing groups, older adults with previous musical background are engaged in performance experiences to foster self-esteem, socialization and group experiences, and physical well-being (Clair, 1996). When

I worked as a music therapist with adolescents who have emotional disturbances, I had a client who was an accomplished pianist. The basis of the therapy was her accompanying me while I played my violin as well as the playing of piano duets. The interactions around our music making and the
musical communication contributed significantly to her ability to relate to
others. Ultimately, we gave a recital. This performance activity as the basis
of the music therapy intervention helped her achieve goals in the areas of
self-worth and self-esteem, frustration tolerance, coping with anxiety, interpersonal relations, and attention to task.

Music Activity Therapy

In music activity therapy (Friedlander, 1994), the client actively responds
musically or nonmusically to the music. The client may clap a beat, do the
actions of an action song, follow the directions given in song lyrics, point to
colors or body parts, or learn skills such as counting or vocabulary words. All
teaching songs used in *Sesame Street*, for example, fall into this category of activity intervention. These activities often emphasize participation in rhythmic responses. Rhythmic chants of the Orff approach, use of rhythm charts,
and rhythm band activities are typical of these interventions. A rhythm band
activity typically used with geriatric clients would involve the participants in
playing rhythm instruments in response to recorded or live music to foster attention span, participation, reality orientation, and physical movement.

Music activity therapy interventions promote goals in a number of areas.
They are often used to achieve goals in cognitive development and functioning, concept development, preacademic skill building, and support to
academic learning. For example, a song like "Angel Band" involves the
participant in counting skills. Social participation, listening skills, and attention span goals can also be achieved. Rhythmic activities also help organize behavior and response. Dr. Oliver Sacks (1990) found that external,
rhythmic music helped his patients "frozen" by Parkinson's disease initiate
movement.

Composing Music and Songs

Songwriting is an effective activity intervention in music therapy (Ficken,
1976; Lindberg, 1995; Robb, 1996). The music therapist assists the client in
creating the music and/or lyrics of a new song. Use of an existing song formula, such as a twelve-bar blues song, can facilitate the process. Music therapists in a hospital setting will often work with patients to compose a "hospital blues" song as an expression of the fear, frustration, and anger that can
accompany a hospital stay. Writing rap songs is currently popular with ado-

lescent clients. A variation on this activity includes song parody in which lyrics of an existing song are changed to reflect the client's ideas, feelings, or memories. In work with geriatric clients, the music therapist might take a song like "This Land Is Your Land" and have the clients insert the states where they were born. This fosters reminiscing and life review.

Other forms of music composition are also used as music therapy interventions. Electronic instruments and computer composition programs facilitate the activity (Nagler & Lee, 1989). Clients are able to create and record their music compositions for future performance. Musical composition techniques work to promote goals in the areas of emotional awareness and expression, identify personal issues, review coping skills, support self-expression and creativity, and foster self-esteem and self-confidence. As Bruscia (1998b) notes, songs and compositions ". . . are the sounds of our personal development" (p. 9).

Movement to Music/Dance

Movement and dance are natural human responses to music, particularly rhythmic music. Though the profession of dance/movement therapy specializes in these activity interventions, there are music therapy techniques that involve movement and dance. Clients can learn and perform simple dances, including square dancing and ethnic dance forms. As a graduate student, I helped lead a square dance group for adult clients with developmental delay. Not only was this an excellent social outlet for these individuals, the group also promoted physical coordination, self-esteem, and leisure time activity. In addition to dance, exercise to music is used as a music therapy intervention. This intervention is frequently used with older adult clients to motivate physical activity, increase muscle tone and joint flexibility, increase range of motion, promote balance and coordination, and support rhythmic flow of movement. These interventions also promote social interaction, interpersonal relations, and relaxation.

Music Combined with Other Art Forms

Some music therapy activity interventions combine music with other creative art forms. A technique used for a client with psychiatric diagnosis includes picking a picture in response to a musical selection or drawing while listening to music. In this activity intervention, music is played, often classical, that has strong emotional content or evokes mental imagery. The client is asked to pick a picture or draw something that best represents the music for him or her. Verbal sharing and processing are then used to help the client gain insight into his or her emotions and reactions. Another combined creative art intervention involves illustrating poems and stories with sound and music. I use story illustration frequently with children. I provide them with a wide variety of musical instruments, often percussion instruments, and ask them to determine what sounds could illustrate the various aspects of a story that will be read. Music can also be combined with the actual writing of poems and stories. In the case of writing a story to music, the music gives the clients ideas for the characters, setting, and plot line. Music can further be combined with craft skills and activities in making musical instruments. These interventions promote the goals of self-awareness and self-expression, emotional awareness, increased creativity, and self-esteem.

Social/Recreational Music

Social/recreational music experiences take many forms (Unkefer, 1990). Musical games such as "musical bingo" or "name that tune" engage people in music for fun and socialization. They also foster goals of improved attention and concentration as well as fostering group experiences and interaction. Musical bingo is commonly used with older adult clients. In this game, the titles of songs are place on the bingo cards. Various songs are then played, and the clients must recognize and cover the appropriate title (Douglas, 1985). Another recreational music activity involves music appreciation groups, which focus on a particular form of music such as opera or Broadway musicals. These groups promote socialization, conversation, and interpersonal interaction. Such recreational music listening can also be used to foster life review and reminiscing. Recreational musical performance groups are performance experiences designed to be immediately successful and enjoyable. In my community, there are a number of such recreational performance groups including a marching kazoo band and a kitchen band.

Recreational/social music groups promote socialization and peer identification, improve self-confidence, and combat isolation and social withdrawal. Recreational music experiences can also be used to develop a client's leisure time skills. Exposure to recreational music groups increases interest in music participation as a positive leisure time activity.

Process-Oriented Music Therapy Interventions

The second category of music therapy interventions is process oriented. In process-oriented music therapy interventions, the emphasis shifts from the results of active music making to the unfolding of therapeutic insights and the intrapersonal and interpersonal processes involved. The musical product achieved becomes much less important, while the ongoing, unfolding experiences with the music or evoked by the music are of paramount importance.

These interventions include improvisation, neurological interventions, music as a reinforcer, music-based discussion, and music and imagery.

Improvisation

Musical improvisation is a spontaneous act of music making where the music is created during the act of playing and not re-created from written music (Bruscia, 1987). Musical improvisation can require highly developed musical skills, such as in jazz improvisation, or no music skill in improvisations that emphasize free exploration of instrumental or vocal sound. Improvisation as a music therapy intervention usually emphasizes the latter. "Clinical improvisation . . . is here-and-now experience where the music of the session is improvised based on the person or persons present in the session" (Hesser, 1995, p. 47). Free, expressive creative movement to music is another form of improvisation. There are numerous, specific improvisational music therapy techniques (Bruscia, 1987). Some require the music therapist to musically improvise in response to client behavior and vocalization (Nordoff & Robbins, 1971); others require the client to improvise, often in a group (Ruud, 1998a). Some approaches have both the client and music therapist improvising (Priestley, 1975).

Bruscia (1987) identifies numerous goals fostered by improvisational music therapy techniques. An improvisation experience allows for self-discovery through the sounds produced. The music that emerges highlights personal and emotional issues of the client. Both the client and the music therapist experience real behavior during the improvisation and not just a verbal memory of the issue or concern. In an improvisational therapy group I conducted, one young man became aware of his disregard for other group members when he consistently played the loudest drum available with no awareness of the other musical events occurring around him. He was able to experience a behavior that directly expressed a lack of empathy for the other group members. After he gained awareness, the improvisational music therapy provided opportunities to incorporate his personal insight into changes in his behavior and his relations with others.

The improvisation experience provides a means to explore and practice new modes of behavior and response. "Musical improvisation, then, is play with musical tendencies and possibilities as a frame within which fantasies and alternative forms of action can be explored" (Ruud, 1998a, p. 119). Improvisation also serves as a form of communication. Sounds produced become signals of communication. As Ruud (1998a) states, through music ". . . we can learn to communicate about communication" (p. 27). Finally, improvisational music therapy interventions allow clients to explore interpersonal relationships and group dynamics. The improvisational group becomes a miniature social system. "Playing music in a group provides an opportunity to explore and more deeply understand relationships in the community, and the changing dynamics of groups as they grow and develop" (Hesser, 1995, p. 49).

Neurological Interventions

Several music therapy interventions directly address problems created by malfunction of the neurological system. Such techniques impact neurological functioning and remediate problems in behavior and functioning by addressing the underlying causes.

Vibrotactile stimulation involves exposing clients to the physical vibrations of sound. Such exposure focuses attention, increases participation, and organizes response of severely impaired clients. Clair and Bernstein (1990a) found clients with Alzheimer's dementia responded better to musical experiences of drumming when a vibrotactile element was involved than when an auditory stimulus was presented alone. Similarly, clients with muscle spasms were found to experience a change of muscle tone when given a vibrotactile stimulation (Sears, 1958).

Another neurological technique is rhythmic auditory stimulation, which is used to remediate gait problems for patients who have had a stroke and others with neurologically based motor difficulties (Thaut, 1997). This technique uses an external auditory stimulus as an entrainment device to rhythmically synchronize motor movement. Sensory integration music therapy, another neurological intervention, engages the client in a series of activities using tactile, vestibular, auditory, and multisensory inputs to assist the client in learning to make successful, organized responses to sensory input (Peters, 2000). An example of a sensory integration intervention would be to have a client sitting on a balance board while rhythmically bouncing a ball and singing a song. Finally, music and relaxation techniques use the ability of music to alter brain wave speed, thus promoting a relaxed mental state. These techniques involve listening to music, often with progressive muscle relaxation exercises. There is a large element of learning and behavioral conditioning involved with these techniques.

Music to Reinforce Behavior

Much of early music therapy research documented the effective use of music to reinforce behavior (Eidson, 1989; Madsen, Cottor, & Madsen, 1968). In these techniques, music is used as a pleasurable experience that will ensure the recurrence of a behavior or response. Music is played after a behavior occurs as a reinforcer for that behavior. Music can also be used as a reinforcer using contingent music listening. If negative or undesirable behavior occurs, the music is stopped. Behavioral change is the primary goal achieved with these music therapy interventions.

Music-Based Discussion

Therapeutic discussion based on a musical experience involves verbal processing of the feelings, memories, and issues evoked by the music. Lyric analysis is an example of this technique. The client listens to a song and, with the music therapist's assistance, responds to the lyric content and musical impact of the song. Verbal processing can be a part of many other music therapy interventions, including improvisation, music combined with other creative arts, and music performance groups. Goals fostered with these techniques include emotional self-awareness and self-expression, development of personal insight, learning coping skills, and social interaction and improved interpersonal relations.

Music and Imagery

Music is known to produce intrasubjective material, especially visual, auditory, and physical imagery (Bonny & Savary, 1990). A number of music therapy techniques utilize this response in creating depth-psychology techniques. Such techniques engage the client in a deep listening experience, where the music evokes the imagery and accompanying emotions.

"Guided Imagery and Music" (GIM) is a specific approach to music imaging developed by Dr. Helen Bonny (Bonny & Savary, 1990). As Bruscia (1998b) notes, GIM ". . . involves the client in imaging to specifically designed music programs while in an altered state of consciousness and also dialoguing with the therapist" (p. 12). The technique is based on Jung's concept of active imagination, which involves the spontaneous emergence of images from the unconscious. In GIM, the music evokes the images and accompanying emotions. This listening experience in a heightened state of awareness generates intense levels of emotional depth and cathartic expression. It allows for increased insight and helps develop problem-solving abilities and coping skills. Through this deep exploration, ego strength is reinforced and unconscious material is accessed and integrated into conscious functioning. This technique is explored at length in chapter 6.

Music Therapy Clinical Applications

Music therapy is also complex in that it can serve a wide range of clients. Modern music therapy is broadly applied as a therapeutic intervention. Several different interventions may be utilized with a client or client group. Music therapy was first used extensively with adult patients experiencing psychiatric problems in veteran's hospitals and in progressive psychiatric facilities like the Menninger Clinic in Topeka, Kansas. It is now also widely used with adolescents and children with emotional and behavioral problems. Individuals of all ages with cognitive impairments and developmental disabilities gain a wide range of benefits from music therapy interventions. Music therapy is now used for children with neurological impairment, including those with learning disabilities and autism. Children with visual and auditory handicaps and orthopedic problems also benefit. Because children respond so well to music even at very young ages, music therapy is a vital part of early intervention and infant stimulation programs. In addition to the patients with psychiatric diagnosis, many adult populations also benefit from music therapy. It has proven to be very beneficial for elderly people, particularly those with Alzheimer's disease and other serious cognitive and medical conditions. Music therapy is successfully used to help rehabilitate patients with strokes and individuals with serious head injuries, and it has come to be an important part of drug and alcohol treatment. There are numerous medical applications of music therapy. Many of these uses contribute to the context of healing—the internal and external environment conducive for health. Work in labor and delivery, surgery and preoperative units, orthopedics and physical therapy, burn units, oncology, and hospice programs provides many examples. Modern uses of music as content of therapy also exist and are explored in chapter 5. In fact, all applications are explored more extensively, and research substantiation of this flexible therapy is addressed throughout this book.

The Phenomenon of Music Therapy

Music therapy practice is based on the phenomenon of music—how we *experience* music. Music therapy is not currently based on the direct impact of specific sounds but on the experience of the highly organized sound combinations called music. The client's emotional state, past experience, memories, social experiences, and previous exposure to music are all vital factors in the music therapy process.

As a music therapist, I am frequently asked, "What music is therapeutic?" When music therapy is approached from a phenomenological perspective, this question is irrelevant. Any music can be useful as the basis for the therapeutic interaction. The experience is most important. So when I begin to work with a client, I determine what music he or she enjoys, if vocal or instrumental is best, what type of music (rock, classical, jazz) will support the stated goals, and what musical elements (scale, rhythm, tempo, etc.) will ensure a response. No music is absolutely beneficial or absolutely harmful. In my practice with adolescents diagnosed with emotional disturbance, I frequently used music that most people would consider detrimental, inappropriate, or negative. Yet I've been able to involve withdrawn children in the activity with me using this music. Once they are involved, I can confront poor attitudes, show them options for their behavior, or help them make better decisions. Sometimes a loud, aggressive grunge rock tune is an important release of emotions for them. In the majority of current music therapy practice, it is the experience of the music and the interactions based on the music that is therapeutic. However, the physical impact of sound combinations is also a factor in the effectiveness of music therapy practice and is largely not considered. This aspect of music therapy is addressed in subsequent chapters.

Having reviewed the current state of music therapy practice, it is time to establish a new theory of music therapy: *music and soulmaking*. To begin, a new scientific paradigm, *complexity science*, is introduced, and the new ideas concerning human functioning based on this science are explored.

CHAPTER TWO

~

Complexity Science:
A New Scientific Paradigm

As a new music therapy intern at Ypsilanti State Hospital, I am assigned to work in-
dividually with a middle-aged woman diagnosed with schizophrenia. Mary is in her
early fifties with graying hair and a sweet face. She loves to sing hymns and gospel
tunes in a pure soprano voice. For the most part, she is quiet, unassuming, and co-
operative. But when she experiences a psychotic episode, she becomes agitated and
aggressive. She grabs my arm and pulls me toward her. As she does this, she pushes
her face into mine and laughs hysterically with a sardonic smile on her face. Need-
less to say this is very unnerving and prompts me to pull away and avoid contact. In
her psychotic state, this is exactly the result she is seeking. The treatment team agrees
that to break Mary of this behavior, all staff members must ignore the negative be-
havior (extinction in behavioral therapy) and reinforce appropriate, positive behav-
ior. My music therapy interventions consist of sitting beside Mary on the piano bench
accompanying her as she sings her songs. When the inappropriate behavior occurs, I
shut down any interaction with her. The music stops, I drop my eyes, and I remain
motionless until the behavior subsides. When her behavior changes, I reward her by
playing her favorite hymn and showering her with attention. After several weeks of
this behavior intervention, Mary completely stops this behavior with me and signifi-
cantly reduces the number of times she behaves this way with other staff members.
Our music therapy session gives me the opportunity to alter Mary's negative behav-
ior, and the music rewards the new, more positive response.

As mentioned previously, modern music therapy is firmly rooted in the
twentieth-century scientific, biomedical method. This effective profession

with its established techniques and approaches is the child of behavioral science. Our approach to music therapy is often behavioral (assessment, goal setting, evaluation, etc.), and a great deal of our research is based on a behavioral approach. As reviewed in depth in subsequent chapters, extensive empirical research has been conducted over the last fifty years to establish music therapy's usefulness with certain clients having disabilities like autism, Alzheimer's disease, and so on; impact on human functioning (memory, emotions, etc.); and affects on physical traits (blood pressure, sweat gland response, etc.). Demonstration of music therapy's effects is not difficult, but an explanation of why and how the effect happens is.

The mainstream scientific community has never really accepted music therapy. It doesn't fit somehow. Modern science is about structure and reducing systems to their component parts. Music therapy is about process and interactions. Controlled, double-blind studies don't reveal everything that is going on in a music therapy session or how a technique is effective. They certainly don't shed much light on how and why music therapy works. Empirical scientific method never had the right tools to completely explain and support music therapy. In expressing this frustration, I often say, "It's like trying to study the stars with a microscope." The tools of the scientific method don't fit the phenomena under study.

As it turns out, this sense of "just not fitting" is not limited to music therapy. Over the last thirty years, scientists from many different disciplines found that empirical science could not explain real-world events like weather systems, turbulence phenomena, and sound production in musical instruments (Gleick, 1987). As they explored these events more fully, it became clear that a new paradigm was emerging—one based on process, wholeness, and nonlinear reactions. This new paradigm holds beliefs that include chaotic movement, wholeness of events, and most important, the inherent complexity of the real world. The new paradigm is now called complexity science. It is the principles of complexity science that will be applied to music therapy in formulating a new theory—music and soulmaking. But in order to understand complexity science and how it applies to a therapy like music therapy, it is important to first review and understand the assumptions of the current scientific method.

The Assumptions of Empirical Science

The word *science* is based on the Latin word *scientia*, which means "to learn" or "to know." But in its current usage, *science* means specific processes and procedures—the scientific method—for making inquiries about nature. The assumptions of empirical science are based on a particular worldview. A worldview is one's total outlook on life, including a concept of the universe, beliefs about the origin and destiny of human beings, and a value orientation (Frame, 2003). Empirical science sees the world as an exterior object that can be analyzed, controlled, and predicted.

From its early application to the physical sciences, the empirical scientific paradigm grew, expanded, and was applied to all aspects of nature including human functioning and health. "It came to pass that the worldview known as *scientific materialism* became, in whole or part, the dominant official philosophy of the modern West" (Wilber, 1998, p. 10). We now live, think, and work in this well-established paradigm. It colors and influences every aspect of our lives—how we think and even how we perceive our world and ourselves. It is important to understand that the empirical paradigm is based on a number of assumptions that are so ingrained in us we probably think they are "the truth" rather than one way to model or map the real world. An assumption is really a guess about how things are—an idea or belief we take for granted. The empirical scientific paradigm holds many such assumptions. These include determinism, control, reductionism, replicability, objectivism, positivism and materialism, and linear development.

Determinism is the belief that absolute truth about reality already exists and is waiting for humans to discover it. Scientific determinism tells us we can know how a process works (curing cancer or decreasing depression with music) and then *prove* the discovery is true. It is believed that a well-controlled, empirical study will prove how things are. Related to determinism are the assumptions of control, reductionism, and replicability. If the laws of nature can be determined, then humans can use those laws to control it. To discover the laws of nature, a reductionistic approach is used. Reductionism is the process of understanding a phenomenon by studying the behavior of its elemental parts (Harman, 1994a). It is assumed that one can understand the whole based on an examination of its parts. This reductionistic approach does not consider a process in its wholeness. The "proof" that a law of nature has been discovered in empirical research is replicability—will the same results occur under the same conditions? Once this information is known, nature can be influenced and controlled. Objectivism is the assumption that the world is an objective place. An observer can, with care, look at a phenomenon from a distance and study things separately from him- or herself. Human contaminates are eliminated. Science also assumes positivism and materialism—the real world is what is physically measurable. This assumption limits what is real to what the human mind can conceive. Finally, the scientific paradigm assumes linear development—complicated processes are made up of identifiable parts. Linear development also assumes progress moves from simple to complex, inferior to superior (Smith, 1989).

The achievements of the scientific approach are many and far-reaching, but there are many problems inherent in relying on this one way of knowing our world. We now need practical understanding of our world, and reductionism hasn't really shown us how our world works. A theoretical understanding gives us little help with our practical problems. There is a ". . . gap between the abstraction of a scientific analysis and whatever it is that is actually out there—a fissure that is inherent, built into the fabric of the cosmos and into the language of mathematics [the world of science] . . ." (Levenson, 1994, p. 236). The gap between what science tells us and what we need to know to survive and cope with our mounting problems grows wider every day. We need practical help. We need answers about the real world—the macroworld. The limited means of knowledge acquisition given us by reductionistic, empirical science can no longer help us deal with an increasingly complex world. We have forgotten that empirical science is only one model of how things are. From beliefs developed in ancient civilizations to modern Eastern approaches, other systems of knowledge acquisition exist. In fact, empirical science is not the only scientific paradigm used in today's world. It is only one of many possible systems of knowledge acquisition.

As I investigated music therapy processes over time, I began to realize that the limitations of the empirical, reductionistic approach to studying music therapy were especially glaring. Clearly, there was much more going on than this approach to science could verify or reveal. The empirical worldview sees everything as composed of objective processes. But what about human experiences, consciousness, values, emotions, interior depth, meaning, spirit, community, and Divinity? These things are very much part of music therapy process. There is also a wholeness to music therapy that the reductionistic approach destroys, let alone acknowledges as important. As philosopher Huston Smith (1989) points out, "It happens, though, that a scientific worldview is impossible. . . . [I]t is impossible in principle, a contradiction in terms. For 'world' implies whole and [modern] science deals with part, an identifiable part of the whole that can be shown to be part only . . ." (p. 144).

The need for a new paradigm is now being recognized. A paradigm that considers a process in its wholeness, that recognizes that natural events (like the weather and getting cancer) are complicated and messy, not simple and neat as science would have us believe, would serve music therapy well. For these reasons, I began to search for a scientific paradigm that would address these concerns and help me study and verify how and why music therapy is an effective treatment modality. And, in fact, such a new paradigm already exists. As Wilber (1998) writes, new paradigms include

> . . . quantum physics, relativistic physics, cybernetics, dynamical systems theory, autopoiesis, chaos theory, and complexity theory. These are all new revolutions, new paradigms in the true sense, with new modes of research, new social practices supporting them, new types of data, new forms of evidence, and new theories surrounding them. (pp. 38–39)

I found that complexity science, with its chaos theory, dynamical systems theory, and theories of self-organization and autopoiesis, greatly informs the full processes I see in music therapy. Let's explore the principles inherent in this new paradigm.

Complexity Science

We experience complex, seemingly chaotic phenomena every day. We just don't realize it. Here are some examples from my own life to illustrate this point:

In the summer of 1993, my husband and I were living in the Florida coastal community of New Smyrna Beach. In early August, a hurricane developed over the Atlantic Ocean. Over several days, we heard the news from the National Hurricane Center that the storm was heading right for us in eastern central Florida. We began to prepare our home and formulated an escape plan. All predictive indications of advanced meteorology showed us getting a direct hit from this ever-intensifying storm. Just as it began to look pretty serious for us, overnight the storm turned northward skirting the East Coast completely and touching the barrier islands of the Carolinas. So what happened? Every indication of sophisticated meteorological science showed the storm moving directly at the Florida coast. Some small factor, which we will never know, dramatically altered the hurricane's path.

I am a tea drinker. Every morning I heat a cup of water in my microwave oven. I always set it to run for three minutes. When it finishes, I take the cup out of the microwave and put in a tea bag. I let it steep four to five minutes, add milk and sugar, and have my morning cup of tea. This is usually a routine, uneventful process. But occasionally, something very odd happens. On these mornings, when I put the tea bag into the cup of water, it explodes into a wild, chaotic boiling movement that throws most of the water out of the cup. It's the same cup, the same type of tea bag. I've microwaved for the same amount of time. What makes the water in my cup break into these violent movements every once in awhile? Why not every day?

I am a violinist and have played in symphony orchestras since I was in high school. Over the years, I have played a number of works many times—Beethoven's Seventh Symphony, for example. With rehearsals and performances, I would say I've played that symphony twenty times. Yet the experience is different every time. Even with the same players and the same conductor playing in the same auditorium, a performance can sound and feel entirely different. What would make such a difference when the room acoustics, the playing of each musician, and the leadership of the conductor should be the important factors in determining the quality of the performance?

The reductionistic, linear scientific paradigm has never been good at explaining such real-world phenomena. For all our efforts at determining causes of events and predicting outcomes, our success is poor, as the simple examples above illustrate. But the beliefs inherent in the current scientific paradigm are pervasive. Challenging them is a difficult and unsettling process of "unlearning" assumptions about our world and accepting new ones. The examples cited above and all real-world phenomena have much in common and give rise to the new assumptions and principles of complexity science.

Real-world phenomena are complex systems in the constant movement of unfolding process. They are *dynamical systems*, which evolve and change in time where each successive state is a function of the proceeding state (Williams, 1997). Because of their nature, these systems are essentially unpredictable and are extremely sensitive to initial conditions. They have emergent properties and are nonlinear, meaning the whole is greater than the sum of its parts. As nonlinear processes, they cannot be cut up into their constituent parts and still be the experience we expect. Their wholeness is important. Real-world events are nonreplicable (Brophy, 1999).

Complexity science, with its emphasis on chaos theory, is a newly developed scientific paradigm related to systems theory that explains these real-world phenomena. It is the science of the global nature of dynamical systems—systems in motion. According to Williams (1997), complexity is a ". . . type of *dynamical* behavior in which many independent agents continually interact in novel ways, spontaneously organizing and reorganizing themselves into larger and more complicated patterns over time" (p. 449). Complexity science recognizes basic underlying interrelatedness and interdependency of the various parts of a whole system (deQuincey, 2002). Complexity is a function of the way things *interact* (Briggs & Peat, 1999). Complexity science focuses on hidden patterns, nuances in complex systems, and the sensitivity of real things. And complexity science establishes the "rules" or constants for how the seemingly unpredictable leads to the new (Briggs & Peat, 1999). Complexity science is the science of the real, practical, messy world.

In this worldview, nature is recognized as a highly complex, interlocking network of nested, dynamical systems. "Relationships between 'parts' are dynamic, ever-changing, because they involve complex networks of feedback and feedforward loops. It becomes difficult, if not meaningless, to identify or isolate individual causes" (deQuincey, 2002, pp. 30–31). Dynamical systems are simultaneously stable and ever-changing. They are in a constant state of renewal. Complexity science also asserts that *everything* in nature is complex—weather systems, economic trends, population growth, the formation of mountains and rivers, the functioning of the human body, and the processes of health and disease. This complexity also includes the functioning of the human mind and its products like consciousness and music. Complexity science sees nature as connected, adaptive, ever changing, and regenerative (Shulman, 1997). Before the principles of complexity science are introduced in detail, an overview of the history of complexity science may help in understanding this new paradigm.

Birth of Complexity Science

In Newtonian or classical mechanical physics, systems in motion, like our solar system, are considered stable—acting in predictable ways and neatly described by linear, mathematical formulas. In the empirical, linear scientific view, very small influences on a system can be ignored since small influences don't have disproportionately large effects. Small variations in a moving system could be approximated, and numbers could be rounded up since small factors would not have much effect in a linear system (Gleick, 1987). But in observing nature, it is clear that systems aren't necessarily neat and predictable. Small things do seem to make a difference. The sudden shift in direction of a hurricane, wind turbulence in a narrow canyon, and all human behavior are all examples of the messiness and unpredictability of the natural world. A fundamental aspect of linear, empirical scientific research is the search for regularity. "Any experiment looks for qualities that remain the same, or quantities that are zero. But that means disregarding bits of messiness that interfere with a neat picture" (Gleick, 1987, p. 41). Science is neat; real life is messy.

Scientists of the nineteenth and early twentieth century either ignored these small variances and unpredictability or assumed they came from outside the moving system. Movement in systems was described by linear differential equations—small changes produce small effects, and large effects occurred by adding up many small changes (Briggs & Peat, 1989). But another kind of mathematical equation also exists—nonlinear equations.

> The term *nonlinear* is defined in the context of relationships between cause and effect . . . where the effect from the sum of two causes is not equal to the sum of the individual effects. The whole is not equal to the sum of its parts. (Scott, 1995, p. 189)

In other words, many small changes in a system may not necessarily add up to big results, but a small change can and often does create a large effect. Nonlinear events occur in our natural macroworld. "Above atomic physics, all levels of the scientific hierarchy are nonlinear" (Scott, 1995, p. 180).

At the end of the nineteenth century, the French mathematician Henri Poincaré discovered problems with using linear equations to describe complex movement. As a scientist and mathematician, he set out to prove the stability of the solar system. The well-established equation for Newton's law of motion predicted the movement of *two* bodies in the solar system. But when Poincaré tried to make calculations for just *three* bodies, complexity and frightening unpredictability ensued. In fact, he found that the solar system should break apart from this seemingly chaotic movement. Poincaré had discovered that a multibodied system (one with complexity) is nonlinear in nature.

> Poincaré revealed that chaos, or the potential for chaos, is the essence of a nonlinear system, and that even a completely determined system like the orbiting planets could have indeterministic [unpredictable] results. In a sense he had seen how the smallest effects could be magnified through feedback. He had glimpsed how a simple system can explode into shocking complexity. (Briggs & Peat, 1989, p. 28)

Poincaré created dynamical systems theory, the theory of systems in motion that vary or evolve over time. However, his discovery went virtually unnoticed until almost a century later when the computer revolution made long, involved mathematical computation possible.

Mathematicians of the late nineteenth and early twentieth century could only calculate the simplest nonlinear equations. But the invention of high-speed computers made complicated, nonlinear equations possible. One of the first scientists to use this new technology was meteorologist Edward Lorenz. In the early 1960s, Lorenz used an early computer to make models of long-range weather patterns. At this time, science assumed if you used ". . . an *approximate* knowledge of a system's initial conditions and an understanding of natural law, one [could] calculate the *approximate* behavior of the system" (Gleick, 1987, p. 15). Lorenz began his experiments using basic nonlinear equations to map and hopefully predict weather change. Graphed patterns seemed to reveal recognizable weather cycles when inputting mathematical data to the sixth decimal point.

> One day . . . wanting to examine one sequence at greater length, Lorenz took a shortcut. Instead of starting the whole run over, he started midway through. To give the machine its initial conditions, he typed the numbers straight from the earlier printout. Then he walked down the hall to get away from the noise and drink a cup of coffee. When he returned an hour later, he saw something unexpected, something that planted a seed for a new science. (Gleick, 1987, p. 16)

Based on the assumptions of linear science, the new run of numbers should have been an exact duplicate of the previous ones. It wasn't even close. In fact they diverged so quickly and completely it was as if totally new numbers were used. "The problem lay in the numbers he had typed. In the computer's memory, six decimal places were stored. . . . On the printout, to save space, just three appeared. . . . Lorenz had entered the shorter, rounded-off numbers, assuming [as science believed] the difference . . . was inconsequential" (Gleick, 1987, p. 16). Clearly, the small change in numbers wasn't inconsequential at all. Lorenz realized there was a fatal flaw in the basic assumption of reductionistic, deterministic science. He also concluded that because of the inherent characteristics of nonlinear reactions, long-range predictions about the weather were impossible.

Lorenz had demonstrated what Poincaré had discovered mathematically— In nonlinear equations, even the smallest effect can be magnified by iterative or positive feedback. Iterative feedback involves continual reabsorption or enfolding of what has come before, like compound interest at the bank. Movement is fed back into itself over and over again (Briggs & Peat, 1989). From this enfolded iterative feedback, a moving system rapidly increases its complexity, the total amount of "information" in the system. The word *information* comes from the Latin word meaning "to form or shape." The movement of a complex system becomes information because it creates new form (Kenyon, 1994). Because of this, nonlinear systems (and, in nature, all systems are nonlinear) have extreme sensitivity to small changes. As Briggs and Peat (1989) write, "A small change in one variable can have a disproportional, even catastrophic impact on other variables" (p. 24). This discovery and additional work in feedback, energy entropy, and the inherent disequilibrium of orderly systems led to the new science of complexity.

Principles of Complexity Science
Complex, natural systems have a number of characteristics in common. To understand complexity science, each of these characteristics is explored in

greater detail, and the terminology relevant to understanding the principles of this new paradigm is introduced.

Deterministic Chaos

Chaos theory is the most famous aspect of complexity science (Larter, 2002). Complex systems display "chaotic movement." It is important to understand what "chaos" means in complex systems. In everyday use, the word *chaos* means "a state of confusion or disorder." It is a total lack of organization or order. This entropic chaos has a negative connotation. It's something to be avoided. As part of complexity science, the word *chaos* takes on a new, positive meaning as *deterministic chaos*. In this context, it refers to seemingly unruly systems that have complicated and irregular movement patterns. Chaos refers to the irregular side of nature, the discontinuous and the erratic. Chaos theory is the study of processes that change dramatically and unpredictably from slight changes or input to the moving system. However, this does not imply complete disorder (Gleick, 1987). A dynamical system is so complex it *appears* random. Chaos actually is an abstract cosmic principle referring to the source of all creation (Abraham, 1994). Deterministic chaos is seen in moving systems with high degrees of order involving very subtle and sensitive behavior. Chaos is about potential, the potential inherent in very complex things. Chaos theory says new order emerges out of the highly complex patterns of natural movement. This order-out-of-chaos processing is explored in detail later in the chapter. All naturally occurring systems, events, and phenomena are complex and, therefore, subject to chaos. "The revolution in chaos applies to the universe we see and touch, to objects at human scale. Everyday experience and real pictures of the world have become legitimate targets for inquiry" (Gleick, 1987, p. 6).

Dynamical systems reach a level of chaotic movement through a special feedback system known as *iterative feedback*. Iterative feedback has a compounding effect, with the movement of the dynamical system folding back on itself in self-reinforcing loops. The effects are then magnified as the feedback influences the system over and over again, adding and compounding the effects. With iterative feedback, the system begins to move or branch in new directions. In chaos theory, these new avenues of movement are known as *bifurcations*. As the movement of the system is compounded through iterative feedback, the effects of a particular iteration create two results instead of one (Van Eenwyk, 1996). As the compounded movement continues, these two branches themselves divide or *bifurcate* into other iterative feedback loops, which continue to bifurcate into more sets of iterative dynamics. "In very short order bifurcations occur so rapidly and generate so many new iterating/bifurcating systems that their dynamics defy analysis" (Van Eenwyk, 1996, p. 332). Bifurcations can develop in a regular fashion over time or in abrupt shifts. A bifurcation is a new path, a new way of life. It is a point of departure at which the system transforms itself and a new order is formed (Briggs & Peat, 1999). The abrupt development of a bifurcation is known as a *catastrophic bifurcation*.

The constantly changing, unstable quality of complex systems involves *edge-of-chaos dynamics*. Systems on the edge of chaos shift between predictable, highly ordered structure and behavior and chaotic activity. As the system shifts, important changes and growth occur. The edge of chaos is the maximum point of creative potential. It is the place where the system begins to evolve (Shulman, 1997). It is also the place of optimum vigor and vitality. A system moving at the edge of chaos can adapt and adjust quickly to change or disturbance without losing its underlying order.

Unpredictability

Unpredictability is an overriding principle of complexity science. "Beyond a certain threshold of complexity, systems go in unpredictable directions; they lose their initial conditions and cannot be reversed or recovered" (Briggs & Peat, 1989, p. 150). Empirical science's deterministic, mechanical view tells us just the opposite. Complexity science now reveals that real-world events are not as predictable as once assumed. Everything in the real world is complex, and once a system attains a small amount of complexity it becomes subject to an exquisite degree of sensitivity to circumstances that make it essentially unpredictable (Polkinghorne, 1993). Where does this unpredictability come from? It derives from several other characteristics of complex systems in motion.

Nonlinearity

Unpredictability in complex systems first comes from their *nonlinear* nature. The term *nonlinear* expresses relationships that are not proportional. As discussed previously, the parts don't add up to the whole. Nonlinearity has to do with the influence of the amplified "small" (Briggs & Peat, 1999). It is about subtle influences. In contrast, linear systems (as assumed in our science) can be graphed on a straight line. A thermometer is a linear graph. Things add up. If it is 50 degrees and the temperature doubles, it is 100 degrees. "Linear equations are solvable, which makes them suitable for textbooks. Linear systems have an important modular virtue; you can take them apart, and put them together again—the pieces add up" (Gleick, 1987, p. 23). Nonlinear systems aren't solvable. They can't be broken apart and added together. If they are, different results are obtained. Nonlinear systems are unpredictable, as Lorenz discovered with his weather calculations.

Sensitivity to Initial Conditions

Unpredictability also derives from a complex system's sensitivity to initial and ongoing conditions. This describes the dramatic effect that small changes, through iterative feedback, can have on large systems through an underlying web of relationships (Shepherd, 1993). In nonlinear systems, where the system has started is of little help in determining where it is going (Van Eenwyk, 1996). This extreme sensitivity to initial conditions is metaphorically called the "Butterfly Effect." This phrase, first coined by Lorenz, says that a butterfly flapping its wings in Tokyo can create storm systems the next month in Texas. This communicates the exquisite sensitivity of complex systems. Let's look at an example. A small stream running through a forest has a very irregular bank. The shape of the riverbank is determined by the conditions along the river's course. Maybe a small tree branch fell into the stream at one point slightly changing the direction of water flow and creating a buildup of sand. The shape of the bank is altered. Perhaps a beaver built a dam in another spot rerouting the stream and making a larger change in the bank's shape. Even the seemingly smallest things can make a big difference in the actual shape of the riverbank. Complex systems, like our stream bank, are unpredictable because of sensitivity to initial conditions—the smallest factor can completely change the whole event.

Wholeness

Unpredictability, nonlinearity, and sensitivity to conditions clearly require complex systems to be considered as a whole. "Though chaos appears to be the opposite of wholeness . . . [Poincaré] realized wholeness lay at its heart" (Briggs & Peat, 1999, p. 155). Complexity science tells us that a natural event in motion—human circulation, a thunderstorm, or a musical concert—must be viewed as an unfolding whole process. Studying an isolated portion of that event doesn't really tell us much about what is actually happening. Unlike empirical science, the principles of complexity science show us that cutting up and examining the parts of a system cannot reveal its true nature. Because the whole is always in a state of flux or transformational change, a phenomenon must be studied in its whole aspect. A good example comes from orthopedic medicine. In traditional medical school training, bones are studied as inert objects separate from other body systems. Because they come from cadavers, they are dead. But living bones, though seemingly hard and unmoving, are actually living, dynamical systems in admittedly slow motion. To truly understand how bones heal, they must be considered in their wholeness—not the bones separate from the marrow and separate again from the joints. When systems are considered in their wholeness, it is acknowledged that a change in any part of the system will always change the whole.

Emergent Properties

Another important characteristic of complex systems is their *emergent properties*. An emergent property is one that is not merely the sum of its components and is not found in previous dimensions (Wilber, 1996). Emergent properties are ". . . novel features of a system as a whole that are not features of its constituent parts separately . . ." (Freeman, 2001a, p. 148). What emerges from the complex movement has features over and above what develops from just adding up the constituent parts. "In a nonlinear system the whole is much more than the sum of its parts, and it cannot be reduced or analyzed in terms of simple subunits acting together" (Shepherd, 1993, pp. 239–240). For example, water has properties that it does not share with either hydrogen or oxygen. When these elements are combined as H_2O, what is created has unique properties not equal to the sum of its parts. These are water's emergent properties (Scott, 1995). Our experience of a complex musical event like a symphony gives us another excellent example. Most symphony orchestras have 150 members playing, on average, fifteen different musical parts and a conductor to coordinate the effort. Playing a symphony is a complex, moving phenomenon (music and sound are movement, as will be explored extensively in the next chapter). Looking at the various parts—the oboe, the second violins, the percussion, and so forth—cannot give you any idea of the musical experience that will emerge when all parts are played together. The *music* is the emergent property of all those performers playing so many different notes in so many different parts. The event, as a whole, is much greater than the mere sum of its parts.

Order and Form

The final general principle of complexity science is the rise of order and form from chaos. As noted earlier, the idea of chaos is not one of confusion and complete disorganization. Chaos and instability are not the same thing in complexity science. In fact, complexity science discovered universal patterns of order underlying the seemingly chaotic movement patterns of complex systems. Chaos is a way of seeing order and pattern where only the random, the erratic, and the unpredictable have been previously observed (Shepherd, 1993). Chaotic dynamics can, in fact, describe stable systems, known as *self-organizing systems* (Holte, 1993). A chaotic system can be stable if its particular brand of irregularity persists in the face of small disturbances (Gleick, 1987). The longer the phenomenon lasts, the more underlying order is revealed.

Let's examine the process of order from chaos. As a moving system (water flow, blood movement, electricity through wires, or whatever) increases its complexity through iterative feedback, bifurcations occur. These bifurcations continue to double, rapidly bursting into seemingly chaotic movement. To understand these complex movement patterns, scientists and mathematicians create a map called *phase space* that uses as many variables as needed to demonstrate the system's movement. Phase space represents all the variables that change in time and completely describes a dynamical system (Ditto, 1996). When countless examples of these maps are studied, it becomes apparent that what seemed like random, chaotic movement displays an underlying, implicit order. There are forces, *attractors*, that organize the movement and provide order. An attractor is a pattern to which a system is drawn or attracted according to its own nature. It is the final trajectory or path of the system. The attractor is a dynamical system's set of stable conditions, a particular pattern of behavior (Williams, 1997). "The attractor underlies and governs the dynamic behavior of a complex system" (Larter, 2002, p. 23). But nature does not take on indefinite forms. It assumes only certain stable patterns. These patterns are the attractors.

There are four general types of attractors that exert influence in different degrees of movement complexity. The first is a chaotic system with no order. The second type is a fixed-point attractor. Seen in simple movement with one vibrating or oscillating body (like a pendulum), this form of movement shortly goes dead. A swinging pendulum vibrates back and forth around the *point of rest* (point of no movement) until it is finally drawn to this point and stops.

A third class of attractor is a *limit-cycle attractor*, which constitutes a regularly repeating path in phase space. Like a ball rolling from a hilltop down to a valley and up the other side, this attractor is *periodic*, recurring at regular intervals. The movement is mechanically repetitive and is independent of what is going on outside it (Briggs & Peat, 1999). The frequency of tone, because it is periodic, is a limit-cycle attractor. Another form of limit-cycle attractor occurs when two oscillating bodies interact. The two previously independent limit cycles get hooked together. Oscillation A is swept into a circle by oscillation B, forming a doughnut-shaped form in phase space called a *torus*. A torus attractor is a chaotic attractor that can collapse multiple cycles of oscillation together into a single dynamic constant (Williams, 1997). The torus is more complex and evolved than fixed-point or limit-cycle attractors. The coupled motion of the oscillating pair is visualized as a line that winds around the torus, making the surface of the torus an attractor itself. If the frequencies of the two oscillating systems are in a simple ratio (expressed in single-digit whole numbers, e.g., 2:3), the twists around the torus join up exactly. The combined system is exactly periodic (recurring at a regular interval). The Cymatics work of Hans Jenny (1972), where frequency creates intricate patterns in various materials, is an excellent example.

As a system increases its complexity, it jumps from fixed-point, to limit-cycle, to torus attractors. But when the system breaks into chaotic movement, a fourth type of attractor, the *strange attractor*, emerges. The strange attractor is the underlying organization of the apparent disorganization of phase space. It is the implicit order underlying the chaos. "A strange attractor is the epitome of contradiction, never repeating, yet always resembling,

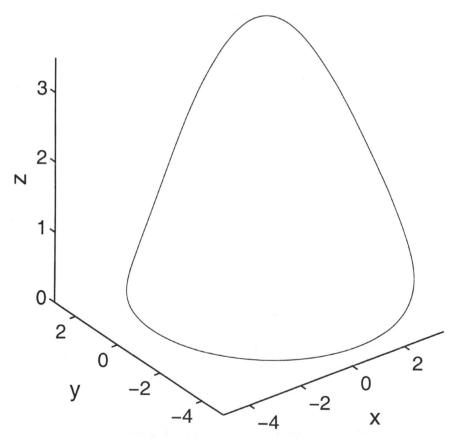

Figure 1. Limit-cycle attractor from the Rössler differential-equation system: $dx/dt = -y - z$, $dy/dt = x + 0.2y$, **and** $dz/dt = 0.2 + z(x - 2.5)$. **Courtesy of Y-C. Lai.**

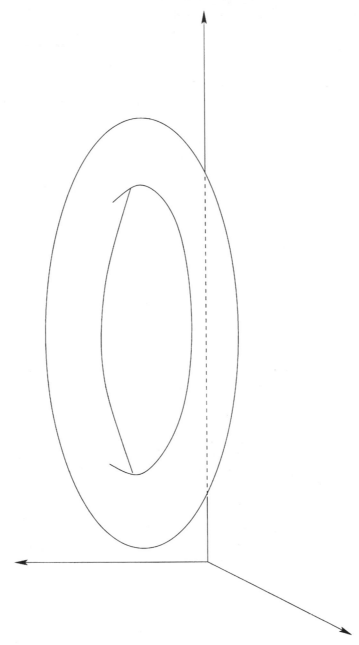

Figure 2. Schematic illustration of a two-frequency torus attractor in three-dimensional phase space. Courtesy of Y-C. Lai.

itself: infinitely recognizable, never predictable" (Van Eenwyk, 1996, p. 333). A strange attractor is an attractor that is broken up. It is also known as *turbulence* in the system. Turbulence is chaotic movement and involves endless divisions and subdivisions at smaller and smaller scales. Each area of movement is moving at different speeds. These are the bifurcations mentioned earlier. The physical shapes that the unpredictability of chaotic form takes are the strange attractors. They are responsible for deterministic chaos, where structure emerges, propagates, grows, splits apart, and is recombined into new patterns (Shulman, 1997). Brophy (1999) notes, "Chaotic phenomena are deterministic in an unpredictable way. Chaotic systems behave according to intricately modeled strange attractors that clearly show relation to real-world phenomena" (p. 118).

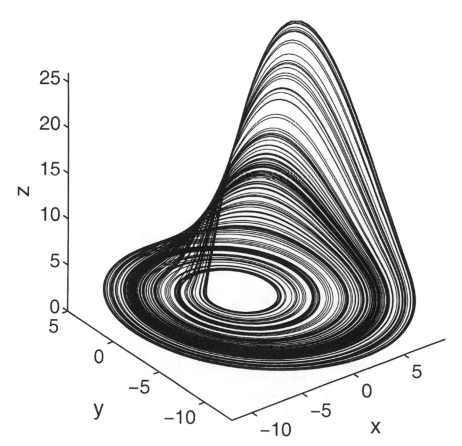

Figure 3.   Chaotic attractor from the Rössler differential-equation system: $dx/dt = -y - z$, $dy/dt = x + 0.2y$, and $dz/dt = 0.2 + z(x - 6.2)$. Courtesy of Y-C. Lai.

The effect of strange attractors acting on a chaotic system is governed by an underlying order to the patterns and predictability of bifurcation development. Richard Feigenbaum, a pioneer in this new science,

> ... discovered, embedded in these systems on the way to disorder, a universal number, a constant as fundamental as π, representing the ratio in the scale of transition points during the doubling process. This constant, 4.4492016090, predicts *when* the splits will occur. He found that when a system works on itself again and again [feedback], it exhibits change at precisely the same point along the scale. Such systems are self-referential—that is, the behavior at one level, or scale, guides the behavior of another hidden inside of it. (Shepherd, 1993, p. 241)

This number, known as the golden section, is universal—different systems behave exactly the same way. The patterns of chaos reveal a universal order inherent in the nature of any dynamical system—water turbulence, animal populations, economic trends, the healthy human heartbeat, and resonance characteristics of musical instruments.

In complex systems, randomness is interlaced with order, simplicity enfolds complexity, complexity harbors simplicity, and order and chaos are repeated at smaller and smaller scales. All this defines their *fractal* quality. A fractal is a pattern that repeats the same design, detail, or definition over a broad range of physical or time scales (Williams, 1997). A fractal is the organization and functioning of dynamical systems, which are the same at all levels of scale, from the largest to the smallest part (Hubbard, 2002). The self-repeating nature of this order is illustrated visually by fractal geometry. These are the traces, marks, and forms created by chaotic systems. This is the geometry of the natural world and is the appropriate mathematical language for describing chaotic, complex systems (Holte, 1993). Derived from the Latin word *fractua*, meaning "irregular," it captures the irregularity that is the signature of nature's creative force. Fractals embrace not only the realms of chaos and noise but also a wide variety of natural forms. "Nature's patterns are the patterns of chaos. 'Fractal' is the name given by scientists to the patterns of chaos that we see in the heavens, feel on earth, and find in the very veins and nerves of our bodies" (Briggs & Peat, 1999, p. 100). Fractal geometry maps all the points in phase space that characterize chaotic movement. What emerges is a picture or form with jagged edges that maps this movement. What is amazing is that this form is self-repeating—the large form is the same as any small portion of the form. This is referred to in complexity science as *self-similarity*. As Eastern philosophies have stated, "As below, so above." Fractal geometry has now proven that adage. But what is unique about the self-similarity of chaotic systems is that the self-similarity is not perfect. There are always slight differences. The term *self-similarity* ". . . includes this idea of individual differences and uniqueness as well as similarities. . . . [In] fractals in nature and art—what is self-similar is infused with what is different in ways that defy description" (Briggs & Peat, 1999, p. 103).

Strange attractors can be mapped as visual geometric forms, but they also have fractal time features. The most common of these fractal time patterns found in nature is the 1/f spectrum. This intermittent bursting behavior in a time series is an unexplainable "noise" variability in a quantity with time. The 1/f spectrum is one of the most common forms of noise in natural phenomena. It is found in earthquakes, volcanic activity, the flow rate of rivers, many levels of the human neural system, and musical melodies (Anderson & Mandell, 1996). Out of this universally organized structure comes form. This so-called chaos is the basis for order, stability, and structure, including

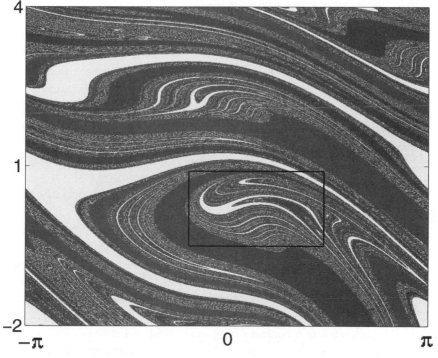

Figure 4. Fractal basin boundaries in the following forced Duffing's system: $d^2x/dt^2 + 0.1\,dx/dt + x - x^2 = 0.06 \sin (0.8t)$. The plane shown is $(x, y \equiv dx/dt)$. The black, gray, and black regions are basins of attraction of three distinct attractors. Courtesy of Y-C. Lai.

life itself (Holte, 1993). The chaos of complex, nonlinear systems is the state of living things. "It is, in fact, difficult to think of a biological 'thing' that does not take advantage of nonlinearity to establish its integrity, its oneness" (Scott, 1995, p. 190).

Complexity Science in Living Systems

There is now abundant evidence that the principles of complexity science are evident in living systems, including the human body and its functioning. Fractal structure is seen in all systems of the body—the branching of the nerves, the folds of the brain, the membranes of liver cells, the human circulatory system, and the structure of living tissue (Briggs & Peat, 1989). Fractal self-similarity pervades the human body. Functions of living systems also follow fractal processing and time scales. The beating of a healthy heart follows fractal rhythms. Each beat is essentially but never completely the same. Optimum heart rhythm stays in the edge-of-chaos dynamic. Too much regularity, and congestive heart failure occurs. Too much chaotic movement, and the defibrillation of a heart attack results.

Other systems in living things also show nonlinear, fractal behavior. Nonlinear dynamics are seen in blood pressure, respiration, and hormone fluctuations and in blood cell variability over time (Goldberger, 1992). From the action potential of nerve firing to the functioning of the immune system, the living body reflects all the principles of complex systems in motion. "Researchers increasingly recognized the body as a place of motion and oscillation—and they developed methods of listening to its variegated drumbeat. They found rhythms that were invisible on frozen microscope slides or daily blood samples" (Gleick, 1987, p. 280). And increasingly, it is believed that healthy functioning is a matter of maintaining and using edge-of-chaos dynamics. Complexity science as it relates to health and disease is explored in greater detail in subsequent chapters.

All biological forms including the human body are examples of special self-organizing structures known as *complex adaptive systems*. Self-organizing structures are those that, though still in a state of constant movement and flux, have self-maintaining features in that flow. They are relatively stable over time, preserving their internal equilibrium while maintaining openness and possible influence from the outside world (Briggs & Peat, 1999). For example, our bodies are in a constant state of renewal and change. The cells of our stomach lining are replaced every three days, and our skin cells are shed and replaced continuously. Although there is this constant movement, the general structure remains the same. The cells of our stomachs do not suddenly develop as a new kidney. In a self-organizing system, it is the ongoing process of re-creation that sustains its identity or preferred state. "The most basic idea of self-organizing systems is that, instead of a single determining agent, there are several interacting forces, which can settle into a preferred state, known as an attractor" (Richardson, 2000, p. 112).

In complex adaptive systems, the order generated evolves as the system learns to regulate itself through iterative feedback. This gives rise to complex adaptation rather than simple, direct adaptation. Complex adaptive systems learn to learn by developing a feedback system to monitor the factors affecting it (Shulman, 1997). This process is the drive in living matter to perfect itself (Kenny, 1989). Survival, growth, and health mean continuing to change from one state to another. To stop changing and adapting to the continuous stream of new information from both inner and outer sources is to die.

The self-creation of complex adaptive systems is known as *autopoiesis*. An autopoieic system's primary function is to re-create itself continuously. Such systems do not simply maintain stasis when confronted by changing external conditions but, rather, dynamically re-create themselves. Autopoieic processes are emergent phenomena of biological systems and move beyond the physics theory of complexity science into a biological principle. Autopoieic systems are thought of as patterns of processes rather than as material structures. "The human body . . . continuously re-creates itself out of new molecular material, while patterns of hormonal, metabolic, and neural activity remain more or less constant" (Combs, 1995, p. 27). It is now believed that life is not a thing but, rather, a process. A living body is a dynamic, ever-unfolding process, not a fixed object (Abram, 1996). Organization of living systems ". . . is such that their only product is themselves, with no separation between producer and product. The being and doing of an autopoieic unity are inseparable, and this is their specific mode of organization" (Maturana & Varela, 1980, p. 49). Anything that continually creates itself is a living entity (Sahtouris, 2002).

Autopoieic self-organizing systems happen not because each individual element has special properties or serves as the determiner of change (such as the genetic code) but because a whole network of individual units reaches a certain state of connectivity.

There is no master control: the organized pattern arises from complex "strategies" of competition and cooperation worked out in response to changing conditions. . . . Outcomes are never predictable in principle, because the number of combinations and changing factors are too large to calculate. (Shulman, 1997, p. 111)

It is the network of interactions going on simultaneously that determines form and functioning of the living organism. In the systems of the human body, this connectivity of interactions results in *recursive organization*.

Recursive Organization

A system is recursive when it has systems embedded within systems embedded within systems (Jibu & Yasue, 1995). Each level of organization is a prerequisite for formation of the next level, and each level is enfolded into the next. Yet each level is a whole entity itself while simultaneously being part of a greater level of organization, which is a new whole entity. For example, an atom is a whole entity, yet it becomes a part of a greater organization, a molecule. A molecule then becomes a part of a great whole entity, a DNA strand (Wilber, 1996). Recursively organized systems evolve and transcend previous levels of organization, but they also include them. They are more inclusive and, therefore, more adequate to cope with the complex world. As Wilber (1998) notes,

> Each higher level possesses the essential features of its lower level(s), but then adds elements not found on those levels. Each higher level, that is, *transcends* but *includes* its juniors. And this means that each level of reality has a different architecture. . . . (p. 9)

So when it is said that the whole is greater than the sum of its parts, it means the whole has a higher or deeper level of organization than the parts alone (Wilber, 1996). Each level in the self-organizing system sacrifices some of its individuality for the sake of the collective. "Yet these hidden degrees of freedom are always present to animate the system" (Briggs & Peat, 1999, p. 134).

Each level of organization in a recursively organized system is important and valued in its own right. "Each stage is true, each succeeding stage is 'more true': it contains the previous truths and then adds its own, emergent, novel truths, thus both including and transcending its predecessors" (Wilber, 1998, p. 207). Input or change on any level of the organization alters the whole system—moving up the organizational ladder and moving down. A change to an atom alters the higher organization of the molecules and the DNA strand. But altering the DNA also affects the organization of its constituent parts, the molecules and the atoms. Higher levels affect the lower levels just as much as the lower levels alter the higher organizational levels. All the building blocks of a recursively organized system are constantly revised and rearranged as the system adapts to new, constantly changing input from the environment. Alter any part of the system, and each component of that whole is affected, and the whole system is changed. This is especially true in the vast interacting systems of the human body. The "hardware" of the human body " . . . is living tissue already organized in a nested hierarchy of information-processing systems. When our human information-processing units solve a new problem, the feedback alters the hardware!" (Shulman, 1997, p. 94).

Biological organisms, especially humans, are composed of numerous series of nested information-processing systems that lead from functioning of the body, to processes of the mind, to emotions, to higher awareness.

> Each senior level in the Great Nest, although it includes its juniors, nonetheless possesses emergent qualities not found on the junior level. Thus, the vital animal body *includes* matter in its makeup, but it also *adds* sensations, feelings, and emotions, which are not found in rocks. While the human mind *includes* bodily emotions in its makeup, it also *adds* higher cognitive faculties, such as reason and logic, which are not found in plants or other animals. And while the soul *includes* the mind in its makeup, it also *adds* even higher cognitions and affects, such as archetypal illumination and vision, not found in the rational mind. (Wilber, 1998, pp. 8–9)

In this recursive organization, then, thought and emotion can influence lower levels of organization (brain, neurons, bodily systems) just as this lower level influences the higher organization expressed as aspects of mind (consciousness, perception, thought).

The recursive organization of biological functioning is also unique in that all these information-processing systems are coevolving. Coevolution involves a striving toward integration so that some parts of the system can be more or less constant, while other parts are freed to be more changing and adaptive. In the human body, certain functioning systems, like breathing and heart rate, are controlled by more or less set structures. But other bodily systems, like the immune reaction and the mental processing of thinking and creativity, continue to evolve and change.

Music Therapy and Recursive Organization

The processes inherent in recursive organization are important when thinking about influencing functioning through a therapy intervention like music therapy. Any part of the structure that is affected by the intervention can and does influence other levels of the organization. As explored in later chapters, music has been found to alter DNA. These changes have effects at higher levels of organization. Yet music can also alter emotional state, an emergent property of higher recursive organization. These changes in emotion can move back down the chain of organization and eventually alter a DNA chain or the molecules of protein that constitute it. However, because of the principles of complexity science, it would be impossible to "prove" what has made the changes or to predictably replicate the results. It will be important to keep these principles of complexity science and recursive organization in mind as the possible ways music therapy has an impact on human functioning are explored in later chapters.

Complexity science is now well established in the scientific community. It is ". . . not just a theory but also a method, not just a canon of beliefs but also a way of doing science" (Gleick, 1987, p. 38). There is, as with all scientific theories, heated debate about its overall validity, principles, and applications. However, complexity science was established in the same way all scientific models have been since the time of Galileo—first through mathematical equations and then through experimental substantiation. This process happened for complexity science through unprecedented interdisciplinary cooperation and research (Gleick, 1987). Traditional science emphasizes narrow specialties and solitary research. But complexity science ". . . breaks across the lines that separate scientific disciplines. Because it is a science of the global nature of systems, it has brought together thinkers from fields that had been widely separated" (Gleick, 1987, p. 5). The principles of complexity science are now applied in many disciplines—biology, human consciousness, economics, cultural development, and, most important to this book, human functioning and the restoration of health (Lewin, 1992). Though complexity science principles are applied to some medical treatments (as will be explored in chapter 6), generally the biomedical model has been slow to make this paradigm shift. A new medical paradigm based on complexity and wholeness is needed to meet the challenges of health and wellness. How does all this relate to music therapy? That is really what this book is about.

What have we learned about chaos and complexity? What does all this mean? We know that our natural world is complex, messy, and, essentially, unpredictable. Dynamical systems in motion (all naturally occurring phenomena, including human functioning) are nonlinear. And we have come to realize ". . . that the complexity of a truly interesting system—a living organism, a mind, a human culture—is awesome" (Scott, 1995, p. 187). It can also be stated that a human invention like music and its impact on human behavior and functioning are also amazingly complex. Because nature is nonlinear, events and processes in our world are sensitive to initial and ongoing conditions. New properties emerge that are greater than and different from just adding up the various parts. The real world must be considered as a whole because the outcome of each process will be different. Exact predictions of what will happen are impossible. The reductionistic dream of our current science has been dashed (Briggs & Peat, 1989). But in complexity science, the underlying equations that determine the dynamics of chaotic systems are quite simple. Therefore, prediction may be lost, but understanding is increased.

If we are to understand complex systems like human functioning and health, we must shift our paradigm and accept new assumptions about the nature of our world. Complexity science offers this new vision.

> This new science makes a strong claim about the world, namely, that when it comes to the most interesting questions, questions about order and disorder, decay and creativity, pattern formation and life itself, the whole cannot be explained in terms of the parts. There are fundamental laws about complex systems but they are new kinds of laws. . . . They are laws of structure and organization and scale, and they simply vanish when you focus on the individual constituents of a complex system. (Holte, 1993, p. 125)

Complexity science is a science of ongoing process rather than of fixed state. It focuses on becoming rather than being (Gleick, 1987). Only the radically new approach of this science ". . . could begin to cross the great gulf between knowledge of what one thing does [as emphasized in current science]—one water molecule, one cell of heart tissue, one neuron—and what millions of them can do" (Gleick, 1987, p. 8). Because of nonlinearity and unpredictability, complexity science is as much about what cannot be known as about certainty and fact. "It's about letting go, accepting limits, and celebrating magic and mystery" (Briggs & Peat, 1999, p. 7). Complexity scientists are working to understand how the real world works.

It is also a paradigm that is very inclusive. Complexity science can and does include information from reductionistic, empirical research. Research from the complexity science standpoint is inclusive of all forms of research yet also has its unique research approaches. As presented extensively in subsequent chapters, empirical research sheds light on how and why music therapy is an effective treatment modality. It is now time to add the new insights and research from complexity science to this knowledge base.

Music Therapy and Complexity Science

Music is a complex, dynamical system in motion. Biological systems, including the human organism, are also complex (Lewin, 1992). The interaction of music and human biological functioning, as occurs in music therapy, must be an even more complex dynamical system. The results of this interaction (the health and therapeutic gains) are emergent properties of this system. The effectiveness of music therapy as a treatment intervention can-not be proven in a reductionistic approach because the process involved must be considered as a whole. There is value, however, in understanding the mechanisms of a system to show the reasons why certain effects might occur (Lewin, 1992). The first step in understanding the mechanisms in-volved in music therapy is to examine the building blocks of music—sound—and how humans perceive this sensory input.

To support the thesis of this book, all the parts of the whole called music therapy are explored in order to understand the immense complexity in-volved. Early Newtonian science, before Descartes' reductionism, acknowl-edged forces in nature that could be experienced without the knowledge of the inner workings (Levenson, 1994). The same approach is used in looking at the power of music to heal. The effects of music therapy interventions are observed and documented with acknowledgment that it is an important healing tool without knowing or understanding all the mechanisms that make it work. Seventy years of clinical practice and fifty years of scientific re-search give us extensive knowledge of the mechanisms involved. In chapter 3, the complexity of sound vibrations, including the energy considerations and the organization of sound known as music, is explored. Music is shown to possess all the criteria for a complex, dynamical system in motion. In chapters 4, 5, 6, and 7, current knowledge concerning the impact of music therapy on the human mind, emotions, body, and spirit is presented.

Because of the principles of complexity science, music therapy will ulti-mately need to be thought of as a whole process. By exploring the complex-ity of the music therapy process, a new theory of music therapy called music and soulmaking will be developed.

~

CHAPTER THREE

Of Sound and Music

I am a new music therapist. I've been in my job at the adolescent psychiatric hospital only six months. David is a small, angelic-faced fourteen year old recently admitted for physical aggression and verbal hostility toward women teachers. Looking at him, it's hard to believe until I greet him on the ward one morning, and he assails me with a barrage of profanity and spits in my face. In our staff meeting, we learn David has been physically abused by his mother most of his life. Now, in adolescence, he generalizes his anger and rage to all women in authority positions. The social worker reports David loves music and is very interested in learning to play drums and guitar. The team decides to use this interest to force him to interact with a female staff member—me, the female music therapist. Scheduling him for two individual music therapy sessions per week, I find David in his room and invite him to our first session. In language I can't repeat here, he tells me he is not going to music therapy with me. He describes me in colorful terms and, to emphasize his feelings, throws a chair at me. Since facility policy requires patients to stay in their room if they refuse a therapy or activity, I retreat to the unit office and wait for the duration of our scheduled time.

This basic routine continues twice a week for three weeks. To motivate David to attend our music therapy sessions, the treatment team agrees to deny him any music or music activity outside music therapy. If he wants to listen to or play music, he has to do it with me. After several weeks, David appears at the office door late in our scheduled time and says, "OK, let's go." We proceed to the music therapy room. He bangs on the drum set completely ignoring me—no eye contact, no response to verbal interaction, no indication I am even in the room.

At this point, normal interaction with David is impossible. But a basic princi-
ple of music therapy is that music is a form of communication and a nonthreaten-
ing form of interaction. I base my approach on these ideas and begin a program
where the music is the only interaction between us. For our next session, I set up
the drum set across the room from the piano. Nothing else is available. As we en-
ter the room, I go immediately to the piano and begin to play as many popular
songs as I know. I say nothing to David and give him no instructions. After a few
minutes, he goes to the drum set and begins to pound wildly and arrhythmically for
the entire hour completely ignoring me personally and musically. This situation
continues for several weeks. Gradually, his drum playing becomes more rhythmic
and patterns appear. We have no verbal interaction, but slowly David begins to
play in tempo with me, start and stop when I do, and repeat rhythm patterns I
play, like the bass line from Chicago's "Twenty-five or Six to Four." David is
aware of me and the music I play. The music is beginning to establish communi-
cation between us.

As the therapy continues, David's general behavior toward me changes—no
more verbal hostility, less tension when we are together, and even some eye con-
tact. The music has changed, too. We play together much more. I nonverbally chal-
lenge him by changing the dynamics, demonstrating a rhythm pattern to use on the
drums, and adding tempo changes. Our playing gets interesting and exciting. David
is enjoying himself, forgetting that he is working with a woman. The shared musi-
cal experience makes interaction nonthreatening. As our musical communication
increases, I begin to give him some basic verbal instruction. This is easily received,
and a new phase of our therapy begins. I can now confront him about his behavior,
and he can share what he is feeling. He begins to talk about his abuse with his psy-
chotherapist. Over the next several months, he makes great progress and is eventu-
ally discharged to return to school (Crowe, 1992).

The first component of the complex, dynamical system in motion called
music therapy is music itself. To understand music, it is necessary to know
about the basic building blocks of music—from basic sound vibration to complex musical forms and devices. This chapter gives a general overview of the
principles of sound production, especially its energetic qualities. To move toward defining music, rhythm is introduced as the agent that takes sound and
organizes it over time to create music. The components of music—rhythm,
tone, timbre, melody, harmony, and dynamics—are the particular parameters
of sound that add another layer of complexity. Other important topics are investigated including how music functions in human society, music performance as a motor skill, and how movement constitutes music and, therefore,
fits the criteria for a complex, dynamical system in motion.

Sound as a Complex, Physical Energy System

The word *sound* is a subjective term used to report aural (hearing) psychological sensation. In a purely physical sense, what our ears pick up as sound is a vibration. A *vibration* is any to-and-fro (back-and-forth) movement—a physical, mechanical energy. Let's use the guitar string to illustrate this point. A guitar string is stretched between two points—the bridge at the bottom and the nut at the scroll. When the guitar is sitting in a corner, the strings are "at rest." To make a sound, someone has to pluck or pull back the string and let it go (*displacement*). The act of pulling back the string puts physical energy into this sound-making system. How far back the string is pulled determines how much energy is put into the system (*amplitude*). The string vibrates back and forth across its *point of rest* until air friction finally stops the movement (Wagner, 1994). There are all kinds of vibrations in our world, but the vibration that produces sound has a special property known as *simple harmonic motion*—when movement on both sides of the point of rest is equal when that string is vibrating. These are sound vibrations.

Sound vibration is mechanical energy and abides by all the natural laws governing mechanical energy. First, sound vibration moves at a particular speed, the *frequency*. This is scientifically measured by *hertz* (Hz) or how many cycles (one back-and-forth movement) occur per second. Musically, our ear hears this as *pitch*. In violin playing, the third string is tuned to A 440 Hz, meaning that the string vibrates 440 times per second and is heard as the tone A. Second, the size of the vibration can vary. We hear this amplitude as *loudness*, measured scientifically as *decibels*. Third, this mechanical energy can influence other things that can vibrate. Have you ever had the experience of playing a tape or CD and at one point in a song have a light fixture buzz? This is *resonance* where one vibrating thing (the CD) causes another body (the light fixture) to start vibrating. All things that can vibrate (and that's potentially everything) have a particular speed or frequency they vibrate at most easily. This is their *resonance frequency* and is determined by the object's size, weight, and density. Resonance is important in perceiving the sound element of pitch and is particularly important for music. Musical instruments are constructed to produce resonance in characteristic ways typical for each instrument (Jourdain, 1997). If all objects have a resonance frequency, then the human body and its structures do too. In chapter 6, the potential healing benefits of sound resonation on the human body are addressed.

So far, these are considerations of *simple* sound. But as already explored, nothing in the natural world behaves in a simple manner, and that is certainly true of sound vibration. Let's return to the example of the guitar string. When the string is plucked, it starts the whole string vibrating. But, by nature, that string moves in a complex fashion. At the same time, the whole string is vibrating, it is also vibrating in half, in quarters, in thirds, and so forth. This produces the *overtone series* and creates *complex sound*. Complex sound is the sound produced by natural phenomena—a violin string being plucked, a person singing a tone, or a tuba sounding a note. Simple sound is never produced in nature. It can only be produced artificially with electronic equipment. Complex sound comes from the complicated patterns of a vibrating body. Though we hear the tone associated with the length of the whole string as the pitch, the tones produced by half, quarters, thirds, and so on are also heard. This collection of tones is *instrument timbre*. The composition of the overtone series (how many overtones are heard, how loud they are, and how they are distributed) gives us the characteristic sound of the guitar, a violin, a trumpet, or a piano. In fact, reproducing the characteristic overtone series of an oboe is how "oboe" key is possible on an electronic keyboard.

Mechanical energy, such as sound vibration, has certain characteristics when it interacts with our environment. The sound vibration has to move from the source (guitar string) to our ear. It has to move or *propagate* through a *medium*. In most cases, the medium to move the sound vibrations is air, but sound can move through water as well as solids like walls (as you learn when your neighbor is playing his or her stereo very loudly). Air propagation is the most common form. When the guitar string is plucked and begins to vibrate, it disturbs air molecules around it. These air molecules, in turn, begin to vibrate back and forth around their point of rest. As they do this, they bump into adjacent air molecules that start vibrating, and those molecules then bump into the ones next to them, until a chain reaction of displaced air molecules begins. This process continues until groups of air molecules bump into something, including your ear. Because groups of air molecules are vibrating back and forth around their respective points of rest, some molecules will bunch together (known as a *compression*) and others will move apart leaving a partial vacuum (known as a *rarefaction*). It is this alternation of compressions and rarefactions moving through the air that is termed a *sound wave*. Sound waves are compression waves. There are several forms of sound waves. *Standing waves* propagate energy in an area 360 degrees around the moving body like a string. These waveforms are likely to be complex with many frequencies occurring because of the nature of the vibrating body. A *transverse wave* moves at a right angle from the vibrating source. And in a *longitudinal wave*, the vibration is propagated in the same direction as the disturbance. This occurs in sound coming from a column of air and in solids.

The environment affects the mechanical energy of sound waves in other ways. When a sound wave bumps into a hard surface, *reflection* occurs. The sound wave bounces off. These bounced waves add to the overall amplitude of the sound and are important factors in room acoustics. Everyone sounds like a great singer in the shower because the hard surfaces in the bathroom give us the added sound of reflected sound waves. The thousands of sound waves occurring simultaneously in a room don't affect the frequency of the sound (how fast the wave is moving) but do influence the amplitude or loudness. This is called *interference*. *Constructive interference* causes an increase in loudness, and *destructive interference*, a decrease. When two tones of slightly different frequencies are sounded together, a fluctuation in perceived loudness occurs. This is *beating* (not to be confused with the beats in music that mark time). Beating is often heard as a roughness or fluttering of the sound.

The study of sound production and the energy considerations in this mechanical energy is a branch of classical physics known as *acoustics*. This basic review of acoustical principles shows the complexity of even simple sound. But the complexity inherent in sound increases as the mechanisms of sound perception are added. This is *psychoacoustics*—the study of auditory sensory responses to the physical stimuli of sound waves (Radocy & Boyle, 1997).

Perception of Sound

The word *sound* is a word of perception. Perception is the human ability to assign meaning to sensory input, in this case, input from the ears. It involves moving the input from the sense organ to the brain where it processes the information, compares it to memories from previous experience, and decides what to label it. Perception requires comprehension. If you do not speak or understand French, you can hear a person talking in French but would not perceive the meaning of the sound combinations. You would be unable to *listen* because that involves perception. Listening is ". . . an active focusing process which allows for a quick and precise analysis of sounds that are heard" (Gilmor, Madaule, & Thompson, 1989, p. 18). The first step in understanding the perception of sound is to understand how the ear works.

Our sense of hearing is very important to us throughout our lives. Hearing is the first sense to develop before birth and the last to leave at death. "In humans the ear . . . is fully functional four-and-a-half months before we are born" (Minson, 1992, pp. 91–92). A fetus in utero can hear sounds at four and a half months. Their hearing world consists mostly of internal body sounds—heartbeat, blood movement, and especially the mother's voice.

> In utero, the fetus is enveloped by the sounds of the enclosed environment. The intra-uterine sound environment, although beyond conscious recall, may leave a wordless and amorphous memory trace which serves as a template for all future rhythmic response and provides us with a lifelong sound and rhythmic symbolic image of security, thereby providing for continuity between intra- and extra-uterine life. (Isenberg-Grzeda, 1995, pp. 145–146)

But recent research shows that before they are born, babies can hear external sounds, and newborns actually recognize songs they have heard before birth (Standley & Madsen, 1990). This occurs because the cochlear nerve is myelinated (able to transmit signals) at twenty-two weeks and extends into the brain so that the temporal lobe is completely myelinated and functioning at birth (Wade, 1996). Newborns are sensitive to music. Infants turn toward music more often than to other sounds. At one month, the baby can distinguish different frequencies and by six months can respond to changes in melodic shape (Jourdain, 1997). Our first awareness is auditory, and we process our world through sound for many months after birth. To develop a comprehensive theory of how music functions as therapy, it is important to understand the basic working of the sensory apparatus of hearing—the ear.

The Anatomy and Physiology of the Ear
The ear functions to gather sound and to *transduce* (change) the mechanical energy of sound waves to the electrochemical energy of nerve impulses. It is divided into three parts—the outer ear, the middle ear, and the inner ear. The outer ear comprises the *pinna* (the folds of skin on the sides of our head), the ear canal, and the *tympanic membrane* or eardrum. The middle ear has three small bones (*ossicles*)—the hammer, anvil, and stirrup—and a membrane, the oval window that is the barrier between the middle and inner ears. The inner ear contains the *cochlea*, the three semicircular canals, and the vestibule, an open chamber filled with thick fluid. With a basic sense of the anatomy of the ear, its function and the complex process of hearing can be explored.

The Outer Ear
Hearing begins when a sound produces a compression wave in the environment. The sound wave travels until it bumps into the pinna of the outer ear. The pinna is the structure, one on each side of the head, which is thought of when referring to "the ear." The pinna, with its folds and channels, functions to gather the compression waves of sound and focus them into the ear canal or *meatus*. The ear canal is a closed pipe—open at one end, closed by the eardrum at the other. Any vibrating body has a resonance fre-

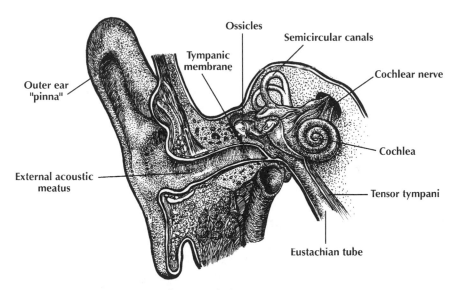

Figure 5.   The ear. Courtesy of B. Brauckman.

quency. The ear canal, actually the air trapped in the closed pipe, has a res-onance frequency range—2,000 to 7,000 Hz. When a tone within this range enters the ear, the amplitude of the wave is increased, and it is heard as louder. This may be why the 2,000 to 7,000 Hz range is the frequency of hu-man speech (Radocy & Boyle, 1997). The ear canal channels air pressure to-ward the eardrum, making the air pressure greater at the eardrum than at the open end. The pressure variations in the sound wave strike the eardrum set-ting it into vibration, just like a mallet hitting a drumhead. The eardrum is very sensitive and will start vibrating with a small amount of pressure change. It is the barrier between the outer and middle ear.

The Middle Ear

The *middle ear* is a bony chamber containing three small bones, the *ossi-cles*. The first of these bones is the *hammer*, which is attached to the eardrum by a *footplate*. When the eardrum begins vibrating, it pushes the hammer. This motion in turn moves the *anvil* and the *stirrup*, which are connected by joints. Collectively, the ossicles act as a piston system. The stirrup is attached to another membrane, the *oval window*, which is the entrance to the fluid-filled *inner ear*. The middle ear functions to transmit the mechanical vibra-tion from the outer ear into the inner ear. But the ossicles have another im-portant function. Their piston action serves to increase the power of the mechanical wave by eighteen times and decrease the physical size of the movement by a factor of three. This protects the delicate structures of the inner ear from loud noises and allows the movement to excite the denser fluid of the inner ear into vibration.

The ossicles are attached by a ligament system and have two small muscles (the smallest skeletal muscles in the body) that control the *acoustic reflex*. This contraction of the *tensor tympanic* and the *stapedius* regulates the ossicles' stiffness and is an important factor in our ability to listen to auditory input. Dr. Alfred Tomatis, a French physician, believes that the functioning of these muscles is, in fact, essential for appropriate perception of sound. He

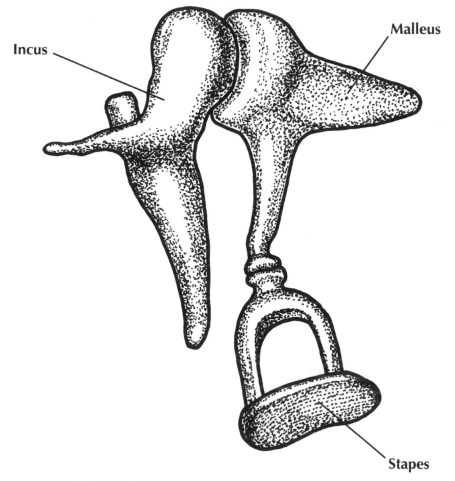

Figure 6.   The bones of the middle ear, the ossicles. Courtesy of B. Brauckman

developed a method to retrain the ear and the brain to perceive sounds appropriately. The electronic ear is a device he developed that transmits sound frequencies to a listener by air and bone conduction. Highly filtered tapes of Mozart's music and Gregorian chant are used to retrain concentration, thought, and communication skills (Campbell, 1992). The music used is highly filtered midrange and high-treble pitches. The shifts in the pitches exercise the stapedius muscle to exert more control over the ossicles, thus improving what the brain perceives. I have done the Tomatis training and found that I could feel those muscles exercise just as much as weightlifting exercises my arm muscles. This type of listening training has wide-ranging therapeutic effects, which will be explored in chapter 4.

The Inner Ear

The *inner ear* is buried deep within our head and is protected by the bony structure of the lower skull. It needs this protection because it is made up of several delicate yet vital structures that make our senses of hearing and equilibrium possible. The inner ear is divided into three parts—the vestibule, the cochlea, and the three semicircular canals. The oval window is located in the wall of the vestibule. This bony cavity is filled with a thick fluid and serves as a transitional area between the semicircular canals and the cochlea. The three semicircular canals give us our *vestibular* sense—balance and orientation to gravity. This is the basis of our spatial (space) orientation. It helps us orient to gravity and tells us where we are in the environment. The vestibular sense, though not part of the hearing sense per se, and hearing sense are controlled by the same spinal nerve. Sound input affects the vestibular sense. Maconie (1997) sees a connection between acquiring a sense of spatial orientation and monitoring high-frequency information in particular: "It is why children squeal with excitement on a roller-coaster" (p. 48). The intense vestibular sensation of the roller coaster ride triggers the high-frequency vocalization of a squeal.

The cochlea is of intense interest in the hearing process. It is the organ of hearing, the place where the mechanical energy of sound waves is changed into the electrochemical energy of the nervous system. When the ossicles push against the oval window, the movement starts the fluid vibrating in the cochlea. The cochlea is a series of bony ducts, membranes, and fluid sacks, and the whole structure is rolled up like a snail. A thick membrane, the *basilar membrane*, divides the sacks of the cochlea. Resting on the basilar membrane is the *organ of Corti*, the place of the transduction of energy. The organ of Corti is made up of hair cells, each having numerous cilia, or small hair fibers, projecting into a fluid-filled space. Another membrane, the *tectorial membrane*, projects just above the cilia.

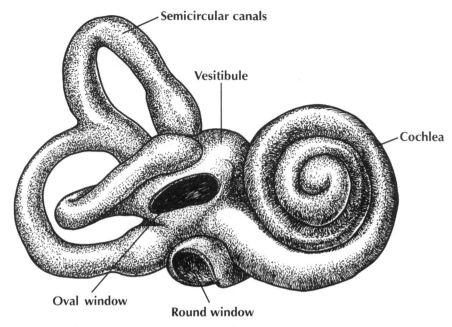

Figure 7. The inner ear. Courtesy B. Brauckman.

When the oval window bulges into the vestibule, it sets the enclosed fluid into vibration and moves the wave into the cochlear duct. The basilar membrane, inside the cochlear duct, begins to vibrate as a whole in response to the wave. This movement pushes the organ of Corti upward, bumping the cilia of the hair cells into the tectorial membrane. Each hair cell is wrapped in nerve fibers. When the cilia are irritated (pushed into the tectorial membrane), the nerves fire. This is the point of energy change. The mechanical energy starts when the guitar string is plucked. It now becomes the energy of nerve firing, an energy of electrical and chemical transmission. The process of nerve firing is examined shortly, but, first, the function of the basilar membrane and the organ of Corti as it relates to pitch and loudness perception needs to be addressed.

The basilar membrane is a thick membrane that runs along the lower side of the cochlear duct. When a vibration enters the system, it begins to vibrate as a whole. But specific frequencies will make specific areas on the membrane vibrate even more. This happens because each area or *critical band* has its own resonance. Because the organ of Corti sits on top of the basilar membrane, the hair cells with the cilia over that particular area will always be stimulated in response to a particular frequency. Over time, we learn to associate that nerve input with the given frequency. This is the "pitch" of the sound. So as

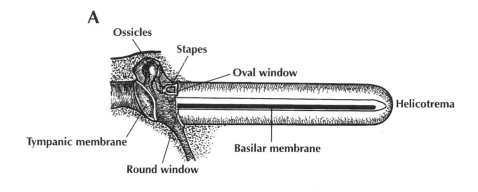

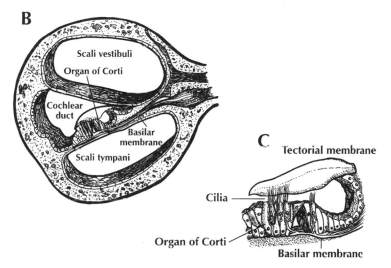

Figure 8. The cochlea: a. "unrolled cochlea," b. cross section of the cochlea, and c. detail of the organ of Corti. Courtesy of B. Brauckman.

a violin player, every time I play the third string of 440 Hz (the frequency) a specific place on the basilar membrane vibrates, causing the hair cells above it to become irritated. The nerve impulses from the irritation arrive in my brain, and I give it a name—the pitch A. This is the "Place Theory of Hearing" (Guyton, 1979). Loudness (amplitude or bigness of the wave) is perceived by the total number of nerve impulses arriving in the brain from the cochlea—the bigger the wave, the bigger the movement on the basilar membrane. Because more hair cells are stimulated, more impulses are added up, leading to our perception of "louder."

What is perceived as "pitch" is really a perception of time—how many sound waves occur in a second or, put another way, how fast the wave is moving over time. Pitch discrimination is frequency discrimination that occurs subcortically, below the thinking brain. It is the result of temporal (time) analysis. Then the naming of pitch becomes a cortical function of sound pattern identification (Wallin, 1991). Hearing is the modeling of relations and patterns including sound occurring over time, total number of neural inputs, and space between tones (Jourdain, 1997). As discussed shortly, music involves perception of deep relations.

This is a basic outline of hearing. However, the actual process is much more complex and not as simple as the above review of ear functioning might indicate. There are many considerations and subtleties in pitch perception alone that are beyond the scope of this book (Deutsch, 1982; Wallin, 1991). To more fully understand the perception of the sensory input from the ear, the workings of our nervous system and brain will be addressed in the next chapter. From this basic understanding of sound, the human phenomenon of organized sound—music—can be explored.

What Is Music?

Great philosophers, theologians, musicians, and composers have tried to define music through the ages. Here are a few of their ideas:

Music is a strange thing. I would almost say it is a miracle. For it stands halfway between thought and phenomenon, between spirit and matter, a sort of nebulous mediator, like and unlike each of the things it mediates—spirit that requires manifestation in time and matter that can do without space. . . . We do not know what music is. . . .

—Heinrich Heine

Music is the art, which is constituted at one and the same time of the corporeal and the spiritual.

—The Arab Brethren of Purity

Music might be defined as a system of proportions in the service of a spiritual impulse.

—George Crumb

Music [is] itself the supreme system of the science of man.

—Claude Lévi-Strauss

I haven't understood a bar of music in my life; but I have felt it.

—Igor Stravinsky

Music is love.

—Hanslick

Music is the art of the prophets, the only art that can calm the agitations of the soul; it is one of the most magnificent and delightful presents God has given us.

—Martin Luther

It has been said since ancient times that the nature of reality is much closer to music than to a machine, and this is confirmed by many discoveries in modern science.

—Fritjof Capra

Defining music can be approached from many perspectives. When the question is asked, "What is music?" several approaches to the answer are really being posed. First, such a question might ask to what experience or to what phenomenon the word refers. What makes up the event called music? A second approach in answering, "What is music?" would be to determine where music comes from or what its origins are. Another answer to this question may be to determine what the purpose of music is or why it exists at all. And finally, an approach can involve what behaviors occur when we're "doing" music. To define music for our purposes, all four approaches to this difficult question are used. As Heinrich Heine wrote, "Music is a strange thing." But it is a truly human thing, a magnificent thing, a pleasurable thing. Let's explore this most human of human behavior.

The Phenomenon of Music
The phenomenon of music is an acoustic event involving specific combinations of sound moving over time.

Whatever else it may or may not be . . . there is no doubt that music is motion. One sustained tone, no matter how beautiful, is not yet music. . . . Musical motion appears in various ways: in melody and harmony . . . in rhythm and form . . . and in counterpoint, texture, and tone color. (Siegmeister, 1965, p. 9)

According to philosopher Suzanne Langer (1953), motion in music is perceived motion since objects are not displaced from one place to another. Yet this perceived motion is very strong in the complex interactions of musical elements. Music theorists and philosophers over several centuries have tried to identify "musical universals" that serve as required elemental building blocks that create the experience we call music. These usually include rhythm, melody, harmony, timbre, form, and dynamics, though all musics do not necessarily contain each element in equal emphasis. "Musical universals place the focus on what music *tends to be like* in order to be considered music, even if not every example has all the features of the majority of musics . . ." (Wallin,

Merker, & Brown, 2000, p. 7). To help us understand the phenomenon of music, let's explore those building blocks, focusing on how they contribute to the sense of movement over time associated with music.

Rhythm

Rhythm is about time and the relationship of tones over time. It is the ordered characteristic of succession. Yet there are no specific sensors for time as there is for light or sound. "There is nothing there to sense. Rather, the psychological experience of time arises from the nervous system's perception of its own interactions with the world. Psychological time is the experience of having experience" (Jourdain, 1997, p. 136). The sense of time passing is in our minds. Patterns of abstract relations are held for long periods, which create a kind of temporal map. Rhythm occurs ". . . when we can predict on the basis of what is perceived [so that] . . . we can anticipate what will follow" (Fraisse, 1982, p. 150). In fact, rhythm perception likely occurs in the thalamus and is a process occurring below consciousness (Wallin, 1991).

The word *rhythm* comes from the Greek word *rhythmos*, meaning "to flow," and implies all aspects of musical timing (Mankin, Wellman, & Owen, 1979, p. 4). Musical timing includes tonal duration, beat, meter, tempo, and rhythmic pattern. "Time is the very essence of music and music experience. Each piece of music is an act of time corresponding to a temporal organization, a tonal flow-becoming—music: it emerges from silence and returns into silence" (Wallin, 1991, p. 2). It is rhythm that allows sound to become music. The Greek word *mousike*, the derivation of the English words for music and muse, included melody, dance, and poetry, whose common denominator is pulse-based rhythmicity (Merker, 2000). "Rhythm is the primordial musical factor, deep-rooted and primitive" (Hughes, 1948, p. 258). It is a cross-cultural phenomenon that is a universal characteristic of all music (Bunt, 1994).

Rhythm provides music's forward movement, making music a dynamic (in the sense of motion and change), energizing force. All nature is rhythmic in the sense of a measured recurrence of things (Hughes, 1948). Understanding rhythmicity is fundamental to understanding the universe (Elliott, 1986). In fact, rhythmic phenomena appear to be all-pervasive in the universe. These include the rhythms of deterministic chaos and fractal time, like the 1/f fractal interval, and the periodic recurrences in the macroworld like the rhythm of ocean tides. The importance of rhythm in nature and especially in living systems is addressed closely in later chapters. Let's now examine the elements of rhythm in music—musical timing.

The first element of musical timing is *duration*. The word *duration* derives from the Latin word *durare*, meaning "to last," and is how long a note is sounded in real time. To hear a pitch at all, a tone must last at least 0.013 seconds. Durations of the tone increase from that fundamental time. In musical notation, duration is measured in half notes, quarter notes, eighth notes, and so forth. But it is the *beat* or *pulse* that is the basic unit of duration. Beats divide duration into equal segments. "Beats are time points on a duration continuum" (Lerdahl & Jackendoff, 1983, p. 117). The beat gives us musical movement over time. Beat provides a regularly recurring perception of our interactions with the world. It gives us the framework on which the musical event occurs. Movement and the perception of rhythm are integrally related.

The second factor of musical timing is *meter*, a musical device for grouping beats, usually in twos and threes. Think of a waltz with its clear grouping of three (boom-chick-chick). *Tempo* is another important factor in rhythm and is the speed at which the beat occurs. Finally, *rhythmic patterns* develop by combining various durations. So a song like "Jingle Bells" can be recognized by its rhythmic pattern alone—short, short, long, short, short, long, short, short, long, short, long. Rhythm is the primary element of the phenomenon of music. Rhythm enlivens music, gives it movement over time, and creates its dynamic character.

Melody

Melody is the movement of tones over time with particular relationships that create shape in space. Melody conveys movement in several ways. It is first the sequential placement of tones of varying durations over time. It is successive movement in pitch, which itself is movement (Maconie, 1997). Tone itself is perceived as motion because the "time-scale of musical pitch is several orders of magnitude finer than the time-scale of conscious apprehension, which is why music can paradoxically be perceived both as instantaneous and as continuous" (Maconie, 1997, p. 10). This occurs because one perception lags slightly behind the other, creating a sense of forward movement.

Melody is also the shape of the movement in space—the pattern of up and down movement separate from the perception of interval relationships. This shape is the *melodic contour*. In melody, the notes move forward along a spatial contour stored in memory. Melodic contour is essential to the perception of melody. This melodic contour ". . . is the discontinuous expression of the continuous curve" (Maconie, 1997, p. 144). The melody is perceived by comparing the discontinuous notes to the melodic shape inherently present or stored previously in memory. Melody perception is trained by cultural conventions for grouping notes into contours. Melodies serve our natural tendency to relate what are actually unrelated tonal events. Each culture develops its own system for creating melodic contour, which then becomes formalized as rules of songwriting or composition (Blacking, 1973). Melody creates a sense of physical movement in space as the notes in the grouping move along the continuous curve of the contour contained in our memories.

Melodies have relationships between the various pitches (notes in musical terms). This relationship is an *interval*. For example, if a note is played and a second is sounded twice as high, it has an interval relationship of an octave. This can be expressed as a numerical ratio of 1:2—the second note is twice as fast as the first. So the octave above a note of 200 cycles per second (cps) has a frequency of 400 cps. These interval relationships give us the sense of forward movement and of a dynamic relationship. "Melody is a musical state in which these relations are harnessed, creating a field of tensions and relaxations, anticipations and surprises" (Rothstein, 1995, p. 102). This movement between tension and relaxation creates continuity, the sense that this group of tones "hangs together." Edward Rothstein (1995) notes,

> This sense of melody suspended over time, of tensions left unresolved and picked up later in order that a surface may be created over the length of a composition, is fundamental to our musical hearing. It is what allows us to speak of suspense in music and what constitutes, in part, the integrity of a composition. This motion of suspension, of extended surface, is one way tonal music addresses the passing of time itself. (p. 107)

In music, we say a melody moves in steps like "Row, Row, Row Your Boat" or in leaps like the beginning of "Somewhere Over the Rainbow." Yet this is a special kind of movement—not a movement from note to note but a flow that has the sense of a gesture. We feel the melodic movement in our bodies. In fact, through gesture, music becomes the language of the body (Ruud, 1998a). "We use our musculature to *represent* music, modeling the most important features of musical patterns by means of physical movements large and small" (Jourdain, 1997, p. 325). When great conductors like Leonard Bernstein or Seiji Ozawa conduct, we see how gesture becomes music. No great conductor just keeps time. They show the orchestra how the music ebbs and flows through the physical representation by gestures and whole body movement. I can remember when I first learned to play the piano as a child, struggling to pick out a melody. It never sounded like the tune I knew. My piano teacher, Mrs. Frank, would wisely have me sing the melody and then say, "Now play it like you sang it. That's the music." The act of singing is in and of itself a gesture since you cannot sing from discrete note to discrete note. The composer Roger Sessions (1971) noted that music ". . . embodies movement of a specifically human type that goes to the roots of our being and takes shape in the inner gestures which embody our deepest and most intimate responses" (p. 19). We experience music as gesture even when we are listening. Khorran-Sefat, Dierks, and Hacker (1996) found that during music listening, the brain structure involved in timing movement in the neocerebellum is activated even though listening is an entirely nonmotor activity. This may be why we experience music as movement and, especially, as gesture. As the great philosopher Nietzsche wrote, "One listens to music with one's muscles" (quoted in Sacks, 1998, p. 5). Music becomes expressive, sensuous movement (Mervin Britton, personal communication, December 15, 1999). In music, this sense of gesture is called the musical phrase—the rise and fall of the music. And the phrasing of music is supported by musical dynamics—the rise and fall of loudness.

The importance of gesture in performing and listening to music is supported by the work of musicologist Manfred Clynes (1977). He links specific emotional states (*"sentic" states*) with expression in the motor system.

> The sentic state may be expressed by a variety of motor modes: gestures, tone of voice, facial expression, a dance step, musical phrase, etc. In each mode the emotional character is expressed by a specific, subtle modulation of the motor action involved which corresponds precisely to the demands of the sentic state. (Clynes, 1977, p. 18)

Clynes argues these sentic motor responses are consistent cross-culturally and are the essence of musical expression. But this kind of gesture is not ". . . simply an expression of an emotion or feeling or thought; it is not a translation of something else" (Rothstein, 1995, p. 208). It is a natural part of how our minds work in relating the sensory information pouring in from our environment. The contour and sense of gesture in melody derive from these cross-cultural, innate movement patterns generated from deep emotional states.

Melody came first in music evolution. Our earliest forms of music were chants consisting of long melodic lines like early Gregorian chant. Children are born with musical behavior, and it is melody that emerges first in very young children. Research shows that infants respond to melodic contour before they can respond to melody per se (Levitin, 1999). Musical contour ". . . is our first musical competence. It has much in common with the prosody of spoken language, in which we are all experts" (Jourdain, 1997, p. 256). Children's early melodies are unstable. They follow no strict beat and waver in pitch (Andress, 1980). Listen to a year-old child singsong a basic melody as he or she experiments with vocal sound making. It has a definite shape but is free-flowing with no true rhythm. Melody is the simplest and most basic of the musical expressions.

Harmony

The third musical element, *harmony*, is closely related to melody. Musical harmony is the simultaneous sounding of tones. It is vertical pitch relations. Harmony gives music depth. The word often evokes thoughts of blocks of pleasant sounds—four-part choral hymn singing, for example. But harmony is about the relationship of notes to each other—pleasant or dissonant, block chords or melodies sounding together like a round. It is the coming together and moving apart of tones. Harmony is never static, never still. It moves over the course of the piece. Western classical music has developed harmony to a fine art. Yet even the earliest musical traditions had forms of harmony in drone tones. A drone tone is a continuously sounding note held while a melody is played. Instruments like the bagpipes and the Indian tambour sound a continuous primary tone against the melody. As harmony moved off one tone, more complex relations developed between simultaneously sounding pitches. Tensions and resolutions between notes emerged, followed by chords. This sense of resolution developed into the system of Western tonality.

The word *tonality* means "loyalty to the primary tone or *tonic*" (Apel, 1969). It is a well-formulated system ". . . of interval relationships of which melody and harmony are transient and partial expressions" (Maconie, 1990, p. 103). Western harmony implies a continuity and coherence of collective movement toward a common goal. Tonality means ". . . the anchor point from which all tones and intervals and chords are measured and compared. It is a constant reference point, a source of pull of gravity" (Jourdain, 1997, p. 105). Over 400 years of development, Western harmony has become a well-established system of procedures for reaching that common goal. It can be thought of as a map of topological space.

> There are rules for moving from one point to another on a harmonic path. There is even a sense of distance and neighborhood. And there is a quality of connection—attraction or repulsion. Some chords increase a sense of tension, others decrease it. There can be a sense of potential energy latent in a given harmony, comparable to the energy we say is latent in a weight when we lift it to a certain height: upon release, there can be a rush to a place of equilibrium. (Rothstein, 1995, p. 109)

Harmony has this sense of movement, gesture, flow, and energy. For example, find a recording of Samuel Barber's *Adagio for Strings* and listen to the opening first phrases. The piece starts with upper strings holding a single note. The lower strings then enter, playing a chord that is in tension with the held note. The chord moves to a resolution of this tension and then holds while the string melody moves in deliberate steps. Each note of the melody has its own tension and release relationship with the held chord. As the phrase builds to a climax, both the melody and the chord move in a growing sense of anticipation, moving toward the final resolution at the phrase's end. It is a dance in space and time, a complex, moving relationship of tension and release. Harmony is the most intellectual of the musical elements. It is inherently the most complex and difficult. Harmony ". . . is the last aspect of musicality to mature in the young, and tests show that many people never achieve harmonic sophistication" (Jourdain, 1997, p. 118). As explored in chapter 6, harmony is the musical element that adds to the overall emotional effect of music (Hughes, 1948).

Timbre

The fourth building block of music is *timbre*, the characteristic sound of a voice or instrument. Timbre is the quality of sound that distinguishes one tone from another even if they have the same pitch and loudness—same note and same loudness, yet the two notes sound different. Timbre is the unique characteristic of the sound. All violins have a characteristic "violin" sound. Even within a range of bad to good tone quality—a student violin compared to a Stradivarius violin—the instruments still sound like violins. A bad-sounding violin doesn't sound like a flute. That is the quality of timbre.

Timbre is first achieved by the distribution of energy among the various harmonic components of a tone. Remember the discussion earlier in this chapter on the vibrational characteristics of complex sound? A vibrating string vibrates not only as a whole but also in half, in quarters, in thirds, and so on. This complex pattern of vibration gives rise to the overtone series, the pitches produced by the string vibrating in half, thirds, quarters, and so forth. But in nature, no vibrating body, like a musical instrument, produces all the pitches of the harmonic series, which also don't have equal loudness when they are produced. Timbre occurs because each musical instrument or human voice varies in the number of harmonics it produces, how these are distributed, and how loud they are. However, timbre recognition is another complex perceptual process. Many other factors contribute to timbre perception, including the initial sound attack and sound wave buildup, vibrato, special resonance characteristics of the instrument, and the person's preparation for the timbre discrimination task (Bunt, 1994).

Our first timbre recognition is the human voice. "A young baby quickly learns to discriminate between the sound of a human voice and other significant sounds, marking out timbre as an early area of differentiation of sound" (Bunt, 1994, p. 47). Copland (1952) found timbre differences are the first sound differences discriminated by the musically untrained ear. Humans are exquisitely sensitive to timbre changes. From voice tone alone, a mother can tell if her baby's cry is one of anger, fear, or attention seeking.

Timbre is a big concern in musical instrument construction. The distribution of energy varies along the harmonic series from instrument to instrument. This occurs because of how the instrument is constructed. "Altering the shape of a wind instrument, or modifying the way in which sound is produced, alters the way in which overtones are enhanced or suppressed, and so changes the timbre of the instrument" (Storr, 1992, p. 58). Only the vibration of certain simple shapes produces true musical tones. It is not often that these shapes occur naturally. Humans have to make instruments to produce sustained musical sounds. The shapes of instruments create the complex, nonlinear vibratory characteristics needed. "It is through nonlinearities that traditional musical instruments, such as violins and wind instruments, produce sustained tones" (Pierce, 1999, p. 277). The human body has such a shape and design, making the human voice our first, and still primary, musical instrument. As Hughes (1948) notes, "Man is a singing animal. Yet he has not been satisfied to make music with his vocal chords alone. From the most remote periods he has sought to adorn or replace vocal melody with the sound of musical instruments" (p. 224). Archaeological evidence now estimates that the first human flute was made as early as 40,000 years ago (Kunej & Turk, 2000). From the development of the first drums and bamboo flutes to our modern orchestral instruments and electronic synthesizers, humans have created instruments with specific timbre to convert the energy and intention of the performer into expressive sound. Musical instruments are transducers (just like the human ear). They convert the performer's energy into another energetic form—music (Maconie, 1997).

Choice of timbre is an important element in music, especially the choice of instruments used. As instrument construction became more complex and varied, the psychological effects of certain timbres became evident. The expression of the performer's emotions, energy, thoughts, and intention became easier and more refined. Choice of timbre became an important part of emotional expression through music. "With some instruments the possibilities of expressive modulation of tone are greater than others: with trumpet the possibilities are limited, for saxophones they are richer, and for violins and cellos they are positively vast" (Maconie, 1997, p. 169).

Form

Form is the overall design of the music—how the composition progresses. A composer chooses a form to convey a musical idea. In Western music, we have sonata form and symphonies with four movements among many types. But most world musical traditions have culturally determined forms for their music. Senegalese drumming compositions have definite forms that involve types of rhythmic patterns played, recurrence of sections, and set endings. When I first heard African drumming, I assumed it was a random event of mostly improvised playing. After I studied Senegalese drumming, I learned that the forms for this music are well established. Form is the broad container for the sounds produced over time. It is a spatial dimension of music. Musical form is not so much something to hear as a way of hearing things. Real musical form is the influence of the total context over the perception of individual parts (Cook, 1990). Perception of form is a high-level cognitive skill. "Form makes itself known through a kind of intellectual discovery that demands a well developed musical memory for sustaining musical fragments over long periods" (Jourdain, 1997, p. 135). But form can be perceived generally without formal education or conscious awareness as we listen because this perception is a function of neural organization (Bregman, 1990). People gain intense enjoyment from music even though they know nothing about it in formal, technical terms. "But when music is heard, the results of all this are somehow synthesized into an immediate and intrinsically rewarding experience that does not, as a precondition, depend upon the listener having any kind of trained understanding of what he hears" (Cook, 1990, p. 2).

Related to form is *musical style*. Music can be identified as Romantic style or in Mozart's style, which is different from Vivaldi's. Style is the language of the composer, the characteristic way all musical elements are treated. It can be a formalized style—the Viennese School of opera—or the composer's personal style.

Dynamics

Dynamics of music are the changes in sound intensity or loudness that give a musical performance its variety. Dynamics range in five increments from *pianissimo* or very quiet to *fortissimo* or very loud. Dynamics also factor into musical *accents* or emphasis on one note that gives a musical passage its edges and points of demarcation.

To conclude the discussion of the elemental building blocks of music, musical notation—the symbols for what notes to play and for how long—must be mentioned. "Standard music notation is a Western invention. It took a long time to evolve, was developed in association with a number of important advances in philosophy and technology, and has survived virtually unaltered through four centuries of cultural and intellectual change" (Maconie, 1990, p. 113). Notation has real practical uses. It allows musicians from different cultures and different languages to communicate easily. It makes large group music making possible. But people can and do appreciate and even perform music without knowledge of notation. "Standard notation is no more and no less than a graph. Notes of music are points on a plane where co-ordinates are pitch and time" (Maconie, 1990, p. 115). Notation is a model from which we construct the real event—musical expression. Notation is useful in limited ways, but it is entirely inadequate in representing the elusive qualities of music expression. "Standard notation resulted in a loss of specification of the very features for which it was devised. In its place emerged a code for managing information and people as dynamic systems" (Maconie, 1990, p. 121). All musical conventions from around the world—scales, notation, set forms, and tuning systems—are arbitrary models placed on the immense complexity of music to make musical performance more practical.

Notation is not the music. Scales are all human inventions, including the Pythagorean scale. Western music uses an equal temperament scale. Temperament means adjustment, and our Western scale has certainly been adjusted to make it practical for music playing and instrument construction. "The tempered scale is the perfect scale—it is perfectly out of tune. The tuning errors of the Pythagorean scale are spread evenly among all keys so that a nearly imperceptible dissonance is always present. . . . A flawlessly harmonious scale is impossible" (Jourdain, 1997, p. 73). It would be a mistake to define music by these musical conventions since they are all limiting factors. Music is much more than a particular form or a collection of notes. Having explored the phenomenon of music, music can now be defined from the perspective of its origins.

The Origins of Music

As detailed in chapter 1, music has historically been regarded as a gift from a Divine source. When the biological basis of music is explored, it is found that music may not be externally bestowed on humans but, rather, is programmed into our functioning from the beginning of our creation and, in that way, is truly a gift from the Creator. "Music is one of man's most remarkable inventions —though possibly it may not be his invention at all: like his capacity for language his capacity for music may be a naturally evolved biologic function" (Clynes, 1982, p. vii). Music first originates in human anatomy and physiology.

In the next chapter, how the brain processes sound is explored, reviewing neuroanatomy and physiology. This is useful information for understanding the biological foundations of music. But the laws of acoustics and the study of psychoacoustics are just the first step in the human organization of sound that constitutes music (Blacking, 1973). Wallin (1991), in his book *Biomusicology*, takes a detailed look at the anatomical and neuroanatomical processes involved not just in sound perception but in *musical* behavior. He argues that all musical behavior is contained in the biology and examines the biology of music making from an evolutionary perspective. He writes that music ". . . is not only a limbic business but also a result of other, more complex functions of the human brain. From this point of view music . . . is an excellent illustration of the evolutionary path taken by the human species" (1991, p. 234). Peretz (1993) and Peretz and Morais (1993) conducted neurological studies demonstrating the brain's specificity for music, suggesting that musical capacity represents a specific biological competence rather than a mere cultural function (Wallin, Merker, & Brown, 2000).

Music behavior meets most of the classic criteria for a complex biological adaptation. "Music is a biological adaptation, universal within our species, distinct from other adaptations, and too complex to have arisen except through direct selection for some survival or reproductive benefit" (Miller, 2000, p. 356). Since music has evolved and endured as a human behavior, it must play some role in biological survival. Music is likely a biological imperative. It is *music*, not individual sounds, that the brain processes, since the cells of the auditory cortex specifically process the aspects of sound that are musical in nature (Taylor, 1997).

Music, then, derives from the human mind, from the fundamental processes of neural activity to the specifics of perception. As Molino (2000) states, "There is no 'music in and of itself,' no musical essence, but only some distinct capacities that one day converged toward what we today call music" (p. 169). Even the simplest musical elements—sensation of tone or rhythm—are psychological constructs.

> The categories in terms of which musicians evaluate pitch and time exist only by virtue of acts of perception that embody culture-specific knowledge; and the same applies to the note itself. Musical sounds do not contain notes in the same sense that lemons contain [seeds]; rather, notes are imaginative entities which have a history and a geography of their own. (Cook, 1990, p. 219)

Only the basic mechanisms for recognizing individual sound are hardwired into our nervous systems. Every other aspect of listening is partly or entirely conditioned by learning (Jourdain, 1997). Music comes from the human mind: not just from the functions of various portions of our brains processing sound but from the complex interrelationships of all those parts. As Leonard

Meyer (1967) puts it, "Music is directed, not *to* the sense, but *through* the senses and *to the mind*" (p. 271).

Singing was the first music, and the instrument of vocal music is the human body. Our bodies are designed as a resonating acoustical instrument. "This groundplan, with its symmetrical, longitudinal architecture around a stabilizing backbone, is the same as that of an acoustical instrument [like a cello or guitar]" (Wallin, 1991, p. 469). We share the ability to make modulated vocal sounds with all vertebrate animals. The first mammals, seventy million years ago, had the basic equipment for producing and perceiving vocal sounds. They possessed the three bones of the middle ear, an epiglottis connecting the lower and upper airway, and thyroid cartilage in folds along the airway where frequency-variable vibrations could be generated. Gibbons, for example, perform complex songs using five different classes of sound (Wallin, 1991). The family dog can make variable frequency sounds to make its needs and desires known, and so could our earliest ancestors. All vertebrates share common nerve structure controlled by similar genes that mediate this vocal response. By 1.5 million years ago, hominid ancestors of humans had the articulatory capacity to form vowels and respiratory capacity to maintain high-volume airflow necessary for singing behavior (Frayer & Nicolay, 2000).

However, it is not specific musical abilities like piano playing or musical forms like a symphony that are inherent in human functioning. Rather, it is the cognitive processes that generate all musical expression that are genetically programmed.

> There is so much music in the world that it is reasonable to suppose that music, like language and possibly religion, is a species-specific trait of man. Essential physiological and cognitive processes that generate musical compositions and performance may even be genetically inherited, and therefore present in almost every human being. (Blacking, 1973, p. 7)

As humans evolved, musical expression evolved beyond the basic biology. "Even the sounds which are the materials of music had to be created. The sustained tone of an opera singer is a most artificial performance resembling nothing in nature or in human speech" (Hughes, 1948, p. 1). As the human brain evolved, so did what we now call "mind." As the mind was able to organize sound and perceive the relations of many diverse musical elements, the complexity and diversity of music developed. The complex organization of sound input gave rise to the complex forms of music known today.

> Music starts in the mind. A sense of music is as individual as the individual mind. Music is the name given to a certain kind of perception of events in the

world of sound. . . . [T]o be aware of sounds as music is to experience something capable of being shared. An experience shared is one that can be verified. It becomes more real. (Maconie, 1990, p. 11)

As humans evolved and began the complex affiliations involved in society and culture, the controlled modulations of vocal sound became an important part of social behavior.

All human perceptions are conditioned by what we are exposed to, and what we are exposed to depends on the culture in which we live. "Without biological process of aural perception, and without cultural agreement among at least some human beings on what is perceived, there can be neither music nor musical communication" (Blacking, 1973, p. 9). It is also correct, then, to say that music comes from human culture, especially the particular forms of music, since our minds are conditioned by our cultural experiences. Musical behavior may have, in fact, derived from the behavior of human groups.

I thus view music in its origins more broadly than as vocalizations, rather as a multimodal or multimedia activity of temporally patterned movements. I also emphasize its capacity not only to attract and charm individuals, but to *coordinate the emotions of participants* and thus promote *conjoinment*. (Dissanayke, 2000, p. 390)

So where does music come from? On one level, it comes from human biology and its relation to sound. On another, music comes from the need for communication and emotional expression, especially exaggerated vocal, bodily, and facial movements (Dissanayke, 2000). On yet another level, music derives from the culture that shapes our perceptions, allowing music to emerge from the human mind. "And, although, different societies tend to have different ideas about what they regard as music, all definitions are based on some consensus of opinion about the principles on which the sounds of music should be organized" (Blacking, 1973, p. 10). Music is about who we are, as individuals, as societies, and even as a species (Wallin, Merker, & Brown, 2000).

The Purpose of Music

Let's now turn to defining music by asking, "What purposes does it serve?" Many people throughout history have written about the purpose of music. The "Why music?" question has endlessly fascinated philosophers, theologians, and, more recently, psychologists.

Aristotle (1958) wrote about the "aims" of music. These included providing pleasure and relaxing and refreshing the mind. He also believed music presented images of character states, like anger and calm, while inspiring the release of emotions. Music could stimulate people to action and profoundly affect the character of the soul. Aristotle also believed music was an object of speculative inquiry, making a contribution to the cultivation of our minds and growth of moral wisdom. The uses of music from the perspective of modern-day psychology and ethnomusicology will be delineated here.

Pleasure

It is important to remember that the first and, perhaps, the most important use of music is for pleasure. Music is an entertainment to be enjoyed. And everyone can enjoy it. Music can be enjoyed without understanding music theory, notation, musical form, or cognitive knowledge. This is true of all music but especially popular music. People can even create and perform music without formal musical knowledge. Paul McCartney is a highly successful musician, songwriter, and classical composer who never learned to read or write music.

When the pleasure music gives is discussed, it is not merely a hedonistic pursuit. Even the experience of musical pleasure has a deeper purpose. There is no such thing as music "just" for enjoyment. The composer Phillip Glass writes, "People love music. It is very nourishing because it takes people out of their everyday mentality and brings them to another level. Making people happy becomes the motivation for the music" (Ehrlich, 1997, p. 22). Similarly, the Tibetan Lama Gelck Rimpoche states,

> All this entertainment has its purpose. . . . [Why do people turn to music?] Because [it] give[s] them some sense of relief. People are tired of always working, being under pressure, tired of life itself, so it's a little relief they're getting. I think it's a great service. . . . (quoted in Ehrlich, 1997, p. xiii)

The pleasure derived from music actually comes from the relations between the notes. "Although pleasure appears to be embodied in the 'sound' of the notes, it mostly resides in high-level relations [among the sounds] that we keenly experience, but to which we bring little self-awareness" (Jourdain, 1997, p. 320). In music, the deepest pleasure comes from the deepest relations. "By providing the brain with an artificial environment, and forcing it through that environment in controlled ways, music imparts the means of experiencing relations far deeper than we encounter in our everyday lives" (Jourdain, 1997, p. 331). Music is so perfectly organized that every tension, every anticipation, is satisfied, giving us intense pleasure. Our brain wants order and organization. It wants disorganization and unrelated sensory input to move to simplicity and order. Music does this. Think of music that doesn't usually give pleasure, such as twentieth-century music or unfamiliar music from another culture. Because the tonal and rhythmic relations expected are not there, it may be intellectually appreciated, but it doesn't give the deep pleasure response, at least until the patterns of those relationships are learned.

Aesthetic Response

Most people think of music as *only* a pleasurable sensation. For them, music is a form of entertainment and nothing else. But music has many other purposes. One such purpose is to create an aesthetic response. Related to the feeling of pleasure, an aesthetic reaction is an intense response to "the beautiful" in art and nature. An aesthetic reaction grabs our whole attention, gives us goose bumps, and makes us cry for the sheer joy and overwhelming pleasure of the experience. Aesthetic perceptions are ". . . moments of at-oneness: with nature, our environment, with other people. They usually happen without prediction and are not necessarily dependent on a reservoir of previous experiential knowledge" (Swanwick, 1994, p. 34). Music gives us intense experiences. "The experience of unsullied order persisting simultaneously at every perceptual level may be taken as a working definition of the word 'beauty'" (Jourdain, 1997, p. 330). Music is perceived as beautiful because it is anticipation perfectly met.

As humans, we seek out the aesthetic reaction. Why do we go to live concerts when recordings are so good and so easily available? Because the aesthetic reaction tends to occur most readily when we are surrounded by live music making. As a performing musician, I know I've had my greatest aesthetic reactions while playing in symphony orchestras. In the orchestra, I am literally surrounded by the sound and am intensely bombarded by the physical vibrations. To play my part, I am moving to the music, creating those gestures that are so significant in musical perception. My complete focus is on the music. If it wasn't, I couldn't play accurately and effectively. For me, the aesthetic reaction comes from the physical impact of sound waves on my body, my intense mental focus, the participation in the deep relations of the music, and the physical movement of playing.

Support to Basic Humanity

As far as is known, an aesthetic reaction is exclusively a human reaction. Many people, including Abraham Maslow (1971) and E. Thayer Gaston (1968b), believe the aesthetic reaction defines the difference between human beings and other animals. Gaston believed the aesthetic experience is ". . . essential to the development of humanness and considers sensitivity to beauty and the making of beauty to be one of humankind's most distinguishing characteristics" (quoted in Radocy & Boyle, 1997, p. 16). The aesthetic reaction is not obviously functional—it does not stimulate action or provide communication. Yet this experience is an essential human need. The real power of music comes from this nonfunctional reaction. Music fosters the aesthetic and serves to develop and reinforce our basic humanness, our essential nature as human beings. Music ". . . is essential for the very survival of man's humanity . . ." (Blacking, 1973, p. 54).

What is our humanity? The very basis of our "person" is a sound concept:

> In Latin, the term meaning "to sound through something" is *personare*. Thus, at the basis of the concept of the person (the concept of that which really makes a human being an unmistakable, singular *per-sonality*) stands a concept of sound: "through the tone." If nothing sounds through from the bottom of the being, a human being is human biologically, at best, but is not a *per-son*, because he does not live through the *son* (the tone, the sound). (Berendt, 1983, p. 171)

But merely *being* a person is not enough. True humanity involves a constant state of becoming. "More so than most other human creative activities, music represents not only the notion of *being* but also—and foremost—of *becoming*" (Wallin, 1991, p. 33). Our humanity encompasses all aspects of our inner life. The relations of tone, rhythm, melody, timbre, and harmony resemble the rudimentary building blocks of this inner life. Our humanity involves the ability to feel love and compassion, to be part of the community, to feel and express emotions, and to have hope and faith in something greater than ourselves. Music provides all these aspects of humanity. According to Kierkegaard (1941), each new generation must learn what is purely human for itself. Development of humanity cannot be passed from one generation to another. "The hard task is to love, and music is a skill that prepares man for this most difficult task" (Blacking, 1973, p. 103). Music explores the deep issues of our humanity. It embodies these characteristics and reflects them back to us. Our aesthetic experiences are an important part of the development of our humanity.

Touching the Divine

Music also serves the purpose of helping touch the spiritual nature of being. As explored in chapter 1, music helps us touch and experience "the Divine" in nature and in ourselves. Through music, we have personal experiences of the spiritual. As a society, we use music in our formal worship ceremonies and rituals. The link of music and spirit is explored at length in chapter 7.

Communication

Another purpose of music is as a form of communication, particularly the expression of emotions. Music is nonverbal communication expressing emotions beyond the power of words to convey. Music provides a subtlety, preciseness, and truth of expression that language cannot approach. "Music mimics experience rather than symbolizes it, as language does. It carefully replicates the temporal patterns of interior feelings, surging in pitch or volume as they surge, ebbing as they ebb" (Jourdain, 1997, p. 296). Proust (1981) called music a means of communication between souls, a communication with the essential nature of an individual. Music evokes the symbols and images of our deepest human responses. Such responses emanate from our limbic system and our nonworded right hemisphere. Our symbolic responses are deeply, essentially human. They predate language by hundreds of thousands of years. The broad forms of these symbols and images are culturally determined (Blacking, 1973). But this expression through music is also deeply personal and individual. "The unique set of an individual's personal experiences may influence which locations, categories, associations, reflections, and evaluations that individual will draw upon in interpreting music as personally relevant. . . . [M]usic is important to human beings largely because they do find it personally relevant" (Higgins, 1997, p. 97). Any given musical element has a variety of personal expressive elements. The expressive power of music comes from this variety within the context of cultural unity of expression. Music is indeed a form of communication, an information-bearing system (Treitler, 1997). The transformation of the sensory signal of music into these culturally and personally relevant symbols is one of music's most important purposes (Wallin, 1991). In chapter 4, the connection of music and speech is explored by trying to answer the question, "Is music a language?"

Effects on Activity Level

Another purpose of music is to affect people's activity level. Certain music stimulates people to action. There is a definite physical response to music. From military bands to aerobic exercise classes, music is used to spur people to move and act. Earliest music took the forms of work songs and accompaniment to dance. The music was used to energize and organize the physical behavior. To accomplish this, stimulative music involves a fast tempo, loud dynamics, and strong rhythm patterns. Conversely, music is also used to suppress behavior. Though any sensory input is stimulating, we learn to associate certain musical features—slow tempo, quiet dynamic, gentle underlying beat—with decreases in general alertness and physical activity.

Sedative music serves to calm us down, put us to sleep, and help us enter a dreamlike state. The lullaby is a good example of sedative music.

Support of Human Culture

Throughout this discussion of the purposes of music, references have been made to its place in culture and society. "Music making is the quintessential human cultural activity, and music is an ubiquitous element in all cultures large and small" (Wallin, Merker, & Brown, 2000, p. 3). In the opinion of many anthropologists, music first evolved from the rhythmic vocalizations of infant–mother interactions or sexual mating into a social activity used to strengthen community bonds and resolve conflicts (Jourdain, 1997; Wallin, Merker, & Brown, 2000). Social touching, deep breathing, rhythmic drumming, swaying, and chanting are fundamentally necessary physical activities to reinforce the social bonding necessary for survival and procreation. Music and accompanying dance became a socially acceptable way to accomplish this (Wallin, Merker, & Brown, 2000). Music, then, became a tool of culture and was emancipated from its earlier functional use (Dissanayke, 2000). Confucius wrote that the superior man tries to promote music as a means to the perfection of human culture (Bonny & Savary, 1990).

The music therapy pioneer E. Thayer Gaston (1968a) wrote that the power of music is greatest in the group. Any group of humans first needs to feel drawn together to be affiliated to each other. Whether a country, a Girl Scout troop, a neighborhood, or a cultural subgroup, a sense of unity is essential for the group to hold together. Music accomplishes this in many ways. First, music is a reason for being together. It gives individuals a common experience and a more comfortable way to interact with others (Sears, 1968). "Being with others through music may thus provide intense experiences of involvement, a heightened feeling of being included, and a deep relationship with others. Through the intimate frame of musical activity, individuals are bound together through common musical experiences" (Ruud, 1998a, p. 64). Second, music contributes to strong emotional bonds among members. The shared experience engenders a sense of unity and belonging to the group. The music elicits shared emotional states, as discussed in later chapters. A third way music promotes the unity of a group is through simultaneous synchronization of movement. Social science research has shown that social bonding is a matter of synchronization of movement and gesture among members of a group (Bernieri & Rosenthal, 1991). The timekeeping elements of music fosters this synchronization of movement. Rhythmic response involves synchronization since our rhythmic movement coincides with the rhythmic stimulus. In most behaviors, a response follows the stimulus, but in rhythm we quickly learn to predict when the next stimulus will occur. We entrain our response to the musical stimulus, allowing us to synchronize our behavior. The steady beat and grouping of beat through meter allow this to happen. "Musical meter is perhaps the quintessential device for group coordination, one which functions to promote interpersonal entrainment, cooperative movement and teamwork" (Brown, 2000, p. 297). This synchronization of movement can occur between two people—a client and therapist, for example—or in larger groups.

Any group needs to share values and ideals. According to Merriam (1964), music serves to enforce conformity to social norms and to validate social institutions and religious rituals. Music, particularly songs, teaches social values. Think of the Barney preschool song "I Love You," which teaches the basic value of caring for friends. Some rap songs communicate and validate beliefs and values that society may find negative but are a part of a particular subcultural group. Gospel music teaches and affirms tenets of faith. Music also gives importance to social and religious events. Music takes the opening of the Olympic Games every four years and creates a ceremony celebrating friendly competition. The use of music in religious ceremonies is one of its most ancient uses. For example, in the Episcopal Church, music validates and cues every aspect of the formal service. There is music to signal the reading of the gospel, to tell the congregation when to kneel and when to stand, and to escort individuals to the altar for communion. Music contributes to the continuity and stability of a culture.

> If music allows emotional expression, gives aesthetic pleasure, entertains, communicates, elicits physical response, enforces conformity to social norms, and validates social institutions and religious rituals, it is clear that it contributes to the continuity and stability of culture. . . . Music is in a sense a summatory activity for the expression of values, a means whereby the heart of the psychology of a culture is exposed without many of the protective mechanisms which surround other cultural activities. (Merriam, 1964, p. 225)

Music not only follows society and reflects cultural norms but shapes, builds, and changes it.

Does music serve a purpose in human culture? Does music matter to humankind? The short answer is yes. From the basic genesis in human biology, to the needs for emotional expression deeper than words, to the importance in society and culture, music simply has to exist. There is no human culture, no humanity, without it. In fact, it is fundamental to all human endeavors. "Music matters because it would have happened anyway" (Maconie, 1997, p. 1). It is an intrinsic part of human functioning, behavior, knowledge, and cultural institutions.

> This is where the ultimate value of music lies. It is uncommon sense, a cele-
> bration of imagination and intellect interacting together in acts of sustained
> playfulness, a space where feeling is given form, where romantic and classical
> attitudes, intuition, and analysis meet; valued knowledge indeed. (Swanwick,
> 1994, p. 41)

It is this fundamental principle of music mattering that ultimately is the basis of music for therapy. The fourth way of defining music, looking at what
constitutes musical behavior, can now be addressed.

Musical Behavior

The musical experience involves both making and receiving music. These
two fundamental musical behaviors are not separate but are a holistic involvement in this immensely complex sensory/motor event. All music behavior is structured by biology, psychology, culture, or the musical processes
involved (Blacking, 1973). From a biological perspective, music making

> . . . is not an isolated skill bound to a separate faculty of mind called "musical-
> ity" but a complex behavior involving perception, cognitive skills, motor per-
> formance, social communicative skills, and emotional, bodily, and symbolic ac-
> tivity. To be engaged in music means to fully use all these development skills.
> (Ruud, 1998a, p. 62)

Different areas of our brains are used when we engage in listening, playing, or
visually reading a piece of music (Sergent et al., 1992). All types of musical behavior are important for music therapy because the therapeutic interventions
involved are based on client's active participation in at least one of them. Let's
begin by looking at the musical behavior of receiving music—listening.

Listening

Hearing and listening are not the same thing. Hearing involves various
parts of our brain receiving and processing sensory input from our ears. Listening is an active perceptual skill. While listening, we engage in an active
process of making sense out of what is heard. "We triumph over this chaos [of
complex sound] by not passively *hearing* with our brains, but by actively *listening* with cerebral cortex, which searches for familiar devices and patterns
in music" (Jourdain, 1997, p. 246). We do not listen to sound waves or even
specific sounds. We listen to *music*. Through exposure to our culture's music,
we learn the form, patterns, and combinations expected from "music." While
listening, we anticipate the sound combinations, preparing ourselves for the
process of perception. Anticipation leads us to prediction and attention. Pre-

diction is the modeling of the deep relations that hold music together. The model thus created forms sound combinations into music in our minds. "As complex music passes before our ears, we incessantly shift focus between its many aspects, always on the lookout for the most crucial features, those that form the 'edges' of musical objects" (Jourdain, 1997, p. 250). For it is the differences, the changes, that create an edge on which our brains focus. What for most of us seems like a passive activity is really an energetic, active cognitive behavior. It is its own kind of performance skill.

In listening, our attention is focused, choosing what features of the sound to attend to and what to ignore. True musical listening involves a whole brain processing. Our right hemisphere's perception of contour and pattern isn't sufficient. Our left hemisphere's ability to perceive and recognize sequence is also needed. We also need the frontal lobe of our brains where short-term memory is maintained. The frontal lobe acts on the auditory cortex to hold the observed events in short-term memory so that comparisons can be made to the previously stored patterns of relationships. "Music is a time art which can only be comprehended by remembering what was heard in relation to what is heard" (Hughes, 1948, p. 5). The frontal lobe holds the patterns just heard long enough for our brains to ask, "Are these relationships of tones close enough to what I've heard before to call it a melody? Does it have a good beat? Can I dance to it?" As we make these comparisons and anticipate what will unfold next, music forms as a process of imagination. An image of the full relationships from what we've heard is created, and music is the result. Music, to be music, involves a form of fantasy. That's why no two people hear music exactly the same way. Our imaginations make it up from the fragments of sound and sound relationships registering in our brains. Music is imaginative perception involving voluntary interpretation of the sound event.

This process of comparing sound relationships to stored memory and fleshing out the experience of music through imagination is achieved not by formal music education and training but by mere exposure to the musical forms of our culture. Everyone can and does actively participate in this listening behavior, since musical literacy is not needed to listen to music. Passive exposure to music is enough. We are all exposed to music from birth and even before. Active, focused listening not only grabs our complete mental attention but takes over our bodies as well. Jourdain (1997) notes, "We use our bodies as resonators for auditory experience. The listener becomes a musical instrument, places himself in the hands of the music, allows himself to be played" (p. 326). Deep music listening becomes a whole body experience, with gestures representing the music.

Performance

Performance behavior often defines music for people. Making music, physically producing the sound combinations—as an opera singer, a violinist, or a country bass player—is the musical behavior focused on the most. Our Western classical music tradition has convinced us that only a select few people become performers after years of study and hours of daily practice. And, certainly, accomplished musical performance is a highly developed perceptual and motor skill. But any organized sound making—a child banging on a pan or people singing hymns in church—is also performance. We all can and do perform music throughout our lives.

Musical performance is a multifaceted behavior involving physical athleticism, intellect, memory, creativity, and emotion (Jourdain, 1997). In traditional performance of Western music, a composer writes notes on paper in a specific combination. The musician reads this score and translates the notation into movement patterns. "A performer by definition is an involved intermediary, through whom notes on paper are realized as actions that in turn influence the production and emission of acoustic images" (Maconie, 1997, pp. 84–85). But as noted earlier, notation is a minimal skeleton of the musical idea. The performer takes this outline and adds the real expression through creativity. The musical meaning is not in the score but in the musician. Each performer brings a unique human dimension to every reinterpretation of the composed music. There are several components of the behavior called "performing," including mental imagery, skilled motor behavior, and sensory involvement.

The importance of holding an image of the music in our short-term memory to the act of listening has already been discussed. Performance involves the same imagery skill plus several others. To play music,

> . . . it is not enough simply to know a piece as a stereotyped action sequence, or as a series of individually known sections, or as a tune supported by harmony, or in terms of how it looks on the page. What is required is a tissue of intertwined, mutually reinforcing imagery. . . . (Cook, 1990, p. 111)

Performance requires the visual imagery to go from printed score to true music. Additionally, *proprioception* (body position) and *kinesthetic* (movement) imagery are also required to place the body in an appropriate posture for sound production to occur. When shifting from first to third position up the violin neck, for example, the performer holds a proprioceptive imagery of the hand position and a kinesthetic imagery of how the whole movement sequence has to unfold to accomplish the shift. Emotional imagery is also needed. We equate this with *musicality* and expressiveness in music. The performers must have an image of the musical phrase, the piece as a whole, and what they intend to express with their playing.

> A truly great performer is able to enliven the music through the sheer intention of his or her consciousness . . . such a performer intuitively expresses into the music essentic forms of human emotion and desire. Such waveforms cannot be captured on a sheet of music. They emerge from the spirit or consciousness of the performer. (Kenyon, 1994, pp. 188–189)

The performing musician represents the music through numerous images, each of which embodies some aspect of the intended whole. These together converge in a manner that allows the production of the music to be played (Cook, 1990). Once the many facets of mental imagery are employed, performance then becomes a highly skilled motor behavior.

Music making is a motor behavior. It is a physical act involving precise, refined body movements designed to create and shape meaningful sound. The physical movement involved in music making is a specific type known as a *skilled motor behavior*. Exercise physiologists define a skilled motor behavior as one that requires sensory integration, memory processing, motor integration, and feedback or knowledge of results (Martinieuk, 1976). Skilled motor behavior is most often associated with highly trained athletes. The precision of a tennis serve or the coordination of a figure skater represents the best of athletic skilled motor behavior. But music performance is also a finely trained athletic skill. Skilled motor behavior involves fine motor skills—the manipulation of small muscles that use a proportionally larger amount of the brain to control. In music, this means primarily the muscle of the hands, arms, and mouth (lips, tongue, and soft palette). To understand the motor skills of a musician, imagine an accomplished pianist who moves both hands in rapid, diverse, and complex coordinated movements or a clarinetist who must use the tongue to subtly articulate a musical passage.

A number of criteria must be met in order for a motor behavior to be considered skilled. Skilled motor behavior is a serial skill. It requires a sequence of movements to complete the task. Watch any musician play, and you'll notice the complex sequences that are needed to perform even the simplest piece of music. These sequences unfold in a physical space and in a precise time organization. Movements necessary to complete the task—changing chords on a guitar, for example—must occur with the right physical spacing and timing to be executed successfully. A skilled motor behavior also has a hierarchy of habits. Learning one component of the skill depends on the degree of mastery achieved in simpler components of the same skill (Martinieuk, 1976). Whether a championship tennis player or a fine musician is training, the only way to master the complex motor skill is to physically replicate the component movements until they become habitual. In other words, it is necessary to practice, practice, practice. To understand music as a skilled motor behavior, a brief review of two essential components of this physical behavior—muscle activity and the neurological control center for movement—is needed.

Skeletal muscle is used for motor movement and is designed to move bones and joints. Muscles are organized functionally to permit mechanical versatility and efficiency of skeletal movement (Wilson, 1986). Skeletal muscle has one job: to change its length. Nerves are attached to the muscle's surface. A muscle moves only when a neural impulse is sent and moves in only one fashion— it gets shorter. Skeletal muscle is made up of many fibers or motor units. These motor units can act individually or in concert, which accounts for the range of force and speed seen in muscle contractions. When a nerve impulse is sent, the smaller fibers contract first with slight force. More stimulation causes more fibers to contract and with greater force. As soon as a muscle begins to contract, it starts another reaction to reverse the effect of the stimulation, allowing rapid alternation of muscle groups. This *ballistic movement* is the precise and rapid adjustment of muscle contraction and relaxation. This very fast movement requires abrupt relaxation of the contracted muscles through an inhibitory mechanism to execute this rapid change. This is important in the motor behavior required for music performance.

It takes a complex system to regulate and coordinate the skilled motor movement of musical performance. This regulatory system comes from various structures in the brain, which will be explored extensively in chapter 4. Clearly, when considering the complexity of music as a motor behavior, this skilled movement is not a simple mechanical activation of required muscles. Every component of the motor sequences must be activated and sent as a *whole* from the brain to the various muscles involved.

> Such observations lead us far from the player-piano conception of motor function, where a discrete neural command moves discrete muscles to bend a discrete finger to play an F-sharp. Many levels of complexity are required to move a three-dimensional body through a three-dimensional world. (Jourdain, 1997, pp. 209–210)

Complex motor action requires anticipation of the whole movement sequence and an activation of the hierarchy of movement before any part of the motor sequence can occur. In our brains, every aspect of the motor skill is intertwined with every other aspect. To add further complexity to this already complex process, one other aspect of musical performance, reading music, is also a perceptual motor skill. Reading music, or any reading, is the motor activity of moving the eyes in rhythmic movements of starts and stops. Eye movements follow the structure of music and center on musically significant turning points. This process engages the visual cortex in musical performance, adding yet another layer of complexity to music.

Music also involves a great deal of sensory involvement. A number of different sensory channels are used in musical performance in addition to the auditory sense. These include haptic sensation, proprioception, and kinesthesia. Generally, our senses essentially give us a map of the external environment. An important sensory input to this map is the *haptic sense*. The haptic sense is our sense of touch but is much more than the mere skin stimulation of our tactile sense. Haptic is a combined sensory system that includes touch, the sense of body position (proprioception), and motion (kinesthesia). Kinesthesia is particularly important because, without movement, true touch cannot be achieved. To activate the tactile sensory apparatus, the ridges on our fingers, those sensory devises must be moved over a surface. A tailor judging the quality of a piece of cloth doesn't simply place a finger on the material. He or she runs it between thumb and fingers, activating the haptic sense. The haptic sensors require movement for sensation to occur. What makes the haptic sense unique is that it requires intentional movement, active touch. This makes haptic sense an issue of the hands. "The haptic system, in addition to the tactile and kinesthetic sensors and somatosensory cortex, includes the active muscles of the arms, hands, and fingers" (Gillespie, 1999a, p. 235). As such, haptic input is a vital part of musical instrument performance, a behavior primarily of arms, hands, and fingers.

After audition, the sense of hearing, the haptic sense is the most important means for receiving feedback from the motor skill of performance. "While audition carries meaning regarding the acoustical behavior of an instrument, haptics carries meaning regarding the mechanical behavior. This mechanical information is quite valuable to the process of playing or learning to play an instrument . . ." (Gillespie, 1999a, p. 229). All instrumental musicians use this information in modifying their performance. A brass player uses haptic and auditory cues to determine if the embouchure (lip position) is situated correctly to produce a certain note. A musician playing an instrument creates a feedback control system. Feedback control exists when the control of an object comes from using information from a sensor like the haptic that, in turn, monitors the behavior of the object (Gillespie, 1999a).

The haptic sense is exquisitely complex because it is a perfect feedback loop. The haptic sense is generated by the act of performance. "The information available to the haptic senses is dependent on the player's actions, or how he/she exerts control over the instrument" (Gillespie, 1999a, p. 230). The actions of the musician make the instrument vibrate. Those vibrations not only produce the auditory sound but produce haptic sensations as well. The movement of vibration activates the haptic sensor. The musician then uses the haptic feedback to modify and refine the performance. A perfect feedback loop is created adding more complex information into the system.

The complexity of hearing and perceiving sound elements alone is immense. Yet, clearly, when active listening and all the elements that go into musical performance are added, the brain activity involved in music is greatly increased, adding to the overall complexity of the process. Two other musical behaviors need to be mentioned since they are used as music therapy interventions—improvisation and composition.

Improvisation

Improvisation is spontaneous music making. In improvisation, the performer makes music without a written score. The improvising musician is creating and synthesizing performance in real time (Cook, 1990). Some improvisation is quite structured, following set patterns and formulas. Traditional jazz improvisation is an example. In this type of improvisation, the musical end product is important. But improvisation can also be free playing without any great concern for how "musical" it is. This form of improvisation is used extensively as a music therapy activity intervention. The musical product is less important, while the process of creative self-expression is paramount. In a group improvisation, sensitive, alert listening is essential. As the group listens to each other and improvises together, it becomes synchronized. It begins to anticipate the musical expressions and move together like a flock of birds or a school of fish might. Jazz musicians call this state "being in the groove." There may also be a process of vibratory entrainment occurring. This energetic phase locking is a fact of physics where one vibrating object moves in synchronization with another over time, first discovered when the pendulums of grandfather clocks in close proximity synchronized. The vibrations of music may also affect the vibrational characteristics of our bodies. This is explored further in chapter 6.

Composition

Composing is a creative activity involving the selection and arrangements of various musical elements into a unified whole. Composers think in sound, creating auditory imagery to be shared with others. The processes of composition are beyond the scope of this book. What is important here is to understand that a composition comes from the mind of a human being. Music begins ". . . as the thought of a sensitive human being, and it is this sensitivity that may arouse (or not) the feelings of another human being, in much the same way that magnetic impulses convey a telephone conversation from one speaker to another" (Blacking, 1973, p. 34). Writing music is about expressing a person's uniqueness and sharing that with others. A composer brings all his or her cerebral activity, feelings, education, musical background, and cultural experiences to the process of composition. Composition is about self-expression at its most basic level. In great music, the whole is always greater than the sum of its parts. It is an emergent property of the musical elements used and the uniqueness of the composer that makes this so.

Thus far, a definition of music was explored by considering what constitutes the musical event, where music comes from, why it exists in human culture, and what behaviors are musical. The amazing complexity of sound, music, musical behavior, and the human processing of all this was explored. Before a more explicit definition of music is formulated, let's return to the basic focus of this book and examine music as a nonlinear, dynamical system in motion.

Music as a Complex, Dynamical System

Human perception of sound and music is gloriously complicated. Sound alone is a complex system. Music is even more so. Add what is known about music's effects on human functioning, and we begin to realize that music may be the most complex system we know. Wallin (1991) states,

> I believe that music as a time phenomenon . . . actually dwells in the center of all this [chaos theory]; that music always incarnates the presence and experience of this specific world that the scientists at the end of this century, and this millennium, endeavor to articulate in phenomenological models. (p. 507)

Music should meet the criteria set for systems to act in a complex fashion, and it does.

Movement

Recall from chapter 2 that in complexity science theory, the whole universe is in a state of constant, chaotic motion. Out of this deterministic chaos, form, order, and life itself emerge. And as explored previously, all aspects of sound and music are about movement. From the movement of vibration creating sound, to the perception of movement in rhythm and melody, to the importance of gesture in music listening and perception, music moves.

Nonlinearity

The complex systems of our world are nonlinear. They do not have straight-line relationships. The responses of these systems are not directly proportional to a given variable (Williams, 1997). Something is nonlinear when the whole is greater than the sum of its parts—small changes can have large consequences. Music may be the most obvious example of something that is greater than the sum of its parts. Let's take a symphony orchestra performance as an example. There are many separate parts that make up an orchestra piece—five string parts, two to three clarinet parts, flute parts, oboe parts, trumpet and trombone parts, percussion parts, and much more. As a violinist, I have spent most of my professional playing career in the second violin section. Second violin parts are often supportive in nature. In other words, alone they can be pretty boring. I once spent an entire Viennese Waltz concert playing the "chick-chick" offbeats to the "boom" of the bass parts in these triple meter pieces (*boom*-chick-chick, *boom*-chick-chick.). Played alone, it was not inspiring music. It wasn't even interesting music. But when we put together the second violin part, the bass part, the soaring melodies of the flutes and first violins, and the interesting percussion touches, something greater was created. It was much more than the sum of all those boring parts. This is basic to all music. This nonlinear aspect of music exists even when considering musical forms that are simpler than a full orchestral piece. A simple sung melody is a greater experience than the sum of the notes it contains.

Sensitivity to Initial Conditions

Recall also that another characteristic of complex, nonlinear systems is their extreme sensitivity to even the smallest inputs or changes. Such seemingly small changes in what we hear can profoundly affect our musical experience. Have you ever had the experience of hearing a piece of music or a song and responding to it immediately and deeply? You like it so much you want to hear it again. But when you hear it performed by a different group or artist or even the same musician but in a different location, you don't have the same experience or the same profound reaction. A classical symphony, for example, has the same notes played by the same instruments. What changes your experience of the piece? The tempo may be slightly different, the musical interpretation may change, or the instrument's tuning may be slightly altered. John Diamond (1981) believes the mental state or intention of the conductor and performers may influence our reaction to the music. Distracted or tired musicians can change the end product of the music enough that we perceive it differently. The Bonny Method of "Guided Imagery and Music," a depth psychology method, takes this factor into consideration when selecting music to be used (Bonny & Savary, 1990). This method concludes that particular performances of the music are critical to eliciting the desired responses from clients. What may seem to be a small factor—the mental state of the performer—exerts a great influence on the dynamical system we call music.

Musical instrument construction is another example of sensitivity to small variables in music. The artisans who make musical instruments know that a slight change in construction (the curve of a guitar body or an almost unmeasurable change in the position of the violin bridge) can completely alter the instrument's sound. The world of violin making gives us our greatest example of this sensitivity. Stradivarius's violins are recognized worldwide as the best violins ever made. For centuries, people have been asking, "Why can't someone make a violin as good as Stradivarius?" With modern technology, every component of a Stradivarius violin can be analyzed and duplicated. Precise measurement of wood thickness, angles of curves, bridge position, total weight, and even the composition of the varnish is possible. Yet when a violin is made to these exact specifications, it is still not as good as a Stradivarius. The best and most likely answer to this puzzle is that Stradivarius—a man with a unique personality, intention for the outcome of his craft, and worldview—did not make the violin. This seemingly small variable may make all the difference in the outcome of the violin construction (Levenson, 1994). It also demonstrates that we cannot analyze the parts of something and expect to reproduce the whole.

The main point about sensitivity to initial conditions in nonlinear systems is that the outcome of complex systems cannot be predicted by the initial variables. Anyone who has attended a musical event and been disappointed with the result understands that knowing a set of variables (the Chicago Symphony is playing tonight, for example) does not ensure outcome. This is especially true in improvisational music. Let's use the supreme live performance group, The Grateful Dead, as an example. True fans heard dozens of this group's performances over its thirty-year history. Some concerts were good; some, uninspired and even a little boring; and some, so outstanding they were transcendent. Yet all the initial factors for each concert were the same—same musicians, same instruments, same songs. It was the small variables—performer's mood, audience size, concert hall acoustics—that made the difference. As in any complex system, knowing the starting place does not allow you to predict outcome. Too many small factors can influence the end result.

Use of Iterative Feedback

Complex systems attain their complexity through iterative feedback. As explored in the discussion of the principles of complexity science, iteration enfolds feedback into the system, multiplying its effects. This becomes another variable that can make large changes. Iterative feedback is how musical performance is possible. Let's explore another example from violin playing. Playing the notes on a violin is not an exact process. When a finger is placed on the strings, there is an approximate placement for a particular note. (For example, to play E above middle C, the finger is placed about half an inch from the scroll on the D string.) But to actually play the correct note involves hearing the pitch produced and getting auditory feedback on whether that is an E or not. The violin is played by receiving instantaneous feedback from the ears and enfolding that feedback into the playing. That iterative process *is* the playing of the instrument.

There is also iterative feedback involved in the muscular adjustments required for playing a musical instrument. The skilled motor behavior of performance requires immediate and instantaneous adjustments of muscle spindles. The feedback comes from auditory and muscular feedback systems that build on themselves as they are enfolded again and again during a musical performance.

Action of Attractors

Complex systems organize through the action of attractors. Recall from chapter 2, an attractor in a nonlinear system organizes the complex movement as the result of its own dynamics. Sound, and particularly music, has a number of such attractors. One of these, a fixed-point attractor, is a region in the system exerting a "magnetic" pull. All systems' movements converge toward it (Briggs & Peat, 1989). In a simple melody like a lullaby, the tones of the cadence (the tone that feels like the point of melodic conclusion) act as a fixed-point attractor. This point of harmonic finality draws all the tones in the system, the melody in this case, to it (Wallin, 1991, p. 343).

A limit-cycle attractor is another possible attractor working in music and particularly in isolated sound, like a single tone. This attractor has a motion that constantly repeats itself periodically—like frequency. It is this periodic repetition of the sound wave that gives us our perception of tone or pitch. The presence of tone, from a singer, a gong, or a tuning fork, may serve as a limit-cycle attractor for other dynamical systems it touches—like Jenny's (1972) sand particles on a metal plate or the beating of a human heart. This idea as it relates to the body is explored in chapter 5. As Wallin (1991) proposes,

. . . at a certain activity level of the developing section of the sonata form or an equivalent structure with a phase space whose dimensions are made up by the parameters pitch, harmony, duration, intensity, and rhythm in different states of coherence, attractors of this type are to be found [in music]. (p. 344)

More research into music as an attractor in complex moving systems will likely show the presence of more complex attractors like periodic and quasiperiodic torus attractors. Torus attractors result from at least two oscillating bodies interacting in phase space. The influence of various intervals (the relationship of two tones) may serve as torus attractors (Steiner, 1983). Even the simplest forms of music have numerous oscillating bodies producing the sound. A singer accompanying him- or herself on a guitar has the oscillations from the vocal chords and the six strings of the guitar interacting in coupled motion. Even a single vibrating string from that guitar likely produces periodic or, possibly, quasiperiodic attractors since the vibrations of the overtone series are up to the eighteen separate vibrations that constitute a complex tone.

Because of the immense complexity of movement indicative of complex sound and the combinations of the complex sound that is music, it seems likely that music is a strange or chaotic attractor in complex systems. The organized disorganization of strange attractors is critical in creating the music itself and in creating order and new form in other systems, like the human body. The most prevalent strange attractor mechanism seen in music is the $1/f$ spectrum. The $1/f$ spectrum or flicker noise is not heard as a sound but, rather, reflects how a particular physical system varies over time. When Richard Voss compared musical melodies to these variations over time found throughout nature, he found that all musical melodies mimic $1/f$ processes in time. When he mapped $1/f$ noise onto sound, he generated a reasonable "fractal forgery" of music because the correlations inherent in the sound mimic the meaning found in natural sounds and music (Voss & Clark, 1975). Voss contends that music represents fractals experienced in time (personal communication, April 2000). Music is fundamentally a nonlinear, dynamical system to its very essence. Voss's experimental measurements of $1/f$ spectra and music ". . . suggest that music is imitating the characteristic way our world changes in time. Both music and $1/f$-noise are intermediate between randomness and predictability. Like fractal shapes there is something interesting on all [in this case, time] scales. Even the smallest phrase reflects the whole" (1989, p. 42). Because music is an intermediate between randomness and predictability, it exists at the edge of chaos, the place in our natural world of optimum vigor, information, and potential. The essence of music is its subtle reflection of nature—from the workings of the mind to the essential nature of the universe. How music as a strange attractor with a 1/f spectra time pattern sitting on the edge of chaos may affect human health and functioning will be discussed in later chapters.

Fractal time is also reflected in musical performance. Great performance is not mechanical but holds its self-similarity while involving what is unique and unexpected.

> The stamping feet of traditional dancers, the drumming of a jazz musician, and the beat given by an orchestra conductor are never totally exact and mechanically metronomic. Computer analysis shows that, like healthy heartbeats, the rhythmic intervals in such music are always slightly irregular. It is this fractal fluctuation within regularity that brings music alive. (Briggs & Peat, 1999, pp. 134–135)

Truly great music and great musical performances reflect the creative, unique self-similarity of our world—in the subtle change of tempos, dynamics, and pitch. It is how the rules are broken, yet maintaining the general sense of self-similarity, that makes music alive, exciting, and exhilarating. "Listening to a great fugue is like listening to the inner movement of existence" (Briggs & Peat, 1999, p. 119).

Emergent Properties
Complex moving systems have emergent properties—increasingly complex levels of order appear over time. Something has emergent properties when many separate events fuse together as a single experience. This clearly happens in music. When we listen to music, we don't hear each distinct part or recognize the chord progression. Even a professional musician trained to hear and recognize a chord sequence or rhythmic device doesn't hear the parts as separate. The music is heard and enjoyed as a whole. A violinist listening to an orchestral piece enjoys the complete musical experience, not just the violin parts. This happens even when we are appreciating a favorite artist or "star." Take a performer like Garth Brooks, whose thousands of fans go to great lengths to hear and watch him perform. They will tell you they are there to see Garth Brooks, but what they really experience as "Garth Brooks" is a multipart event perceived as a unified experience. In addition to Mr. Brooks's singing and stage presence, there is the bass guitar part, the slide guitar player, the backup vocalists, the drummer, and a fiddle part. And there is the staging, the lighting effects, and the energy of the audience. All this together is the musical experience, the emergent phenomenon we call "Garth Brooks."

Wholeness

Finally, one of the basic principles of nonlinear, complex systems is that they must be considered in their wholeness as process, movement, and flow (Briggs & Peat, 1999). From the previous discussion, it seems obvious that music, to be music, must be experienced as a process in its wholeness. Analyzing parts of this system can give us some understanding of underlying processes. But to be appreciated—to be music—it must be a unit. A time-honored tradition of a formal music education is analyzing music. This involves cutting it apart, breaking down its chordal structure, identifying melodic devices, and determining musical form. This process helps us understand how the music is put together, but it does not contribute to a better performance or to greater musical appreciation. This analysis process does not help us really experience or appreciate the *music*. I had a college music history teacher who announced to our class that if the class was ever analyzing a piece of music we loved, we could leave class—no questions asked. I realize now this was a very enlightened teacher who understood and acknowledged the importance of wholeness in music. He didn't want the analysis process to destroy our true experience or love of the wholeness of the musical experience.

All theorists of complexity science emphasize this need for wholeness, including Dr. David Bohm, the noted quantum physicist. He (1980) based his nonlinear quantum theory on the importance, in fact necessity, for a theory of wholeness. He called this theory the "implicate order." This is ". . . a process of movement, continuously unfolding and enfolding from a seamless whole" (Shepherd, 1993, p. 245). According to this theory, all that exists unfolds out of the implicate order becoming explicate (matter). It implies that what we term "reality" is actually a process. Bohm (1980) writes that ". . . not only is everything changing, but all *is* flux. That is to say, *what is* the process of becoming itself, while all objects, events, entities, conditions, structures, etc., are forms that can be abstracted from this process" (p. 48). Bohm is speaking of quantum movement. Later he also states that ". . . this enfoldment and unfoldment takes place not only in the movement of the electromagnetic field but also in that of other fields, such as the electronic, protonic, *sound waves*, etc." (1980, pp. 177–178, emphasis added).

Music is a "whole" in which there is "a process of movement continuously unfolding and enfolding." Bohm (1980) himself states,

> In listening to music, *one is therefore directly perceiving an implicate order*. Evidently, this order is *active* in the sense that it continuously flows into emotional, physical, and other responses, that are inseparable from the transformations out of which it is essentially constituted. (p. 200)

Music therapist Dr. Charles Eagle goes further when he states, "One may assume that music *is* the implicate, enfolded order of the universe, from which all products and/or processes can become explicate" (1991, p. 59). Music is unlimited process expressed in—but not restricted by—form and structure. It is process, it is form, and it is whole. If, as Dr. Eagle theorizes, music with its specific sound combinations is the implicate order out of which all matter and process emerge, everything we need to know and understand should be revealed by studying it—including human health. With this extensive investigation of the process and phenomena of music, it is now time to formulate a definition of music relevant to the theory of music and soulmaking.

Defining Music

By exploring music from so many different perspectives, a definition of music as it relates to the music therapy theory of music and soulmaking can be formed. Music is first and foremost a product of humankind. Music comes from the intentional endeavors of people. "Music is a meeting between sound and human consciousness. . . . [M]usic had to be created by man. It did not antedate him. It developed with him" (Hughes, 1948, p. 1). Sound is an experience of physical motion. Music is the totally unique interaction between sound and people, the relationship between sound and human beings. It is the idea behind or beyond the sound. Human consciousness is ". . . what enlivens sound into information" (Kenyon, 1994, p. 188). Music forms in the human mind to express and meet our deepest needs—to express emotion, to create a sense of belonging to the group, to touch the Divine. Though the forms of music are culturally determined, the urge to create music and its various roles and functions are universal elements. The basic physiological structures needed for musical behaviors are "hardwired" in our brains, but it is not an artificial invention of humans. Terhardt (1995) writes, "The picture emerges that music not only obeys the basic and general principles of sensory acquisition of information but that it even provides an archetype of those principles, i.e., exhibiting them most purely" (p. 81). Music comes from us as part of us. It is a product of human uniqueness. Music sets us apart from other animals and fundamentally reflects who we are.

Music is unique in human creations. It is simultaneously product and process. The product is the musical event, the combinations and organizations of tones, rhythm, loudness, and tone quality. It is a "thing" of immense complexity. Yet the product is also a process. "In music, though, the product is a process: it occurs through time and in time" (Rothstein, 1995, p. 98). The product, the musical event, spins out over time as a transitory event. It must be created anew every time—whether as a new performance or as a creation of individual imagination as we listen to a recording. Unlike a painting or a sculpture that has permanence, the true musical product exists only when performed and experienced. As already discussed, a score, though permanent, is not the music. It is only a skeleton. The flesh comes from individuals performing the composition for others to perceive and experience. It is the process of performing and listening that creates music. Music is an ". . . information process working simultaneously on many different levels, generating a complex of responses from the most basic and physical to the most elusive and abstract" (Maconie, 1990, p. 3). It is this information exchange on so many diverse levels of human functioning that makes music such a unique human endeavor. Music is highly structured and organized (rigidly so in many compositional styles), yet it allows—in fact demands—unrestrained process and creativity. Music is created out of a dizzying array of diverse and complex elements, yet it is understood and appreciated with no formal knowledge of those elements. It is natural for us to understand music. It reflects the very nature of our world including how our minds function. As higher brain functioning developed in the neocortex (the new cortex found in humans), the forms of Western and Eastern music emerged as reflections of the patterns and timing of the brain at work (Leng & Shaw, 1991).

Music is a self-organizing stream of energetic information (Moses, 2000). It is an open energetic system. "By definition, an open system is non-linear even if its infrastructure might contain linear events [like rhythm or musical form] . . ." (Wallin, 1991, p. 17). This constant flux of energy/information builds the system to new states of complexity through iterative feedback. As a nonlinear dynamical system in motion, music is a system of evolving structures that are in constant transition that is nonequilibrium in nature. The influx of energy increases complexity until a new bifurcation or new order of structure emerges. So not only is the musical experience itself an emergent property of this open system, but the various aspects of that experience—musical style, emotional expression, and so forth—are emergent properties in and of themselves. The emotional state or musical style emerges from the increasing complexity in the system. As Wagner stated, "Music does not express the passions, love or longings of this or that individual in this or that situation, it *is* passion, love and longing" (quoted in Hetlinger, 1989, p. 4). "Music gives back the actual vibratory message, not the symbol in writing or the representation as in painting. Music touches the original essence" (Maman, 1997, p. 41). The complex processes and relationships that interact in musical behavior transcend their individual features and emerge as an entity greater than the sum of its parts—music.

As a self-organizing system, the phenomenon of music is vibrant and alive (Metias, 1985). It has presence, a life force all its own. It is living in the sense that it has an animated existence. It is full of energy and activity because of the dynamic flow and ambiguity that spring from its complexity (Rider, 1997). Music is a living, though transitory, entity because it is self-organizing. "Nonlinear dynamics now offer a mathematics of self-organizing systems that appear to be on the borderline between living organisms and nonliving media" (Hunt, 1996, p. 265). Music is an entity because it has a distinct, independent, and self-contained real existence. As Wallin (1991) states,

> Natural systems [like music] . . . are fed by positive feedback as a main characteristic. They are self-organizing and therefore, in a general sense, equivalent to "living systems" such as cells in organisms, and exchange energy with their environment—"energy" includes its non-physical equivalents "motivation," "emotion," "information," etc. (p. 142)

Because of the sensitivity to initial conditions and the feedback inherent in complex, moving systems, they are unique and nonrepeatable in a fashion usually associated with organic behaviors (Hunt, 1996). In this sense, music becomes a "living" energetic system. Energy is the capacity for vigorous activity. To be energetic is to be forceful, powerful in action, and effective. No wonder music has played such a pivotal role in human concerns.

Throughout this chapter, the phenomenon of music was explored from many perspectives. It is clear that music is a complex energetic system that potentially affects human functioning in many ways. Let's now turn to current music therapy practice to illustrate this power of music to heal and speculate on new ways that this energetic system is used as a therapeutic tool. To accomplish this investigation, something that complexity science says cannot be done—break human functioning up into four parts—is presented. This is done only as a means to organize a vast amount of material and because these divisions of functioning are in keeping with current terminology. The four aspects of human functioning explored include the brain and mind, the body, emotions and feelings, and spirit. Obviously, these divisions are somewhat arbitrary. How can mind be separated from emotion or, for that matter, from the body? How can spirit be truly separated from mind? But maintaining these standard distinctions enhances understanding. In order to understand reasons why music is an effective tool for therapy, human functioning in these areas must be investigated using current information from many types of research and from music therapy practice. Once accomplished, the parts are integrated again in a holistic theory of music therapy—music and soulmaking.

~

CHAPTER FOUR

Music Therapy and Problems of Brain and Mind

My music therapy colleague and I are participating in a weeklong community event demonstrating the uses of music therapy interventions, particularly with older adults. We challenge the nursing home staff to bring us their most difficult residents. They comply, and we work with small groups and individuals, most with diagnoses of Alzheimer's disease. This terrible condition strips the brain of its ability to function. Patients lose memories and become agitated and aggressive. Near the end of our time, we hear Lucy, another Alzheimer's patient, coming down the hall toward our room. She is screaming, highly agitated, and obviously frightened. She enters the room, and the extent of her fear and panic is clear. Her face is strained and distorted. Her yelling and cursing gets louder and more aggressive. She strikes out trying to hit us. We give her a rhythm instrument, and it flies across the room. My colleague picks up his guitar, begins to strum rhythmically, and we sing "You're a Grand Old Flag." Instantly, Lucy changes. She joins in the singing, and the yelling disappears. Her face relaxes. She smiles and even laughs. She sings the whole song with us. When it is over, she remains calm and teases my colleague about his guitar playing. The observing nursing home staff is in tears. They've never known Lucy to do anything but yell and hit. I see this reaction to familiar, rhythmic music all the time with patients with Alzheimer's disease. It is the basis of music therapy work with these individuals, emphasizing quality of life, reduction of agitation, and normalization of personality.

The investigation of the effectiveness of music therapy begins with the brain and nervous system and its creation—the human mind. The brain is the master control center for all aspects of human functioning—from aspects of mind like perception and memory, to control of bodily behavior like motor movement, to generation of emotion, and to the affiliative behavior of spirit. If something affects the brain, it causes changes in reaction, function, or behavior. In other words, it is therapeutic. Unquestionably, the human brain and nervous system are the most intriguing biological entities in the animal kingdom. They are probably the most complex structures in the universe (Rose, 1998a). What this structure can produce—from simple perception to the great mystery of consciousness—is astonishing. The brain and mind have fascinated scientists for centuries, but since the late 1970s there has been an explosion of interest in brain structure and functioning fueled by major advances in the technology needed to study the brain. Theories of brain organization and physiology are as numerous as the number of scientists studying all the questions inherent in investigating the brain and mind. Yet with all the remarkable information that has been gathered, less is known about the human brain than about the surface of the moon. Science has only a dim idea of what is happening in the human cortex or even in mammals. But this activity ". . . is at a level of complexity, of dynamic complexity, immeasurably greater than anything else that has ever been discovered in the universe or created in computer technology" (Popper & Eccles, 1977, p. 243).

In this chapter, brain functioning and aspects of mind from the perspective of complexity science are reviewed and the impact of sound/music on the structure and functions of the brain is explored. How sound/music can affect different levels of brain organization—from the increased chemical secretion, to the rhythm of the binding phenomena, to nonlinear global functioning of the products of the brain and aspects of mind—is addressed. It is shown that the brain is a fluid, recursively self-organized system with nonlinear, dynamical characteristics. From this overview of brain and mind, the influence of music on this highly complex system is demonstrated, and the effectiveness of music therapy interventions with problems of the brain and mind is explored.

Though the theory of music and soulmaking is based on the physics theory of complexity, physics principles alone cannot explain the how's and why's of a living, biological system. Brain science is vastly more complicated than the study of physics (Edelman, 1992). Another layer of complexity must be added, namely, the uniqueness of biological systems. Biological systems have unique characteristics compared to other systems addressed by pure physics. Biological systems require "biological thinking." First, biological thinking is population thinking, which considers individual variation in a population as a source of diversity not an error. These variations must be accounted for in a biological system. Second, biological organisms contain recognition systems. Recognition is the ". . . continual adaptive matching or fitting of elements in one physical domain to novelty occurring in elements of another, more or less independent physical domain, a matching that occurs without prior instruction" (Edelman, 1992, p. 74). For example, the immune system is a recognition system. During immune system functioning, one physical domain (the human body) reacts to novelty (a new invading virus) without prior instruction. Our brains are also selective recognition systems. Because recognition systems are by their nature biological and historical systems, they are not strictly governed by the science of physics. "But all the laws of physics nevertheless apply to recognition systems" (Edelman, 1992, p. 79). To continue the development of the theory of music and soul-making, the biological principles explored in the next two chapters are added to the physics theory of complexity science.

The Brain and Nervous System

The basic anatomy of the brain and nervous system is immensely complex. A detailed overview of this is not possible here. To provide a basic understanding of brain anatomy, fundamental components of the brain and its structure as they specifically relate to music perception and musical behavior are presented.

Like all our biological systems, the human brain and nervous system initially develops from the construction codes of DNA found in the genes. DNA is the chemical component of genes. The building blocks of DNA and all matter are atoms. Researcher Joel Sternheimer (1983) discovered that atoms have a musical nature. He found that each atomic particle has a corresponding frequency, which is inversely proportional to its mass and creates a harmonic relationship. "This 'music' of the elementary particles means that we, who are composed of these elementary particles, are also composed of musical frequencies" (Maman, 1997, p. 15). DNA has acoustic (periodic) oscillations due to the vibrating and undulating motion of the helix itself (Swicord & Davis, 1983). Even at this basic level, musical principles are evident. Though there is still a common misconception that quantum effects are not relevant to macroscopic systems like DNA and brain formation, the principles of complexity science show that these small effects, including quantum properties, can have large, macroscopic consequences (Brophy, 1999).

Researchers Ohno and Ohno (1986) also found musical principles in gene replication. They discovered that regular repetitions occur in gene duplication. In their research, they took the coding base sequences of genes and transformed them into musical scores by assigning two musical notes to each of the nucleotides on the DNA code to create melody and based rhythms on the distances between the nucleotides' bases. Familiar melodies were produced (Rider, 1997). Conversely, musical scores can be transcribed into DNA coding base sequences. In 1988, Ohno concluded that the coding sequences of genes constitute fundamental and derived repeating units. All these complex interplays between fundamental and derived recurring units that characterize each gene coding sequence can best be appreciated by their musical transformations. Researcher Fabian Maman (1997) has actually altered DNA using specific sound input. As he writes, "We are music deeply, to the smallest particle of our being. We are music in the nucleus of our DNA, in our molecular structure" (1997, p. 15).

Anatomy and Physiology of the Nervous System

In the development of the brain and nervous system, the DNA initially codes for development of the specialized cells of the nervous system, the *neurons*. Our brain is composed of 100 billion neurons and their supportive glial cells. Neurons are unlike anything else in the universe. They have varied shapes, electrical and chemical function, and connectivity—the ability to link with other neurons (Edelman, 1992). Structurally, each neuron has a cell body with a *nucleus*, many *dendrites*, and one *axon*. The dendrites are input fibers for the neuron and extend from the cell body in numerous branches receiving signals from other neurons and moving them toward the cell body. Each neuron has one axon, which functions to send signals out from the cell body to dendrites of other neurons. There is a gap between the axon of one neuron and the dendrite of another known as the *synapse*. Synapses have many different shapes and multiple connection networks that change over time from sensory input and experience with the environment (Brophy, 1999). The end of each axon has an enlarged bulb, the *presynaptic terminal*, containing sacks of chemicals called *neurotransmitters*. The ends of dendrites also have an enlarged end, the *postsynaptic terminal*, designed to react to the chemical irritation of these neurotransmitters (Tortora & Anagnostakos, 1987). There are over fifty different neurotransmitters—substances including acetylcholine and amino acids such as glutamate and neuropeptides. "We are still trying to guess why the brain uses such a diversity of substances. The probable answer is that diversity provides a rich grammar of interactions between neurons which optimizes the range and tuning of responses available in different situations" (Robbins, 1998, p. 35). There are 100 trillion synapses in the nervous system and a much larger number of combinations of connections—ten followed by a million zeros (Edelman, 1992).

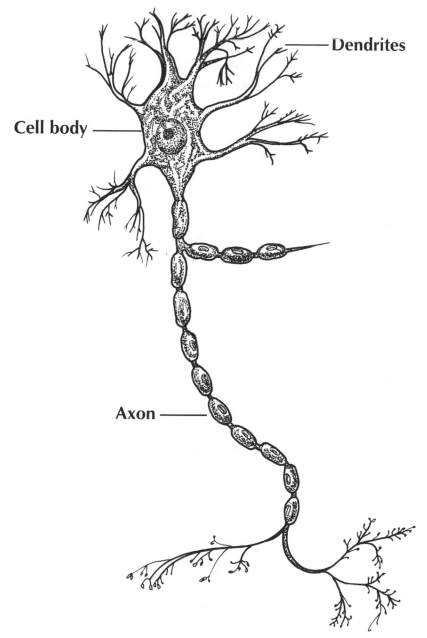

Dendrites

Cell body

Axon

Figure 9.   The neuron. Courtesy of B. Brauckman

When a nerve is activated or fired, a *nerve impulse* is generated. The nerve impulse involves electrical and chemical processes. A nerve is at rest until it is irritated or stimulated in some way. When the nerve is irritated, exchange of potassium and sodium ions occurs across the cell membrane. The irritation allows sodium ions to rush into the nerve. This alters the internal membrane from a negative to a positive charge creating an *action potential* or spike of electrical voltage. The flow of ions through the cell membrane creates electric currents (Wallin, 1991). As one area of the cell membrane reaches an action potential, it irritates the next section of the membrane. This creates a chain reaction in the cell membrane moving the electrical charge along the neuron. As soon as a section of the cell membrane is changed by the influx of sodium, it becomes more potassium permeable. Potassium rushes back into the membrane to move the cell to its resting state. This causes a short period of time called the *after potential*, which is close to a normal potassium balance. The after potential constitutes a downswing toward the state of rest or readiness for another action potential to occur. Recordings of this process show that ". . . the afterpotential and the return to rest look like a melodic cadence with a major leading tone before the tonic!" (Wallin, 1991, p. 335). This basic level of brain organization demonstrates a musical quality.

When this electrical potential arrives at the presynaptic terminal, the irritation causes a sack of chemicals to open. The chemical floats across the gap, irritating the postsynaptic terminal and causing the whole process to begin in the next neuron. This is the chemical part of the electrochemical energy of the nerve impulse.

The basic process of a nerve impulse is obviously complex, but the actual system is far more intricate and complicated. For example, Wallin (1991) points out that the ion pumping action has its own rhythm:

> There exists a combination of potassium-calcium channels (pumping ions in and out of cell body membrane) that makes the cell body function like an oscillator with a slow basic wave; the action potentials are thus "inoculated" on this slow oscillation of the membrane of the cell body. The slow wave reflects a spontaneous activity of the cell itself—its rhythm is intrinsic. (p. 336)

The basic process of neural transmission is a wave with a measurable rhythm. Neural transmission is a complex system in motion. As such, it is nonlinear. The action potentials appear in sudden bursts with an explosive quality and then are coupled in positive feedback (Wallin, 1991). These nonlinear dynamics are explored in detail later in the chapter.

Neurons make up the brain, spinal chord, and peripheral nerve system that send signals throughout the body. There are two nerve systems that the brain activates. The first is the *sympathetic* nervous system that activates response and directly energizes behavior. The second is the *parasympathetic* nervous system that allows for inhibition of excitement and promotes calmness in the face of stress. It controls energy and the conserving processes of sleep, rest, and healing (Janov, 1996). It also regulates behavior and emotions (Schneider, 2001). As explored later, music affects brain structures that connect to both nervous systems, allowing music to, at times, arouse us and at others to inhibit behavior and express emotions.

Brain Structure

A classic approach to studying brain structure is to partition it according to task. In a theory first postulated by MacLean (1973), the brain is envisioned as being roughly divided into three levels (the triune brain) corresponding to specific types of information management. The most primitive portion of our brain, the *brain stem* or reptilian brain, mediates the most basic life functions. The paleomammalian brain, the *midbrain*, encompasses the brain structures that feel and generate emotions. Finally, the neomammalian brain, the *neocortex*, processes higher brain functions like language, reason, and logic (Kenyon, 1994). This "upper brain" receives much attention for its control of specifically human functions, including music, but all levels of brain functioning seem to be involved. "An impressive body of research suggests that a significant amount of neonatal mental functioning is carried out by lower brain centers, and that these evolutionarily earlier parts of the brain are the foundations for some complex human behaviors" (Wade, 1996, p. 66). The three parts of the triune brain are separate but interconnected complex adaptive systems that control all aspects of human functioning (Shulman, 1997).

Structurally, the cortex, the gray matter of the brain, is divided into two hemispheres by a large fissure, and each hemisphere is divided into four lobes roughly based on general functions. It has a fractal shape in its folded, craggy fissures, turns, and bends (Briggs & Peat, 1999). Each lobe is responsible for particular functions. The occipital lobe processes vision, and the parietal lobe handles sensory processing. Hearing is mediated in the temporal lobe, while the frontal lobe deals with long-term planning, movement control, and speech production (Hodges, 1996b). The cerebral hemispheres are connected by a thick band of neurons, the *corpus callosum*, which keeps both hemispheres of the brain in constant communication. To introduce specific structures and areas in all three levels of the brain, let's look at several specific brain processes related to music and musical behavior and the brain anatomy associated with each—sound and music perception, impact of sound on the brain,

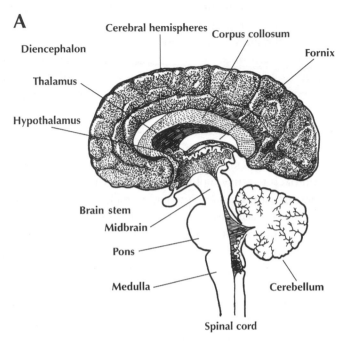

A

Cerebral hemispheres   Corpus collosum

Diencephalon   Fornix

Thalamus

Hypothalamus

Brain stem
Midbrain
Pons
Medulla   Cerebellum

Spinal cord

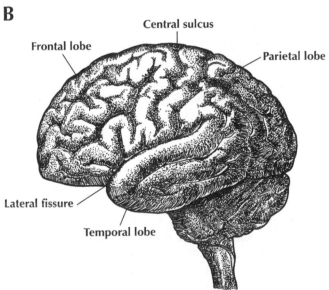

B

Central sulcus

Frontal lobe   Parietal lobe

Lateral fissure

Temporal lobe

Figure 10.   The brain: a. cross section and b. three-dimensional illustration. Courtesy of B. Brauckman.

music and the neurology of emotional response, and coordination of motor behavior.

Sound and Music Perception

To review the path of the auditory nerve to the brain, a simple overview of what is in actuality a very complex process will be presented. Auditory input to our brain involves specific neuron groups affecting five portions of the brain—two portions of the brain stem, the midbrain, and both hemispheres of the cortex. Each neuron group responds to specific qualities of a tone such as pitch, tone quality, and so on. In addition to these *afferent neurons*, the auditory system has *efferent nerves* that go from the brain back to the ear in three descending pathways—one to the thalamus, a second to the midbrain, and a third to the lower brain stem and, eventually, to the ear. This creates reciprocal information in the form of short feedback loops, allowing the ear to make adjustments and to select particular sounds for attention (Wallin, 1991). With all this information going up and down the central nervous system, the simple act of hearing engages large amounts of our brain. That occurs with just hearing simple sound. When listening to music, which is much more complex, more of our brain is activated. Add the act of playing music, and the brain is then engaged in processing touch and controlling motor function. Music, especially playing music, engages more of the brain than any other single activity. Positron-emission tomography (PET scan) research supports this contention (Mazziotta et al., 1982).

Let's review the auditory pathway from the ear to the various parts of the brain. The auditory nerve has synapses in five areas of the brain, creating more chances for sound to affect neural functioning (Guyton, 1979). The first synapse of the auditory nerve is in the brain stem, the most fundamental part of the brain. The brain stem is an extension of the spinal cord and contains all ascending and descending nerve tracts that communicate between the spinal cord and various parts of the brain. The auditory nerve enters the brain stem and branches to innervate three divisions of the *cochlear nucleus*. These cell groups possess various kinds of neurons situated in different parts of the structure. Some groups respond only to low and middle frequencies, while others respond to high frequencies. Some neurons specialize in reproducing repetitive low-frequency stimuli (like repetitive drumming), while others respond to steady-state sounds such as vowels (Wallin, 1991). Neural physiological research shows that incoming *sound* is extensively processed in the brain stem before conscious awareness occurs.

The next auditory synapse is also in the brain stem—in the *olivary complex* of the *pons*—the bridge from the spinal cord to other parts of the brain. This is where the nerve pathways from the ears cross. To add complexity to the process of hearing, we have two ears. Each ear has two pathways to the brain—one that goes up without crossing to the opposite brain hemisphere and one that does cross. This creates four auditory inputs to the various structures in the brain, providing even more stimulation and complexity.

From the brain stem, the auditory nerve next synapses in the main station of the *diencephalon*, the *inferior colliculus*, a midbrain structure essential for attention to auditory input. The diencephalon is the relay center to other parts of the brain from the peripheral sense organs. It functions as a pacemaker to drive all our biological rhythms. The auditory nerve also impacts the auditory receiving areas of the *thalamus*, the *medial geniculate body*, and the *hypothalamus*. The hypothalamus is involved in the *autonomic nervous system* (brain activities processed below consciousness awareness), homeostatic processes, endocrine system regulation, and mediation of survival behavior. Musical stimuli have a strong effect upon the neurological firing patterns of the hypothalamus (Taylor, 1997). From the thalamus, two branches of the auditory nerve separate. One goes to the *amygdala* and *hippocampus*, which are responsible for fear states, startle reactions, and general arousal. The other branch goes to the auditory areas of the *cerebral cortex* for perceptual processing. "Selection and analysis [of sound] take place in the auditory cortex; 60 percent of the cortical cells there respond to specific tones" (Ornstein, 1991, p. 174). The frontal lobe of the cortex, especially the *orbitofrontal cortex* and *cingulate gyrus*, is also activated to provide subjective evaluation of the sensory input. The orbitofrontal cortex exchanges information with the limbic system and is responsible for translating judgments about social situations into action and emotional response. It communicates with the cingulate gyrus, serving as an interface among the frontal cortex for decision making, emotions of the limbic system, and brain structures controlling movement (Carlson, 1992).

Because there are four pathways from the ears, both hemispheres of the cerebral cortex are involved in perceiving sound. We know that the two hemispheres of our brain process information differently. Our left hemisphere is characterized by linear, analytical, logical, temporal thought (Blackeslee, 1980). Numbers, speech, and sequencing come from the left hemisphere. Holistic processing with emphasis on relationships and comparisons comes from our right hemisphere. "The right hemisphere processes information in a connected way that minimizes in harmonious elements. It works in an intuitive, synthetic, spatial, holistic, and symbolic manner" (Wade, 1996. p. 151). Because auditory pathways connect to both hemispheres, the two forms of processing are used in perceiving music. Wallin (1991) gives a good example of this. In his review of the research literature, he reports that tones of short onsets and low stability of a tone are preferred by the right ear/left hemisphere, while normal onset and high-stability tone perception is a left ear/right hemisphere preference. It is a common misconception and too simplistic to say music perception is a right hemisphere process only. The two cerebral hemispheres are also specialized for emotional processing related to music like they are for information processing. "The left hemisphere responds to the verbal content of emotional expression and the right to tone and gesture" (Ornstein, 1991, p. 81). A song with words and the tonal/gestural qualities of music would stimulate both. Much research has tried to localize various musical responses in a particular hemisphere with mixed results (Radocy & Boyle, 1997). It is important to remember that lateralization, the dominance of one hemisphere over the other, indicates that each side of the brain manages certain activities, but dominance does not mean absolute control of a particular function (Jourdain, 1997). It is likely that specific elements of sound perception occur in various areas of the brain but that processing music involves the whole brain working in concert.

The brain's cortex is where thinking and talking about music occurs and where meaning is assigned to auditory input. It is in the upper cortex where perception of the highly complex stimulus of music finally happens. Sound arrives at the primary auditory cortex situated on the temporal lobe at both sides of the brain (Jourdain, 1997). The complex network of connecting neurons in the cortex is organized as a honeycomb of columns a few neurons wide that stretch from top to bottom through six layers (Edelman, 1987). In the primary auditory cortex, individual columns respond most strongly to specific frequencies of sound. Interestingly, the brain is activated differently when pure sound versus music is used. Music activates parts of the frontal cortex and the temporal lobe (Jourdain, 1997).

It is a mistake to assume that the cortex can actually process all the input it receives as separate and distinct bits of information. The auditory cortex processes sounds by ". . . detecting starts and stops, following frequency contours, and assembling overtones into unified notes, all without a smidgen of conscious effort" (Jourdain, 1997, p. 63). Ultimately, the brain focuses on two things—change in the stimulus and the relationships between sounds. Final perception of music comes from the work of the secondary auditory cortex, which reassembles the sound components detected by the auditory cortex. The brain models relations between the various sound features it receives and then models relations among these relations, and so forth, in a complex web. Modeling deep relations among sound components constitutes our final comprehension of music (Jourdain, 1997).

It's these relations—intangible, resistant to observation, difficult to describe and classify—that *are* music, not the atmospheric vibrations that jiggle out of musical instruments. The vibrating molecules that convey music from an orchestra to our ears don't "contain" sensation, only patterns. When a brain is able to model a pattern, meaningful sensation arises. (Jourdain, 1997, pp. 4–5)

Impact of Sound on the Brain

This general overview of the auditory pathway to the brain hints at the amazing complexity of this process. Other brain structures in the four general divisions of the brain are also affected by sound, adding even more complexity. There are three times more nerve connections between the ear and the brain than between the eye and the brain (Tomatis, 1987). This shows the tremendous impact that sound input has on the brain and its functioning.

The first effect of sound on the brain is the ability of tones in the 3,000- to 8,000-Hz range to resonate or set the brain as a whole into vibration. This potentially affects cognitive functioning (Kumar, 1997). Second, the direct innervation of various brain structures gives rise to physiological effects created by sound input. Let's look at the most important brain areas for these effects.

The *reticular activating system* (RAS), located in the oldest part of our brain, is a brain region that runs from the medulla oblongata, just above the end of the spinal chord, to the top of the midbrain, just below the thalamus (Damasio, 1999). It is a network of loosely connected nuclei and fiber systems that influence alertness and arousal. It includes the reticular formation of the brain stem and the reticular nuclei of the thalamus. The RAS, important in our perceptual and behavioral alertness, contributes to body position as it relates to survival and helps maintain internal stability (homeostasis). The RAS is the brain area primarily concerned with managing the life process and representing the organism in the brain. It is associated with wakefulness and sleep, with emotion and attention, and with consciousness in general (Damasio, 1999). The RAS receives data from the ascending sensory pathways via the fifth cranial nerve and projects axons to the cortex, thalamus, and spinal cord, providing activation and modulation of output.

The auditory nerve has connections, some indirect, in a number of the structures constituting the RAS. Sound input is especially important in being alert and aware. It is an essential part of our survival. When we hear a crash outside our bedroom window at 2:00 a.m., we are instantly awake and on our feet ready to fight or run long before our brain tells us what we heard. This is the RAS in action. Sound's influence on this part of the brain creates many specific physiological effects and responses.

Certain physiological reactions elicited by sound and music have been verified by research dating back to the 1930s (Radocy & Boyle, 1997). These *autonomic nervous system* effects include impact on heart rate, pupil dilation, sweat response, and respiration. In fact, ". . . a group of cells [of the reticular formation] discharge in synchrony with the rhythm of respiration. Presumably they function as the pacemaker for that rhythm" (Nauta & Feirtag, 1986, p. 187). Sound, particularly strong, regular rhythmic input, influences this rhythm of bodily functions. However, the research shows that this influence is unpredictable and inconsistent (Radocy & Boyle, 1997). There is a common misconception that music of a certain tempo (say sixty beats a minute) will consistently slow your heartbeat to that rate (Harrer & Harrer, 1977). This is untrue. The body is set up to maintain homeostasis within a dynamic range we consider "normal." The body isn't going to let an outside stimulus like music drastically alter something as important as heart rate.

Music and the Neurology of Emotional Response

Perhaps the most recognized effect of sound on the brain is the stimulation of emotions—biologically determined complex patterns of chemical and neural responses. They are engaged and processed automatically and are generated in the midbrain region of the brain (Damasio, 1999). James Papez was the first to identify this "emotional brain" with various structures metaphorically identified as the *limbic system* (Purves et al., 1997). The limbic system includes structures and areas in the limbic lobe: hippocampus, amygdala, portions of the hypothalamus and thalamus, cingulate cortex, and fornix. Many scientists are challenging the limbic system theory as an explanation for the emotional brain and questioning whether the limbic system exists at all (LeDoux, 1996). Current research shows that some of these structures are involved in some emotional responses, but not all. There may not be one emotional system in the brain but, rather, many (LeDoux, 1996). Each class of emotion is mediated by separate neural systems that evolved for different reasons. This is another example of the complexity inherent in brain structure and processes.

There are two limbic structures that are particularly important in emotional reaction to music: the amygdala and the hippocampus. The amygdala is the specialist for emotional reactions because it colors our experiences with emotions (Goleman, 1995). When sound input enters the brain, it first travels to the thalamus and then crosses with a single synapse to the amygdala, thus receiving input from the lower portions of the brain. However, the amygdala also receives input from the brain's higher centers. It then sends signals to every part of the brain, including the decision-making center, the frontal lobe (Pinker, 1997). This is why emotion is important in thinking, learning, memory, and consciousness (Wallin, 1991). The thalamus and amygdala serve as bridges between the body and sensory input and the functions of mind. The amygdala and hippocampus ". . . control access to our emotions, influencing what is experienced and what is not, what is learned and what is not. When input is too charged, painkillers are released and the message doesn't get through to conscious awareness" (Janov, 1996, p. 194). This release of brain chemicals, which is addressed in greater detail in chapter 5, is why highly emotionally charged experiences can block out memories.

As mentioned earlier, signals from the amygdala to the hypothalamus trigger autonomic nervous system responses (Parker, 1998). They also influence endocrine system functions and organize survival behavior. Musical input affects the neurological firing patterns of the hypothalamus. Music thus has a direct effect on the various emotional processing centers in the brain. "What seems certain is that there is a closer relation between *hearing* and emotional arousal than there is between *seeing* and emotional arousal" (Storr, 1992, p. 26). Music's direct impact on the thalamus and connections to most limbic structures may broadly account for emotional reactions to music.

There is also a chemical mechanism of emotional transmission. Candace Pert discovered this chemical mechanism of emotional transmission in her work on *neuropeptides* (Pert et al., 1985). Neuropeptides are forms of endorphins common to the central nervous system and immune system of the body. These chemical informational substances have receptors on every cell in the body (Pert, 1997). The receptors are single-protein molecules found on the surface of cells in the body and brain. Receptors are scanners looking for their compatible chemical substances, the *ligands*, floating throughout the body. The ligand binds to the appropriate receptor like a key in a lock. When this binding occurs, the receptor molecule, made up of a chain of amino acids, rearranges itself, thus "unlocking" the cell membrane and allowing information to enter the cell (Pert, 1997).

What is interesting to the exploration of music therapy's impact on the functioning of the brain is the behavior of the receptors and ligands. Receptors and their ligands are ". . . constantly moving, dancing in a rhythmic vibratory way" (Pert, 1997, p. 23). This constant movement sits at the edge of chaos, creating optimum potential for receptivity. As the ligand and receptor bind, they change shape. As Pert (1997) describes it, they ". . . wiggle, shimmy, and even hum as they bind and change from one shape to another . . ." (p. 22). The receptor "recognizes" the appropriate ligand by the particular vibratory characteristic of the carbon chain that constitutes it. Rather than a lock and key, this process is ". . . two voices—ligand and receptor—

striking the same note and producing a vibration that rings a doorbell to open the doorway to the cell" (Pert, 1997, p. 24).

At this basic level of communication in the body, vibration at a particular frequency is the mechanism. This ligand–receptor communication system represents a second nervous system, another and older means of communication compared to the electrical system of the central nervous system. As Pert (1997) writes,

> These receptors and their ligands have come to be seen as "information molecules"—the basic units of a language used by cells throughout the organism to communicate across systems such as the endocrine, neurological, gastrointestinal, and even the immune system. Overall, the musical hum of the receptors as they bind to their many ligands, often in far-flung parts of the organism, creates an integration of structure and function that allows the organism to run smoothly, intelligently. (p. 27)

This new theory of information exchange in the nervous system focuses on a purely chemical, nonsynaptic communication between cells. The means for this communication to happen is the vibration characteristics of these chemicals. Emotions are not the receptors/ligands themselves but are emergent properties of the oscillating coupling of the receptor/ligand dynamical system. Emotion is a simultaneous field shift over the whole body/mind interaction. Emotions can no longer be seen as being held in the head. Emotion, and in fact all aspects of mind, is located throughout our entire body, in all places at once. Such a system is ever changing, dynamic, and entirely flexible.

> In the old paradigm, we saw the body in terms of energy and matter. Hardwired reflexes, caused by electrical stimulation across the synapse, ran the body in a more or less mechanical, reactive fashion, with little room for flexibility, changes, or intelligence. With information added to the process, we see that there is an intelligence running things. It's not a matter of energy acting on matter to create behavior, but of intelligence in the form of information running all the systems and creating behavior. (Pert, 1997, p. 185)

Emotion is the energy of this system. It is possible to say that both physical and energetic environmental information could affect it since biological behavior is dynamically linked to the environment. Music can potentially be an important part of that energetic environmental information. It is first a physical energy, which is explored at length in chapter 5. It is also a direct environmental stimulus to emotions as a vibratory input.

Coordination of Motor Behavior

A large portion of our brain is involved in movement, including the complex movement patterns of musical performance. "The whole point of a brain is to move. . . . Movement is the concern of the whole brain" (Jourdain, 1997, pp. 206–207). To get the body to move, a vast amount of our brain must work in a huge cooperative effort. For example, the control mechanism just for the hands alone, so important in musical performance, is tremendous. "The muscles in our hands are supplied more densely and finely with nerves . . . our spinal chords more thickly channeled for rapid communication between brain and hand, and most important, our brains more ingeniously designed to generate elaborate hand movements" (Jourdain, 1997, p. 205). Let's look at the numerous brain structures involved in the complex process of moving.

The neural impulses sent to the muscles come directly from a structure in the spinal chord called the *anterior horn*. The anterior horn is a "smart" relay station. It is under the control of higher brain centers that actually initiate the needed neural impulses. But every signal going out to our muscles comes through the anterior horn. It monitors the motor activity, gathers and interprets sensory information, and modifies the outgoing signals so the movement is as accurate as possible. That's why it is "smart."

In the upper brain, the *motor cortex* is very important. Running from ear to ear across the top of the midbrain structures, the motor cortex functions as the hub of the motor system. It contains the largest neurons in the central nervous system and is in direct contact with the cells of the anterior horn and with a wide variety of other brain structures. The motor cortex is the command center for motor movement. The *cingulate* cortex is also instrumental in motor movement. This structure has ". . . an odd combination of sensory and motor roles. The cingulate is a massively somatosensory structure which receives input from all divisions of the somatosensory system . . ." (Damasio, 1999, p. 261). It receives signals from the internal environment and the muscoskeletal areas while being involved in the execution of complex movements including vocalization. The cingulate is also involved in the processes of attention, emotion, and awareness.

Motor movement depends on the function of the *basal ganglia*. This midbrain structure regulates the cooperative efforts of muscle groups relating to body posture and controls the execution of a sequence of motor programs. The basal ganglia help regulate movement in a motor program by coordinating sensory and motor responses. However, they also help direct what is to be done according to a *motor plan*. "This appendage works over longer time scales and helps correlate whole sequences of gestures in a plan" (Edelman,

1992, p. 106). The basal ganglia assist movements by arranging groups of muscles into a body posture appropriate to the intended task. They also have an important role in initiating movement.

> The basal ganglia are hard at work in music making, for they have much to do with managing long sequences of postural adjustment. . . . [G]ood musicians work in motions that are much larger and longer, motions that encapsulate all the details of a long passage. It is these large motions that imbue music with line and balance, and the basal ganglia are likely to have much to do with them. (Jourdain, 1997, p. 212)

The *cerebellum* is another important structure for motor control. It works with other parts of the motor control system to initiate and improve the smoothness and timing of muscle contractions. It is the cerebellum that regulates the contractions and inhibitions of muscle needed for ballistic movement so necessary for musical performance. "The cerebellum appears to be crucial in carrying out movements that are *ballistic*, that is, too quick to be adjusted by feedback. Once initiated, a ballistic movement follows its course, and only afterward does the brain learn what has happened" (Jourdain, 1997, p. 214). The cerebellum stores numerous subprograms of movement. These details of ballistic movement must be worked out in advance, allowing the movement sequence to be executed with absolute accuracy in a nearly automatic way.

A skilled motor behavior, like music performance, is also very dependent on *feedback*—knowledge of results. Feedback allows for instantaneous adjustment in the motor performance. Performance is not just a flow of commands from brain to muscle. Feedback from muscles back to the brain is vital for this complex movement pattern to occur (Jourdain, 1997). Sensors embedded in the muscles called *muscle spindles* accomplish this. The muscle spindles create a self-contained reflex subsystem, which acts directly on the anterior horn. When feedback arrives in the anterior horn from the muscle spindles, the signals sent out from the anterior horn are adjusted to create smoother and more precise movement. "Accurate movement requires that the brain monitor every result of its efforts in a perceptual loop of feedback and adjustment" (Jourdain, 1997, p. 202).

The *parietal cortex* plays another important function in the motor control system. Here the brain assembles incoming sensations. Information from sight, hearing, touch, movement, and body position are drawn together. "In the parietal cortex, a map of the body meets a map of the world. The coordination of these two maps gives rise . . . to motor plans, which play out as actual movements" (Jourdain, 1997, p. 219). The complex motions of musical performance are launched only after the parietal lobe prepares maps of the body and the external environment. What is noteworthy about the brain's control of motor movement is not that it controls muscles but that it actually controls the *movement*.

Brain Functioning

Having addressed neural anatomy from the perspective of musical perception and behavior, brain functioning is now addressed. As with any complex system, looking at the various parts of the brain doesn't reveal how the brain actually functions. Even the most detailed neuroanatomy does not really explain how processes like perception or memory occur. As LeDoux (1996) writes, "The identification of brain regions associated with specific functions should not be taken too literally. Functions are mediated by interconnected systems of brain regions working together rather than by individual areas working in isolation" (p. 77). Looking at isolated areas of function can give us some reasons why certain things might occur, but the neuronal prerequisites for perception, memory, and so on do not explain these phenomena. The processes involved, how the brain actually works, and how it is organized for function must be examined with particular emphasis on its nonlinear, fractal processing. A good introduction to brain function is to explore how the brain develops.

Neonatal Brain Development

Brain development is *ontogenetic*, which by definition is the ". . . product of continuous exquisite interplay between genes and environment" (Rose, 1998a, p. 3). It is, in fact, our interactions with our environment, our experiences, that ultimately "wire up" our brains. Nobel Laureate Gerald Edelman's (1987) theory of "Neural Darwinism" states that neurons select themselves and form connections early in life as a function of their stimulation. "Through neuronal selection in infancy, the cells in the brain that strike a match with the environment thrive; those that do not, fall into disuse. These are the thousand potential forms of mind" (Ornstein, 1991, p. 123). We are born with an oversupply of neurons and potential connections between them. Those that are not used are lost. In fact, many researchers now believe that experience with the environment actually solidifies connections already present in the brain rather than develops new ones. Current research verifies that connections in the brain are more widespread at birth than later in life. As the infant learns, the number of neural connections in the brain are selected. The connections that are important to the individual are activated, and the ones that rarely are used eventually atrophy (Burke & Ornstein, 1995).

Not only are certain neurons selected, but, more importantly, vast connections between neurons are formed. "In the embryo, each individual develops a specific pattern of neural connections inside the brain. After birth, at different fixed periods in different organisms, new patterns of neural connections develop" (Ornstein, 1991, p. 124). In the first two years of life, 30,000 new synapses are formed *every second* under *each* square centimeter of the brain's surface (Rose, 1998a). The potential connections are inestimable.

Donald Hebb (1952) first postulated vast networks of neurons that organized themselves as "reverberating circuits" based on mutual activation. Based on his ideas, learning involves the rewiring of the brain through a process of neurons firing together. "What you do and what you think can change the patterns of connections with the neural networks of your brain" (Robertson, 1999, p. 101). Experience molds these connections—whether creating new ones or breaking old ones—so that our brain remains a shifting, responsive organ over the course of our lives. The brain and nervous system are in continuous structural change. They have plasticity (Maturana & Varela, 1987). But skills and abilities created by these connections exist not in rigid connections but in the *patterns* of the connections between neurons. "Experience, in short, is sculpted into the *pattern* of connections between neurones, not necessarily into specific connections between particular pairs of neurones" (Robertson, 1999, p. 11). So even if some of these connections or individual neurons themselves are destroyed, the pattern can still remain, preserving the skill or memory. "On the other hand, if more than a critical number of cells in a circuit are lost, then the pattern of connections cannot survive and that particular brain circuit will permanently lose its ability to do what it used to do" (Robertson, 1999, p. 95). A certain level or critical mass of cells and connections must exist in order for the pattern to survive. In other words, there must be a certain level of complexity present for the pattern that constitutes the skill or memory to exist.

Neural connections are created through the various experiences of life. This process actually begins long before birth and is based in large part on sound sensation and rhythmic, intrauterine movement experiences (Ayres, 1979). A fetus is able to hear and cognitively process sound in utero by five and a half months since cochlear function, basilar membrane response, and development of both inner and outer rows of hair cells in the organ of Corti all occur by the fifth to seventh month of pregnancy. This allows transmission of acoustic information to the eighth cranial nerve. This is the first of the cranial nerves to develop in the fetal brain (Taylor, 1997). Research by Shetler (1990) shows auditory evoked response exists in the fetal brain, indicating that the stimulus is transmitted to the brain where it can be perceived and stored in memory. This is likely due to the fact that the auditory nerve has its myelin sheath or covering prenatally, allowing the neurons to transmit a signal to the brain (Campbell, 2000). Other sensory nerves in the body do not develop this covering until after birth, preventing full transmission of sensory input to the brain until later development. Woodward et al. (1992) conducted research that showed the normal third-trimester fetus perceives and responds to externally presented music. The range of usable musical frequencies is 40 to 4,000 Hz and corresponds with the hearing range of the fetus in utero (Maconie, 1997). The early ability of newborn infants to respond to parameters of sound indicates prenatal exposure and learning (Blum, 1993). Infants respond to changes in frequency, intensity, duration, and temporal and spatial patterns of sound (Papousek & Papousek, 1981) as well as in the prosody—the emotional/intonational aspects of the human voice (Locke, 1993; Schore, 1994). By two months, they respond to rhythmically presented facial and body movements (Beebe et al., 1982; Trevarthen, 1984).

Because auditory receptors develop early in the developing fetus and acoustic input in the intrauterine environment is extensive and varied, ". . . the auditory tract may well be the fetal brain's primary source of stimulation for formation of the cognitive structures to be used initially for postnatal intellectual development" (Taylor, 1997, p. 20). The rapid mental progress noted in human babies is based on the prenatal sensory experiences that begin the process of building cognitive structures (Ward, 1993). This prenatal structuring makes the newborn infant able at birth to receive and perceive sensory information, process perception, and shape experience (Taylor, 1997).

As a child continues to develop, connections are strongest when experiences are strongly rooted in culture and have a strong emotional element. "For among the different types of experience we can have, all of which change the brain to some extent, emotional events can have the most dramatic effects on the trembling web [of connections]" (Robertson, 1999, p. 170). An emotionally charged experience serves to activate a broader and wider sampling of neurons. More of the brain is connected together, making the pattern harder to destroy. Robertson (1999) goes further by stating, "Some types of emotional learning happen best if we aren't aware that it is going on" (p. 177). The first and most profound cultural connection is the child interacting with a parent. These interactions are based on sounds, timbre, movement, facial expression, and gesture. All these interactive factors are a part of music and musical interactions (Bunt, 1994). Music is an experience deeply rooted in human culture. Though music is a deeply emotional event, its impact on emotion is often not overt. We aren't necessarily aware that the strong emotional connections are occurring. Music, especially music linked with a learning event, provides these important types of experiences.

From the fetal period on, infants are able to structure acoustic space (Mehler & Fox, 1985). They can locate sound sources in three-dimensional space, distinguish speech from background sound, and recognize sound from different sources (Wade, 1996). Music has great potential for providing experiences that create and maintain deep networks of connections in our brains and supporting learning and memory, as is explored later in the chapter. In fact, music is more fundamental than language for making connections in the brain (Wallin, 1991).

In addition to reinforcing neural connections, experience with the environment can make structural changes to the brain. Research reported in the March/April 1999 issue of *Psychology Today* demonstrated that strong emotion from traumatic experiences can negatively affect neural anatomy and functioning. This research showed that early emotional trauma in children impacts the size of the prefrontal cortex (involved in decision making and judgment) and the amygdala (involved in emotion generation, especially anger). Positively, children who have experience playing musical instruments before age eight show an increase in the size of the corpus callosum, indicating increased communication between the cerebral hemispheres (Amunts et al., 1996; Picone et al., 1997; Schlaug et al., 1995a). The corpus callosum has a hundred million nerve fibers. An increase of as little as 15 percent constitutes a vast increase in information flow (Jourdain, 1997). What we learn as children physically molds our brains and allows them to work in different ways (Robertson, 1999). This effect is so prominent that musicians' brains are structurally different from nonmusicians'. Robertson (1999) notes,

> The left half of the brain known as the "planium temporale" is bigger in musicians than in non-musicians. This part of the brain is important in verbal memory, and musical training before the age of twelve is now known to lead to better verbal memory. In other words, musical training not only expands the body-area of the brain used by the musical instrument, but also stimulates more general physical changes in the brain, benefiting other faculties. (p. 29)

With the overview of neonatal brain development, the overview of *neurophysiology*, or brain function with a particular emphasis on the nonlinear nature of how the brain works, can be addressed.

Neurophysiology

Neuroscience and the study of neurophysiology have progressed rapidly in the last thirty years due in large part to improved tools for investigation.

The PET scan gives scientists information on the metabolism of brain activity, while fMRI (functional magnetic resonance imagery) provides data concerning the brain as it works in real time. ERP (event-related potential) and MEG (magnetoencephalography) are newer technologies that show us that the brain is not ". . . an orderly fixed pattern of cells and their connections, but [is] in constant dynamic flux, with different areas 'lighting up' at different times depending on the mental challenges being faced" (Rose, 1998a, p. 10).

Brain function has been a fascination of science for hundreds of years. From the mechanistic views of Descartes, to the functional location theories of Penfield and the neural network model of Globus, to computational models that see the brain as a highly organized information-processing system like a computer, theories of brain function abound (Jibu & Yasue, 1995). Neuroscientists

> . . . have masses of data and lots of limited theories at different levels, for instance about how nerve cells propagate information or which of the regions of the brain are responsible for encoding speech, but we still lack any grand unified conception of what it means to be a brain, and how it does what it does. (Rose, 1998a, p. 5)

Many scientists now use a globalist approach to brain functioning. This approach sees the brain working as a single, integrated whole as opposed to a localization approach, which assigns mental functions to specific, different parts of the brain (Kosslyn & Koenig, 1995). Approaching brain function from a perspective of wholeness begins with its recursive organization.

Recursive Organization of the Brain

The brain is a recursively organized structure that has an immensely stratified organization. Each level of that organization—from the quantum to neural networks—is important in and of itself. Each level is iteratively folded into the next layer of organization, shaping and informing the new organization and its function. The new levels of increasing complexity will not be identical to the previous ones or mere *additions* of their properties. An emergent system is always greater than the sum of its parts. And this is certainly true of the immensely complex human brain. The human brain and its aspects of mind are extraordinary examples of self-organizing structures. Not only do basic levels of organization influence the more complex levels, but the higher levels also change and influence lower levels. For example, the global organization for consciousness can and does influence the chemical, neuronal, perception levels as well. The neurologist Roger Sperry (1993) pictures consciousness as a high-order emergent property stemming from holistic neural properties that will, in turn, exercise a "downward control" over lower neural functioning.

The brain and mind, then, are complex dynamical systems because they have evolved in a physical world that is chaotic and fractal in nature. The brain carries the internal process patterns that match the primary organization of the world itself. It ". . . is the nonlinear product of a nonlinear evolution on a nonlinear planet" (Briggs & Peat, 1989, p. 166). The organizing principles of mind and the physical universe are ultimately identical. The search for "how the brain works" is rooted in a study of chaotic, nonlinear physics. To understand a nonlinear, dynamical system like brain/mind, it is important to examine the various layers and their functioning. This is overviewed next, but this alone does not explain the global, high-order functions like learning, consciousness, and music. For that, a look at the human mind as a self-organizing system emerging from the nonlinear dynamics of the brain is needed.

The recursive organization of the brain begins with neurons. The billions of neurons of the brain are organized into local circuits by synaptic connections. If these circuits are arranged in parallel layers, they are *cortical regions*, and if grouped in nonlayered collections, they are called *nuclei*. Both types of circuits are interconnected by axon projections to form *systems*. These systems link at higher levels of complexity into systems of systems or *networks* (Damasio, 1999).

Brain functioning is usually equated with the cerebral cortex. The cerebral cortex is organized into networks, known as cortical columns. The cortex is organized as a

> . . . honeycomb of columns a few neurons wide that stretch from top to bottom through six layers. . . . [I]n the primary auditory cortex, individual columns respond most strongly to specific frequencies of sound. Columns may well be the most basic units of information processing in the cortex. (Jourdain, 1997, pp. 52–53)

However, neural function is not based on monolithic neural networks. Instead, brain functioning is based on a metaorganization principle. Just like everything in the complex natural world, neural function is stratified.

> Stratified neural networks are networks with multiple scales of organization. Unlike monolithic neural networks, a stratified network can be comprised of interconnected units which themselves are pre-existent neural networks. . . . In highly stratified networks, this subdivision may continue iteratively to a

great depth until individual neurons are finally reached. (Alexander & Globus, 1996, p. 34)

Each scale of organization in the stratified system performs very different tasks in many different ways, but they combine to create the next level that, in turn, has its own unique properties and functioning. A supersystem, like memory or music appreciation, arises out of the functioning of the interconnected parts—from neurons, to sensory perception, to networks. This stratification leads to the simultaneous presence of vastly different processing styles.

> On the one hand, we have the relatively unmodifiable connections that enable sense data to be decoded. . . . On the other, the subtle changes in cellular connections that form the brain representations of learning and memory enable us to modify our thoughts and actions as a result of experience. (Rose, 1998a, p. 4)

A simple, basic function may, in fact, be localized in a particular brain region. However, a complex mental activity may actually emerge in a number of ways. "Thus, we can have it both ways: some functions are localized but the brain works as a whole to produce Functions [complex activities] that are not localized" (Kosslyn & Koenig, 1995, p. 12).

Complex brain functions are a product of the *interaction* of neural and chemical signals and the relationships between and within multiple regions of the brain. Edelman (1992) believes the dynamic *arrangement* of brain structures create mental processes, not their actual composition. In this view, neural networks enfold multiple forms of information that exist simultaneously in any number of cortical regions. "Inverse transformation unfolds these patterns from any portion of the cortex—making neural networks something like the harmonic resonators of music instruments" (Hunt, 1995, p. 53). It is the *relationships* that create complex brain function. In this way, the brain really is more like a symphony than a computer because music, in general, and a complex musical form, like a symphony in particular, emerge from the complex relationships of tone produced over time. The highly stratified organization of the brain working as a whole gives the brain its high degree of plasticity. This makes our brains open, not closed, systems.

Higher Brain Function

A highly evolved, human cortical function is called *higher brain function* (HBF). HBF requires a major portion of the cortex plus input from various subcortical areas, especially the thalamus. Human mental capacities, such as mathematics, reasoning, problem solving, and musical behavior, are HBF. Such complex tasks require tens of seconds to minutes to complete without necessarily requiring new sensory input (Leng & Shaw, 1991). HBF requires spatial organization and extremely accurate timing for the organized firing of groups of neurons over large regions of the cortex. Spatially, the cortex is organized into columns, which are made up of process subunits or mini columns called trions (Mountcastle, 1978).

Columns have structure connectivity in three types of units. Vertical connections among cortical areas create mini columns. Mini columns are connected horizontally to neighboring mini columns, creating a second type of unit. The third unit involves the long-range connection between distant columns. These extensive networks of connectivity have nonlinear dynamical processing, as does each mini column itself. The response of the functional unit is not simply the linear sum of the individual neuronal responses (Leng & Shaw, 1991).

In addition to spatial organization, the timing of column activity is also a vital component to HBF. Each column has an inherent, quasistable periodic firing pattern. These patterns exist prior to any stimuli being present and constitute a basic repertoire of such firings (Boettcher, Hahn, & Shaw, 1994). The subunits or trions have three possible firing patterns. According to Edelman's (1987) selection principle, learning occurs because a stimulus selects out a particular response from this repertoire rather than the brain being instructed in response to that stimulus. This provides the basic repertoire of spatial-temporal firing patterns onto which stimuli and internal processing are mapped (Leng & Shaw, 1991). This pattern of spatial and temporal firings of HBF is the language of the brain. As Boettcher, Hahn, and Shaw (1994) state,

> . . . These inherent firing patterns are related by specific *symmetries* and form the internal neural language of the cortex. . . . Although different "mappings" representing the information in the cortical firing patterns will be involved in each higher brain function, the internal neural language of the brain is the same for the various higher brain functions. (p. 54)

In some interesting research, Leng and Shaw (1991) mapped computer-generated spatial-temporal sequences of memory patterns of the trions or subunits onto musical pitches and possible instrument timbres and produced recognizably human styles of music: minuet, waltz, Indian ragas, and other forms of Eastern and Western classical music. "Different mappings gave different recognizable styles of music!" (Shaw, 2000, p. xiv). The researchers concluded that since all HBF processes have the same "language," music could provide a window into HBF. "The trion model is a *viable* cortical model for the coding of certain aspects of musical structure and perception. Thus, it will be useful in understanding other higher creative cognitive processes" (Leng & Shaw, 1991, p. 229). It is the complexity and relationship patterns of *music*, not single tones, particular intervals, or rhythms alone, that express this inherent language of HBF.

> Music composition, performance and listening all involve the evolution of this inherent repertoire of spatial-temporal patterns. . . . *We suggest that what is involved here is the perfect use of these inherent spatial-temporal patterns common to our species. As listeners, we need only appreciate the result of having these inherent patterns excited in our brains.* (Leng & Shaw, 1991, p. 252)

Those inherent patterns are likely the 1/f frequency spectrum mentioned previously.

Extensive research now supports these conclusions on HBF (Shaw, 2000). Of particular interest are the studies by Rauscher, Robinson, and Jens (1998), which exposed rats to various music-listening/learning experiences. In one study, rats were exposed to Mozart music, music by composer Phillip Glass, white noise, or silence for twelve hours before learning to run a maze. The rats exposed to Mozart learned the maze faster and with fewer errors than any of the rats in other conditions. Since rats cannot exercise musical preference or emotional reaction to the sounds heard, exposure to a particular music that possibly resonates with the internal neural language is doing something physically to the brains of these animals. This again illustrates that the brain is working musically. Lewis Thomas (1974) believes that music is the effort we make to explain to ourselves how our brains work. Based on this research evidence, an assertion can be made that the forms of human music are reflections of the patterns and timing experienced as we think, reason, and calculate.

Binding

One of the big questions of current neuroscience is how all the various factors of neural processing hold together as a unified perception, memory, or experience. This is the binding problem. Binding requires ". . . some form of time-locking of neural activities that occur in separate but interconnected brain regions" (Damasio, 1999, p. 335). Many neuroscientists now speculate that this binding function is a pacing rhythm, ". . . a widespread, oscillating electrical signal that could entrain many different neurons to dance in rhythm with each other" (Baars, 1997, p. 72). These oscillations are coherent waves of a particular frequency (Edelman, 1992). The brain, in fact, is a mass of such oscillating patterns at different scales of organization because sensory channels send multiple messages, and each of these messages is encoded as an oscillating process at different time scales. Neurons and neural masses in various spatial organizations are bound by the oscillatory message appropriate to their own scale of organization (Alexander & Globus 1996).

Neural systems have several types of global oscillating behavior. These include periodic, semichaotic, and chaotic behavior. Mathews and Strogatz (1990) postulate that limit-cycle oscillators (periodic oscillation) provide proof that wavelike processes are capable of sustaining the recursively embedded dynamics of brain function. HBF has its own oscillatory processes. A fast coherent EEG rhythm of 40 Hz is postulated as the binding frequency of cognition since it may play a role in binding together features of objects (Traub, Jeffreys, & Whittington, 1999). This rhythm, known as a *gamma rhythm*, indicates the speed of electrical activity and is an audible tone of 40 Hz, like the E string on a bass guitar or the lowest notes of a pipe organ. It may be possible that the oscillation of frequencies in music or its rhythmic pulse could affect this binding process in brain functioning. Like in the trion model, music may reflect or resonate with this inherent brain process. If verified, the application of music could serve in remediating problems in this area. For example, Traub, Jeffreys, and Whittington (1999) report that disruptions in the gamma rhythm are present in people with Alzheimer's disease and may contribute to the cognitive dysfunction characteristic of this disorder. Research is needed to explore the connections of auditory input from music on the rhythms of the binding process and the possible application of music therapy to remediate such dysfunction.

Electromagnetic Field Generation
Finally, in exploring how the brain works, it is important to note that all the movements in the brain—the oscillating activity, electrical potential of neurons, and oscillating coherence between cortical columns and lower brain structures—create an energy field that projects beyond the body. This energy is an electromagnetic field. MEG, mentioned earlier, ". . . exploits the fact that . . . whenever there is an electric current, there is a magnetic field at right angles to it. The brain's language of communication is electric, and so every region of the brain is surrounded by a fluctuating magnetic field . . ." (Rose, 1998a, p. 11). In particular, J. C. Cowan (1991) believes the source of this coherent energy in the brain is the vibration of parts of the axon's membrane that connects the neurons in the thalamus to the cerebral cortex. The activity in the cerebral cortex shifts quickly, and the periodicity of the thalamic pacemaker changes more slowly. This generates an extremely complex field that extends throughout the brain and into the space

outside the brain. A discussion of the importance of energy fields for healing is presented in the next chapter.

From this basic overview of brain functioning, it is clear that the brain works in a highly complex fashion. "Simple calculations show that the number of humanly graspable sentences, sentence meanings, chess games, melodies, seeable objects, and so on can exceed the number of particles in the universe" (Pinker, 1997, p. 137). The immense variability and diversity of brain functioning and the enormity of the recursively organized brain connections can only result from the dynamic processes at work. To have a true picture of brain function, we must now look at brain processes as dynamical, nonlinear events.

Brain Function as a Dynamical, Nonlinear Event

Having briefly overviewed current neuroscientific knowledge of brain structure and function, let's return to the idea that the brain, on all levels of organization, functions through nonlinear dynamics and that the product of brain function, aspects and properties of the human mind, are emergent functions of those nonlinear dynamics. "With the advent of the research on the nonlinear dynamical systems it seems that we 'finally' have a formal key to the way the brain/mind performs" (MacCormac & Stamenov, 1996, p. 8). There is now substantial, though not entirely conclusive, research evidence of chaotic mechanisms in all levels of neural dynamics (Basti & Perrone, 1989; Freeman, 1992). This avenue of study is now identified as nonlinear psychophysical dynamics or the study of nonlinear dynamics in human systems (Gregson, 1996).

Nonlinear dynamics are first seen at the level of the neuron. The neuron, as a cell, is itself a physical fractal form both structurally and functionally in terms of dendrite axon trees (King, 1996). The neuron is an integrated field-processing unit capable of chaos and unstable bifurcations. Mpitsos, Burton, Creech, and Sonila (1988) demonstrated chaotic patterns in the spike trains of individual neurons. Ion pumping, the essential function of neurons, shows a number of dynamical features, including period-doubling bifurcations and chaotic movement. The firing patterns of neurons also show nonlinear aspects. There is considerable evidence that both the firing of individual neurons and the activation of patterns of neurons are nonlinear dynamical systems (MacCormac, 1996). Nerve impulses are a form of nonlinear diffusion. "Nonlinear diffusion entails abrupt, wavelike impulses of activity that travel along the axon with constant speed and shape, carrying information reliably from one point to another" (Scott, 1995, p. 49). The actions of strange attractors have been verified in the electrical activity of the olfactory lobe of rabbits (Freeman, 1992), in the spontaneous firing of squid axons (Aihara, Matsumoto, & Ikegaya, 1984), and in human neocortical EEG rhythms (Frohlich, 1986). Arnold Mandell (1983) found individual rates of firing for dopamine receptors, serotonin receptors, and single-cell EEG activity have fractal self-similarity. Additionally, synaptic connection patterns also show dynamical properties. As King (1996) notes, "This is supported by the obvious complexity of typical central nervous system neurons, with up to 100,000 synaptic junctions having a variety of anatomical forms . . . unstable bifurcations across threshold, and other nonlinear features . . ." (p. 206).

The organization of brain connectivity—the neural networks or information loops—also show nonlinear processing. Freeman and Barrie (1994) found general chaotic activity in the cortical circuits. "The loops heighten the possibility that bifurcation and the amplification of some input will take place. . . . [T]he brain is a nonlinear feedback device . . ." (Briggs & Peat, 1989, p. 166). As noted earlier, the brain is a recursively organized system where multiple scales of neural structure are organized into modules at many different scales of the nervous system, each "nested" in the next more complex system. It is a stratified structure. Each level of the stratification uses edge-of-chaos dynamics (Alexander & Globus, 1996). As explored in chapter 2, "edge of chaos" refers to a dynamical balance between highly ordered and highly chaotic structure at multiple scales.

> Chaotic dynamics makes it possible for microscopic sensory input that is received by the cortex to control the macroscopic activity that constitutes cortical output, largely owing to the selective sensitivity of chaotic systems to small fluctuations, and their capacity for rapid transitions. (Freeman, 1992, p. 452)

Flexibility and vigor in neurological processing thus are created because nonlinear dynamical systems allow for an interrelated network of neurons that move abruptly from chaos to stable patterns (MacCormac, 1996).

Edge-of-chaos dynamics is important in understanding how brain function leads to aspects of mind. "In the case of a brain system, movement to a slightly more *ordered state* constitutes as recognition, engaged, unreceptive mode of interaction whereas movement to a slightly more *chaotic state* constitutes an alert, ready, receptive mode of interaction" (Alexander & Globus, 1996, p. 39). For example, Pellionisz (1989) did research on edge-of-chaos dynamics in cortical perceptual systems. He found that cortical dynamics ". . . poised at the edge-of-chaos function to integrate incoming sensory stimuli into neural dynamics. . . . *[T]he cortical area begins in a slightly chaotic trajectory and then relaxes into a more ordered metrical space as the sensory input is successfully recognized*" (Alexander & Globus, 1996,

p. 41). In other words, the sensory area, say for auditory input, maintains a readiness to respond to auditory input through edge-of-chaos dynamics. A sound entering the ear and activating various brain areas actually creates a new order. This constitutes the recognition of the input. As Alexander and Globus (1996) note, "*The edge-of-chaos dynamics is self-similar across multiple scales of neural organization, utilizing a limit-cycle attractor for recognition, participation, engagement states and utilizing a chaotic attractor for ready, receptive, disengaged brain states*" (p. 57). Neural mechanisms poised at the edge of chaos have a real advantage since the chaos can be turned on and off instantly through a bifurcation. It is a very energy-efficient system (Alexander & Globus, 1996). Only a slight shift in dynamics can move the brain from a ready state to a brain function like recognition and back to a ready state.

These shifts to increasingly complex processes are fractal in nature, particularly the form of fractal time known as the *1/f spectrum pattern* or flicker noise, discussed in chapter 2. This 1/f phenomenon creates fractal correlations in time allowing vertical integration over all levels of neural processing from the neuron to supersystems. The 1/f spectrum is an oscillation that binds the neural activities into a whole. Through this binding, a living system self-organizes. How can time patterns originating in the medulla reticular formation enable the self-organization of behavior?

> 1/f processes seem to provide the cement binding the elements of cortical dynamics together. . . . 1/f-like spectra in the EEG result from correlated activity between cortical and subcortical sites over a broadband frequency range and may be indicative of brain self-organization during attentional states. (Anderson & Mandell, 1996, p. 102)

Musha (1981) was the first to postulate a relationship between a higher-order activity, perception, and 1/f-like fluctuations. As noted by Anderson and Mandell (1996),

> Fractal time patterns seem to be recurrent in evoked and spontaneous activity on multiple levels. . . . [F]ractal time processes may underlie human perception. If 1/f processes have properties of convergence in nervous systems, then a profoundly new view of the dynamics of neural organization and the neural basis of sensation and perception is created. (p. 90)

These patterns are present during a variety of highly activated mental states, including behavioral orienting, REM activity, sexual behavior, and stress (Anderson & Mandell, 1996).

The 1/f spectrum time events in the nervous system seem to be generated and disseminated by the reticular formation (Anderson & Mandell, 1996). These processes begin in the developing fetus.

> 1/f patterns generated by the consolidation of 1/f processes on many scales in the developing nervous system may have the unique ability to provide *in utero* fractal forgeries of the sensory world which the fetus will encounter at birth. Thus, endogenous self-generation of 1/f activity patterns in the developing CNS [central nervous system] and in spontaneous activity patterns in the developing body of the fetus would provide organizing information to coordinate developmental processes on many temporal and spatial scales. (Anderson & Mandell, 1996, p. 91)

The intervals of these 1/f spectra time events in the nervous system vary depending on the chemical neurotransmitter involved (Anderson & Mandell, 1996). Thus the basic organizing factor in our neural system is generated beginning with our chemical makeup.

The 1/f spectrum is one of the most common time fractals found in nature, in general, and in the nervous system in particular. In both neurobiology and neurophysiology,

> ... 1/f patterns in time are profound in their recurrent appearance across many levels of organization in the nervous system, from the underlying cellular dynamics of ion channels and intermittent firing patterns of neurons to developmental phenomena occurring during the organization of breathing to global dynamics in the nervous system such as sub-cortical, transcortical and scalp EEG defining behavioral states of consciousness. (Anderson & Mandell, 1996, p. 77)

For example, Teich (1989) found the 1/f spectrum in the spike trains from the auditory nerve in cats, while Lowen and Teich (1993) identified long-term fractal fluctuations in the intervals that constitute auditory nerve action potentials. They speculate these action potentials may originate in the 1/f bursting patterns of the cochlear hair cell ion channels. The cochlea of the inner ear gives us hearing. Because many low-frequency sounds have the 1/f spectra, patterns of low-frequency activity contained in the auditory system may be able to match and efficiently sample natural sounds, providing a mechanism to detect the structure of correlations in sound (Teich, 1989). The ear mechanism and naturally occurring sounds both contain this particular fractal time, making the auditory mechanism of the ear, auditory nerves, and brain particularly effective at processing the sound stimulus. It also makes musical input, which is full of 1/f spectral changes, a potentially useful tool in impacting the neurological functions that also include these time spectra.

The process of self-organization in a living system is by definition a nonlinear, dynamic process. The brain is an outstanding example of a self-organizing system because a self-organizing system maintains its shape while in a state of open exchange with its surroundings. As previously noted, it is input from the world that starts this process going, but it is the self-organizing dynamics of the brain that construct the knowledge of that world. There is no "real world"— only our construction or perception of that world. The ". . . only knowledge that animals and humans can have of the world outside themselves is what they construct within their own brains" (Freeman, 2000, p. 414). It is literally true that perception is reality, and that reality is constantly changing as new input alters the neural connections. Each exposure to a stimulus changes the brain's synaptic structure so that it cannot respond identically over time, although it may appear subjectively to be so. As Heraclitus remarked, "One cannot step twice in the same river" (Freeman, 2000, p. 414). This may be the strongest evidence for the dynamical, nonlinear dynamics of the brain. Even the smallest things can profoundly influence brain functioning and the product of this functioning—the mind. "Gaining access to new information, even accidentally, changes the mind; this is one reason small changes can make large differences in the way we operate. The immediate access to information shifts our ability to recall and our judgment" (Ornstein, 1991, p. 108). MacCormac and Stamenov (1996) even suggest it is fractal or fractal-like patterns that may function as a computational interface between brain and mind.

This basic overview of brain anatomy and function provides initial information on how sound/music influences functioning in this area. It is now time to consider in more detail the specific functions of mind and how music therapy interventions affect this level of human functioning.

The Functions of Mind and Music Therapy

Mind requires brain functioning, but is more than just the activities of the brain (Dossey, 1992). Mind is a process running parallel to the physical processes in the brain, not a "thing" (Pribram, 1991). Goertzel (1995) believes the mind is a self-generating process dynamic rather than a physical process. Most neuroscientists would support this broad position, though many would include the entire nervous system—in the brain and in the projecting neurons throughout the body—as the genesis of mind (Brophy, 1999). Wilber (1998) sees the brain and mind as connected but not the same thing since they possess profound differences. The mind can do things the brain cannot. One prominent current theory of mind is based on a computational model. In this model, the factors of mind are seen as merely highly or-

ganized patterns of activity over sets of neural units. This model assumes
that, much like a computer, mind is programmed through experience
(Pinker, 1997). However, other researchers envision mind as more than just
programmed cognition (LeDoux, 1996). They believe aspects of mind are basic original productions that cannot be predicted or foreseen by inherent
neural structure. "Neuronal processes are a necessary but not sufficient condition for cognition and consciousness. One cannot, however, predict the
contents of cognition by fully understanding the organization of neuronal
patterns as these activations are nonlinear and self-organizing" (MacCormac,
1996, p. 136). In this view, aspects of mind are emergent properties of biological brains resulting from the arrangement and chemical communication
among nerve cells, which is continuously formed by and changed by sensory
input from the environment (Johnston, 1999). Mind, then, is an emergent
flowing together or coalescence of the senses (Hunt, 1995). It is a ". . . self-
organizing nonlinear physical process with a reflexive property allowing it to
modify its own process" (MacCormac, 1996, p. 149). The processes we identify as mind—sensation, perception, learning, memory, consciousness, and
more—emerge out of the action of these recursively self-organized brain systems. Mind is ". . . the self-organization of a chaotic system arising from the
interactions of millions of changing connections. Under certain conditions,
these connections produce what seems to be background noise (chaos) and
under other conditions meaningful activities like perception or thinking (=
ordered patterns)" (MacCormac & Stamenov, 1996, p. 26). Though Mac-
Cormac (1996) sees that functions of mind, such as cognition and consciousness, are dependent on neuronal processes for their existence, they still
have an emergent independence from the brain.

In this view, a mind facility like perception does not actually begin with
casual imprints on receptors but, rather, starts with the internally generated,
self-organized neural activity, which lays the groundwork for processing of future perception. "Perception is a self-organized dynamic process of interchange inaugurated by the brain in which the brain fails to respond to irrelevant input, opens itself to the input it accepts, reorganizes itself, and then
reaches out to change its input . . ." (Skarda & Freeman, 1990, p. 279). The
major sensory structures develop as a dynamical system creates new bifurcations (King, 1996). "Studies of the nonlinear dynamics of the primary sensory cortices show that patterns that are constructed by chaotic nonlinear dynamics in cortical neoropil replace stimulus-driven activity" (Freeman, 2000,
p. 411). Vandervert (1996) even claims that the ultimate attribute of mind,
that of consciousness, does not emerge from dynamic processes but is itself
continuously generated entirely of the fractal holonomic representation of

the body in the brain. This makes our conscious state directly accessible in the form of fractal-like patterns (MacCormac & Stamenov, 1996).

Other researchers, though in the minority, do not locate the mind in the brain or body at all. No neurophysiological research conclusively demonstrates that the higher levels of mind are located in brain tissue (Hunt, 1996). Candace Pert (1997) believes that mind cannot be explained in physical terms alone. In her view, it must also consist of a nonmaterial substrate, composed of the information that is flowing in and around it. The physical brain would be like a radio receiver, while the information that constitutes the mind is like the radio waves around it. In this view, mind becomes, or at least generates, energy as information. According to Benor (1992),

> Mind exists outside of the brain or overlaps several dimensions to include the brain, which is a transducer for mind across the boundaries between dimensions. . . . In this view, mind resides on some non-physical plane(s) but expresses itself via transformation of energy or of information through the brain. . . . [I]t may be that aspects of mind function as an energy field, with the brain being a transducer for this field. (pp. 85–86)

This topic is addressed in chapter 5, when human energy states, including the possibility of consciousness, are explored.

Whatever its genesis or constitution, it is the mind, not the brain, that makes decisions, asserts the will, takes the initiative, interacts in the world, and is ultimately aware of what is happening. The mind understands, comprehends, reasons, and pronounces judgment. Most functions of the mind are the focus of various therapeutic interventions, including music therapy. They support cognitive development in young children and in individuals with learning disabilities, developmental delay, cognitive impairment through head injury or Alzheimer's disease, and other conditions that affect functions of the mind. These functions include sensation, perception, discrimination, and concept development; cognition, reasoning, and HBF; behavior, motivation, drives, and volition; learning, memory, and intelligence; imagery and creativity; language and speech; and consciousness. Let's briefly overview these functions of mind related to sound/music and, in particular, to music therapy practice.

Early Cognitive Skills

Early cognitive skills are the building blocks of all mental processing. They include formation of sensation, perception, discrimination, and concept development.

Sensation

When our sense organs interact with the world, simple sensory qualities make neural patterns in nerve cell circuits and turn those patterns into an image of the real-world experience. These simple sensory qualities are known as *qualia*. How these images are formed in our neural structure is unclear. A neurobiological account of simple sensation impressions is incomplete (Damasio, 1999). Qualia are sentient experiences. Sentience is our capacity for sensation—the power of perception by the senses. Because each of our experiences is unique, our sense of "how the world is" is individual and unique.

> Qualia constitute the collection of personal or subjective experiences, feelings, and sensations that accompany awareness. . . . These sensations may be very precise when they accompany perceptual experiences; in the absence of perception, they may be more or less diffuse but nonetheless discernible as "visual," "auditory," and so on. (Edelman, 1992, p. 114)

Our first diffuse sentience comes from experiences of movement—our own movement in the womb, our first movement in the world after birth, and sound, which is the world moving around us. The Greek root for the word *sensation* is the Greek word for movement (Hunt, 1995). For young children or clients with severe cognitive deficiencies, music therapy interventions provide these first sentient experiences through the movement of sound. For an infant or individual with infant-like capabilities, the barrage of sensation is a blur. These experiences must be brought into focus through the mirroring activities done with an involved adult (Robertson, 1999). As explored later, musical sharing is a dialogic mirroring event that can provide the feedback needed by infants to make sense of the sensations they are experiencing.

Music also floods the brain with 1/f spectrum fractal time patterns that help to establish normal functioning. "If a technique was available to reestablish fractal time patterns in these [brain damaged] infants, therapeutic intervention for these and other developmental disorders might be possible" (Anderson & Mandell, 1996, p. 93). Music therapy may, in fact, be this intervention. A disorder like autism, characterized by an inability to process sensation, responds well to music therapy interventions (Edgerton, 1994; Mahlberg, 1973; Nelson, Anderson, & Gonzales, 1984; Saperston, 1973).

Perception

According to the great visionary psychologist William James (1890), sensation and *perception* are alternative organizations of the same material—sensory input. Perception is the process of assigning meaning to sensation through involvement by all aspects of the organism. Meaning involves the interpretation of events (Winkelman, 2000). Perception requires abilities in identification, discrimination, labeling, and categorization. It requires memory because perception comes from comparing previously received and stored sensations to the new input.

Perception is an ongoing dynamic process of interaction between the organism and its environment. It is an open activity involving a dynamic blend of receptivity and creativity in the act of orienting to the world (Abram, 1996). Hunt (1995) sees perception as a sense of awareness "with." The "with" is the world in which it occurs. This world is shared with others inhabiting it. Specifically, that interaction has to do with movement. According to Hunt (1995), there is no perception outside of the movement capabilities of organisms. Sentient organisms must locate themselves through movement and respond to surfaces in the environment valued in terms of approach and avoidance. Similarly, Gibson (1966) believes that perception involves ". . . the complexity of the patterning offered directly to the peripheral senses, constituting a dynamic flow of gradients and textures around the organism—most especially when it is in motion" (Hunt, 1995, p. 64). Though much of this movement required for perception comes from moving into the world, the dynamic flow of movement can also come to us in the form of sound and the organized sound of music.

There is another way in which music can aid in the organization inherent in perception. This involves large-scale rhythmicity inherent in grouping phenomena (Elliott, 1986). "Perception . . . is an attunement or synchronization between my own rhythms and the rhythm of the things themselves, their own tones and textures . . ." (Abram, 1996, p. 54). Organization is simplification, and simplification allows very complex information to be perceived.

Piaget (1977) theorized that early cognitive development comes as a result of sensory/motor experiences. The physical manipulation of sound-making instruments can be an important part of this process. Because of its multisensory nature, participation in music can also contribute to *sensory integration* (James, 1984). Sensory integration is the organization of sensation for use. It is a process of locating, sorting, and ordering sensation arriving in the brain from all sensory channels. This process then leads to the formation of perceptions. The sensory integration process turns sensations into perceptions through integration. Sensory integration is developed when a child is engaged in adaptive response behaviors—behaviors that are purposeful, goal-directed responses to multisensory experiences (Ayres, 1979). Music therapy activity interventions provide these multisensory adaptive response behaviors for clients. For example, a child who is bouncing a ball in rhythm while singing a song is receiving multisensory experiences of locating, sorting, and ordering sensory input with motor response. Engagement in the goal-directed, purposeful active response to music is a sensory integration activity.

The final way music may influence perception is through emotion. Pert (1997) notes that perception is colored by emotion. Emotional content of music can support development of perception through its strong emotional input. In these ways, sound/music exposure contributes to the development of the basic cognitive skill of perception.

Discrimination
Contrary to popular assumption, the mind does not register every detail of a sensory event as a separate piece of information. Instead, it receives sensory signals and interprets them as a whole (Ornstein, 1991). Basic to perception is *discrimination*, the ability to compare perceptions and be aware of similarities and differences. In fact, perception *is* discrimination since our brains pay attention to changes. "Neurons fire when something different happens and don't respond significantly when they are continuously stimulated" (Ornstein, 1991, p. 105). Neurons adapt to constant sensory input and stop firing. This accounts for the perceived decrease in the loudness of a fire alarm over time. The mind responds to signals of change, signals of beginnings and endings, and signals generated from new circumstances. If the pitch of the fire alarm changes, we perceive an increased level of loudness because we are re-oriented to the overall sensory input. Well-composed music is constantly changing to provide the novel stimulus needed for ongoing perception and awareness to occur. Various music therapy interventions provide clients with a wide variety of sound discrimination tasks to teach and exercise this ability. For example, I may create a game where the client must discriminate between the sound of a shaker, a bell, and a drum. The constant changes inherent in music provide for the development of discrimination skills.

Concept Development
From discrimination, *categorization* occurs as our first true cognitive skill. Categorization occurs when ". . . the continuous variable, and confusable stimulation that reaches the sense organ is sorted out by the mind into discrete, distinct categories whose members somehow come to resemble one another more than they resemble members of other categories" (Harnard, 1987, p. ii). Categorization is at the heart of all mental activities, including all forms of music behavior. This cognitive skill involves both complex identifications (like when we recognize a category of objects known as drums by the

similarity of how sound is produced and the object is used) and position or relative groupings. The musical scale is a great example of categorization by position.

> Our brains subdivide a range of possible frequencies . . . into a number of compartments. Rather than keep track of a very large number of discernible positions along the range [of frequencies], our brains economize by tracking on a small number of sub-ranges (notes in the scale), each a "category." (Jourdain, 1997, p. 63)

Categorization occurs through connections among various networks in the brain. We need categories to cope with an overwhelming and confusing sensory world. Since we cannot possibly store information about every detail of every sensory experience that we encounter, categories help us draw inferences (guesses) about the world from the few details we do perceive. We can observe *some* of the properties of the object, assign it to a category, and then from that category predict properties we have not observed (Pinker, 1997). Categorization of music is a good example of this. We categorize different types of music into a *genre*, such as country and western. As we have experience with this genre, we store properties of the music like the instruments used, vocal quality, and lyric topics. When we hear an unfamiliar piece of music, we quickly compare what we hear to determine if it fits our category, and we then predict what we will actually hear.

From categorization, it is an easy step to *concept development*. A concept is a general mental representation that does not refer to a single item but, rather, to a whole category of items. Concepts help us predict more attributes of a thing than we could get from current sensory information alone (Richardson, 2000). Concepts include things like loud and quiet, big and small, and near and far.

Neurologically, concepts occur when different portions of the brain map past sensory experiences so that parts of past activities can be reconstructed and recombined for current use. To do this, the brain must have extensive connections among the frontal, temporal, and parietal cortices and to the hippocampus and basal ganglia (Edelman, 1992). Because music behavior as an experience uses these same areas, it is a means for creating these connections. Music therapy goes beyond rehearsing linguistic concepts to becoming a means to rewire the brain so the ability to form concepts is developed. Exposure to music with a reasonably complicated structure facilitates the establishment of neural networks and improves cerebral functioning (Storr, 1992).

Initial concept development occurs through bodily activities and sensory input. When teaching the concept of up and down during a music therapy intervention, high sounds are sung while having the child stretch up high, and the child moves down toward the floor in response to a low sound. Hearing the sound and moving their body in correspondence to the concept helps them understand and learn.

Concept development is also a basic social behavior. The influence of social regulations, as an important part of the environment, actually changes cognitive processes. "In fostering concept formation, then, social regulations radically alter cognitive regulations, and this process unleashes enormous cognitive powers in people as concepts become extended in vast knowledge networks" (Richardson, 2000, p. 154). One of the most powerful social influences on concept development is language. The word *concept* is generally used in connection with language. We begin to label our perceptions (the music is very loud) and categorizations (trumpets are very loud) with language. Concepts, therefore, are not ultimately dependent on immediate sensory input. "Unlike the brain areas mediating perceptions, those mediating concepts must be able to operate without immediate input. . . . [I]n forming concepts, the brain constructs maps of its *own* activities, not just of external stimuli, as in perception" (Edelman, 1992, p. 109). Use of songs in music therapy helps develop the language for concepts and develops the internal maps needed for ongoing use of the concepts.

Higher Brain Functions

With the development of concepts, the mind now has the building blocks for the development of those processes of mind associated with HBF. These complex, "large" functions of mind involve activities of the cortex, especially the neocortex, in cooperation with all structures of the brain. "But the greatest amount of new cortex, as shown by our bulging foreheads, is not sensory or even linguistic; it is the part that involves abstraction, planning, and control of self in action" (Baars, 1997, p. 64). These processes include thinking, reasoning, problem solving, learning, memory, behavior, language, and overall intelligence. These also include specific human endeavors like artistic expression, ritual formation, and music behavior.

The characteristics of HBF were discussed earlier in this chapter. However, to access and utilize HBF, the higher-order cortical areas of the frontal, temporal, and parietal cortex must be connected to lower brain structures like the hippocampus and basal ganglia. This is critical to understanding these higher-order faculties of mind because much of brain function occurs well below the level of thought or conscious awareness. Vast amounts of neural processes and contents, including core or waking consciousness, remain subconscious. They are not known to our extended, self-aware consciousness. These subconscious processes are extremely important in all aspects of our mental functioning. There now exists research evidence ". . . that for most conscious events we can find unconscious ones of comparable complexity. Nonconscious routines are believed to be involved in all mental tasks, though they seem to lack the unity, coherence, and accessibility of conscious experiences" (Baars, 1997, p. 17). These subconscious processes are not random events but specific functions of great importance. They are the building blocks of more complex forms of mental functioning. According to Hunt (1995), "Perception, semantic recognition, and verbal thought can all remain 'implicit' or 'unconscious' and are capable of expression independent of any conscious awareness system" (p. 35). Listening to music is a good example of this process. As the CD player begins to play a Brahm's symphony, I am aware of the music, recognize the composer, remember having played the piece in college, and enjoy and appreciate the experience. But I have no awareness of the auditory perception of all the notes bombarding my ear or the memory process that compares the arrangement of notes to the array of melodic contours stored in my memory. Nor am I aware of what elements constitute all the processes of mind involved in this experience. And whether these subconscious processes ever reach awareness or not, the results of their activity can and are stored in memory (LeDoux, 1996). These stored subconscious processes are vital to cognitive functioning because they give us natural comparison conditions to judge new input and experiences.

Thinking and Reasoning

Thinking is a cognitive operation that involves the generation of innumerable possibilities in response to environmental cues and the need for survival. Decisions are made when our emotional value system (*hedonic sense* of relative pleasantness or unpleasantness) selects a particular possibility and implements it. *Reasoning* depends upon the ability to simulate a variety of alternative scenarios that are possible in the current situation and to make a decision based upon their probability of occurrence and their expected hedonic consequences (Johnston, 1999). The more information we have—the greater the complexity—the more choices we can generate in our reasoning. It is our emotions that guide which of the possibilities we will choose. "Our feelings influence our reasoned decisions, and the more intense our feelings, the greater their impact" (Johnston, 1999, p. 171).

Involvement in music is as important to a child's cognitive development as any other mental activity including language. As mentioned earlier, Leng and Shaw's (1990) research showed that music is a form of inherent prelanguage that is available from an early age and allows access to inherent brain patterns, enhancing the ability of the cortex to develop these patterns and improve other higher brain functions. Music provides exercises for the brain to develop HBF. Research (Rauscher, Robinson, & Jens, 1998) using music to help rats learn complicated maze patterns supports this contention. Rats exposed to music learned to run a maze faster and more accurately than those not exposed to music. The researchers theorize that some aspect of the organized patterns of sound and silence influenced brain development in the areas of higher brain functioning. Pinker (1997) sees the basis for abstract thinking as the concepts of space and force. As explored in chapter 3, music is an experience in the relations of space—melody, intervals, and movement—and force—dynamics and physical impact of sound waves.

Behavior

Behavior is activity and response to internal and external cues. It is the observable responses we have to our environment and other relationships. Behavior has many components. It first derives from actions of the brain/mind but must be manifested as action in the environment. To manifest behavior, we must be alert and attentive to stimuli in our surroundings. We must react (behave) in a manner appropriate and adequate to the context presented. As Pinker (1997) states, behavior is a ". . . complex interaction among (1) the genes, (2) the anatomy of the brain, (3) its biochemical state, (4) the person's family upbringing, (5) the way society has treated him or her, and (6) the stimuli that impinge upon the person" (p. 53). Behavior is actually an integrated whole emerging from the complex interactions of many components. Antonio Damasio (1999) uses the metaphor of a symphony performance in the following quote to describe this process:

> The principles I wish to highlight here are: First, that the behavior we observe in a living organism is not the result of one simple melodic line but rather the result of a concurrence of melodic lines at each time unit you select for the observation; if you were a conductor looking at the imaginary musical score of the organism's behavior, you would see the different musical parts joined vertically at each measure. Second, that some components of behavior are always present, forming the continuous base of the performance while others are present only during certain periods of the performance; the "behavioral score" would note the entrance of certain behavior at a certain measure and the end of it some measures later, just as the conductor's score notes the beginning and the ends of solo piano parts within the movements of a concerto. Third, that in spite of the various components, the behavioral product of each moment is an integrated whole, a fusion of contributions not unlike the polyphonic fusion of

an orchestral performance. Out of the critical feature I am describing here, concurrence in time, something emerges that is not specified in any of the parts. (pp. 87–88)

Behavior, then, is an emergent property of the interaction of the various brain functions, inputs, and influences. Altering, changing, or modifying behavior could involve input at one level—such as the chemical or perceptual—and/or the interaction of all its layers.

Music and Behavior

Music potentially influences behavior because it can affect each level of the organization needed and influence the integrated activity of the various components as a whole that stimulate behavior. Music has a ". . . biologically meaningful effect on human behavior by engaging specific brain functions involved in memory, learning, and multiple motivational and emotional states" (Thaut, 1990a, p. 19). A large body of music therapy research has focused on the use of music therapy to alter behavior (Bellamy & Sontag, 1973; Jorgensen, 1974; McCarty et al., 1976).

For behavior to occur, something has to prompt the action or response. That prompt is a *drive*—an internal energizer of behavior (LeDoux, 1996). It is emotions that serve to drive behavior like they drive reasoning and decision making. "Emotion and the biological machinery underlying it are the obligate accompaniment of behavior . . ." (Damasio, 1999, p. 58). As discussed previously, emotions are generated in the limbic area of the brain and are not learned. Johnston (1999) notes that congenitally blind and deaf children exhibit the same facial expressions in response to emotions as other children, indicating that emotions and emotional expression are part of our biological system. In fact, emotion involves more aspects of mind than we realize.

We think of emotions as *feelings* of sadness or anger. Though there is disagreement as to definitions, emotion and feeling are not the exact same thing. For the purpose of this book, emotion refers to a collection of physiological changes occurring in the body and brain (Damasio, 1994). Related to emotion is *affect*, which involves the sensory feelings directly related to specific sensory input. "Emotions differ from affects in that they possess distinct qualities that are not a function of sensory inputs" (Johnston, 1999, p. 80). Emotion and affect occur in the absence of any complex cognitive process. Feelings are conscious events that attach memory to emotional reaction and do involve complex cognitive processes. Feelings and problems of feelings are addressed in chapter 6.

As explored earlier, emotion is the basic component and chief organizing system of all mind processes. Emotions do this by giving value to our choices. This value is based on the hedonic tone—the pleasantness or unpleasantness—of a choice.

Pleasantness/unpleasantness relates to our basic survival. What is pleasant tends to support survival—the sweet taste of ripe fruit or bitter taste of poisoned food. This hedonic tone is the basis of our motivational reactions so that emotion is basic to survival, growth, and adaptation (Johnston, 1999). Emotions influence all aspects of mind, and they do so subconsciously.

Motivation

From the basic drives and attention derived from emotion, *motivation* arises. Motivation is ". . . a behavioral state in which activity is directed toward satisfying needs" (Thaut, 1990a, p. 12). Motivation is behavior characterized by an increased general arousal and by organization through the action of affective behavior moving toward maximum positive emotional state. Motivation and emotional state are the same processes along an intensity continuum since the same brain structures are linked to both—limbic forebrain, hypothalamus, and brain stem (Thaut, 1990a). As explored previously in this chapter, the auditory nerve also affects these same brain structures so that music arouses and expresses emotion. Music perception, then, can provide ". . . rewarding arousal states that will be actualized as motivated behavior to maximize emotionally satisfying, rewarding, and pleasurable experiences" (Thaut, 1990a, p. 13).

Music and Motivation

Research has verified this link of music and motivation. Contingent music listening (allowing music listening when certain behavior is displayed) significantly motivates children to alter their behavior (Eisenstein, 1974; Hanser, 1974; Jorgenson, 1974). McCarty, McElfresh, Rice, and Wilson (1976) found that contingent music listening decreased inappropriate bus behavior. The change in behavior was virtually instantaneous, showing that the music affected their motivation to change their behavior. We are all more motivated to exercise when music is added to our routine. Gfeller (1988) found that 97 percent of research subjects indicated that music improved mental attitude toward the exercise activity, while 79 percent indicated that music aided in pacing, strength, and endurance. Aerobics and Jazzercise programs rely on this ability of music to motivate behavior. Oliver Sacks (1990) recounts the use of familiar music to motivate "frozen" patients with Parkinson's disease to walk and dance.

Music also influences another aspect of motivation: *volition*. Volition is self-initiated behavior coming from a decision or act of will. This type of motivation requires no external stimulus. It comes from a deep sense of desire, from the emotion of satisfaction and personal fulfillment. Music is valued and esteemed in cultures and is often the only activity that an individual voluntarily joins. During my clinical practice with adolescents with emotional disturbance, it was not uncommon for the music therapy sessions to be the first therapeutic effort in which the clients would engage. Music gives us that deep sense of fulfillment and personal satisfaction. It is emotionally gratifying and thus can positively affect volition.

Music Therapy and Motivation

In music therapy practice, we routinely see how music motivates behavior. In my own clinical experience, I have witnessed how a child with a cognitive impairment will refuse to participate in an activity when invited. This same child will suddenly join in the singing once it starts. The rhythm and melody pull them into the activity. They cannot help themselves. I've seen this happen numerous times in nursing home facilities. Residents who refuse to attend a session suddenly appear at the door once the music starts. Numerous research studies have shown that music, compared to other "activities," motivates participation in older adults including those with Alzheimer's disease (Clair & Bernstein, 1990a, 1990b; Clair, Bernstein, & Johnson, 1995; Pollack & Namazi, 1992).

Learning

Learning is an adaptive process that allows us to fine-tune our behavior to increasingly rapid environmental change (Johnston, 1999). Learning can be defined as the acquisition of knowledge or skill. For example, I learned the chord progression of the opening bars of Beethoven's Fifth Symphony. From a psychological perspective, learning is the modification of behavior through practice, training, or experience. For example, I learned to play an F minor scale today. It requires paying attention or becoming consciously aware of some material (Baars, 1997). In neuroscience, learning requires some alteration in the brain—neurochemical, structural, or activity level—so that the newly learned pattern of response (scale playing or memorizing the multiplication table) can be repeated at a later time in response to an environmental cue. Learning depends on a vast array of neurodevelopmental functions As Levine (2002) notes, "Our minds make use of different clusters of neurodevelopmental functions to learn specific skills and to create particular products" (p. 28).

Again, emotion plays a key role in learning as it has in other cognitive processes. Learning . . . is not a general-purpose mechanism that allows all environmental relationships to be acquired with equal proficiency. Instead, it is a constrained mechanism that depends upon an affective value system that provides an immediate appraisal of only those events that have important [species survival] consequences. (Johnston, 1999, p. 75)

Learning is governed by two cognitive arousal systems, each controlled by emotion. The first arousal system explores small, random variations of stored information by generating temporary changes to the synaptic connections between nerve cells (Johnston, 1999). "The second arousal system provides the necessary feedback for evaluating the hypothesis generated by the first system. . . . These feelings of reward activate the second arousal system that will retain the synaptic weights that led to that behavior" (Johnston, 1999, p. 77). The hedonic pathway—the pleasant/unpleasant sensation—is generated in the brain in the medial forebrain bundle. This structure is also central to learning. McGaugh (1994) did research that documented that the recall of new facts is enhanced by the presence of certain degrees of emotion during learning.

Music and Learning

There has been considerable popular media interest recently questioning whether music affects learning. Does music make us smarter? Is there a "Mozart effect"? Does involvement in music increase mathematics test scores or IQ tests? Controversy has arisen among researchers about whether music supports certain elements of learning, like spatial learning (Rauscher, Shaw, & Ky, 1995; Shaw, 2000), or not (Carstens, Huskins, & Hounshell, 1995; Newman et al., 1995; Steele, Brown, & Stoecker, 1999). One research project, for example, shows music does affect a learning task, while another definitely shows it does not. This may be an excellent example of the limitation of reductionistic research in describing a complex process. It is more than likely that each piece of research is, in fact, accurate under the initial conditions that were present when the experiment was conducted. So what does this show us about the impact of music on learning, memory, and intelligence? Probably very little since this type of research misses the point of what constitutes a highly complex process like learning.

The impact of music on learning may come from its complex interaction with the brain. Learning is a complex process of mind and is not reducible to a simple process or experience. In learning, development of one ability strengthens all other abilities (Ornstein, 1986). The principles of complexity science support this contention. To judge whether involvement in music can influence our ability to learn, we must look at how music affects the larger processes of learning and not make judgments based on the effects on test scores or specific learning tasks. Since developing any skill strengthens all abilities, learning music has general applicability to learning. As Levine (2002) notes, "The brain's toolbox is vast, the total number of neuro-developmental functions inestimable. On top of that, the range of different combinations of functions called upon to accomplish academic tasks is mind-boggling" (p. 29). Based on the principles of complexity science, impact or change to any of these functions, no matter how small, could have a major impact on the ability to learn. Gardner (1983) theorizes musical intelligence as one of nine forms of learning needed for full intelligence. Developing this intelligence through learning to perform music would thus support all other learning abilities. There are a number of specific ways music may affect learning.

The importance of making neural connections for brain formation and the role experience with music may play in this have been discussed previously. Without adequate neural connections, mind and certainly learning cannot occur. Those connections are made through experience with our environment. They must be stimulated. "What you stimulate, grows: think of thousands of neurological connections that take place in the smallest instant, the neurological changes that are constantly happening, which give you the capacity, the framework, for new types of transferred information" (Sornson, 1993, p. 120). A key role for music in learning may be in the amount and complexity of stimulation provided by the experience of music. The musical stimulation to so many parts of the brain creates the neurological "framework" on which learning eventually occurs.

Music may affect learning in a second way as a means of focusing our attention. Neuroscientist Bernard Baars (1997) points out that the content of learning is unconscious. In order to learn we need to focus attention, to become conscious of some material. Music provides a multisensory input to alert the brain and focus awareness. The novelty generated by the changes and edges in melody and complex rhythms provides the needed neural arousal. "Novelty and unexpectedness merely arouse the nervous system, but this arousal is the necessary and sufficient condition for learning to occur" (Johnston, 1999, pp. 103–104). When information accompanies music, like songs that teach counting or word recognition, the spotlight of consciousness is focused on that information, making learning more likely. *Sesame Street* teaching songs have been using this principle for over thirty years. Music therapy research (Gfeller, 1983; Madsen et al., 1975; Wolfe & Horn, 1993) supports this contention.

A third way in which music may influence learning is in the formation of basic stimulus response or conditioned learning (Combs, 1995). Conditioned learning occurs when a positive experience follows the learning task (a dog receiving a treat after performing a trick). Because of the pleasurable, enjoyable aspects of music, music has been found to be an effective reinforcer for behavior (Cook & Freethy, 1973; Dorrow, 1976; Wilson, 1976).

As mentioned earlier, a fourth way in which music may have an impact on learning is in the importance of emotion. McGaugh (1989, 1990) documents that recall of new facts is enhanced by the presence of certain degrees of emotion present during the learning process. It seems that very particular visceral input is vital for the generation of emotions that assist learning (Damasio, 1999). According to Johnston (1999), that emotional state is pleasant sensation. Music likely assists learning because it is intrinsically pleasant and gives the learning task affective value. As previously noted, emotion informs our values, which, in turn, become motivation. According to Richardson (2000), optimal conditions for this linkage of learning and value are tied with a meaningful cultural activity, like music. Music is a culturally valued event that, by its nature, links sensory input with emotional content.

Finally, there has been much attention recently on the importance of brain synchronization or cortical integration to overall effectiveness of learning. Brain synchronization refers to the entrainment of the brain wave activity between the two hemispheres of the cortex. Entrainment refers to the coupling of two or more oscillators into a common frequency. Considerable research on this phenomenon has been conducted at the Monroe Institute (Russell, 1993). According to this research, poor cortical integration causes problems in learning.

> Good learning is whole-brain learning; good communication is whole-brain communication. Good mathematics involves spatial and pattern recognition together with good memory and symbolic use. Every aspect of learning that works well involves both sides of the brain; so cortical integration is especially important. (Sornson, 1993, p. 119)

In particular, research has focused on bilateral synchronization of brain waves as a superperformance learning state (Bullard, 1993). In techniques developed by the Monroe Institute, known as Hemi-Sync, frequency has been used to create this synchronization of brain waves. This is currently a very speculative area. Further research is needed to verify that this phenomenon occurs and how and if sound or music might positively contribute to establishing this superperformance learning state.

Memory

It is impossible to discuss learning without investigating *memory*. Nothing is ever learned without the use of some component of memory (Levine, 2002). Scientific understanding of human memory has changed dramatically in the last fifty years.

Early research on memory focused on physiological processes and neural changes as *memory itself*. Physiology is important in understanding memory, but physiology itself is not memory. Edelman (1992) contends that a physiological basis for memory, such as synaptic change, is often mistakenly equated with memory itself. Brain circuitry of memory involves the higher-order cortices, especially the temporal lobe and prefrontal cortex of the brain (LeDoux, 1996). These cortical areas have close network relations with the subcortical areas of the limbic system, including the thalamus, amygdala, and hippocampus, and with other important sensory and motor areas of the brain (Damasio, 1999).

Of the subcortical systems involved in memory, the hippocampus and amygdala are particularly important. The hippocampus plays a vital role in relating short-term memory to the establishment of long-term memory. Extensive research has shown that the hippocampus is essential for the ability to lay down or *encode* memory (Squire, 1998). The role of the hippocampus is to help order events that have been immediately categorized by the cortex and then ensure that these categorized events support the synaptic changes in the cortex that create long-term memory (Edelman, 1992). Additionally, there is a definite time element in memory formation tied to the function of the hippocampus. This brain area seems to determine what experiences or parts of experiences we remember over time. The role of the hippocampus in regulating sleep and especially REM sleep is also important in memory formation. Preliminary research (Karni et al., 1994) has looked at the importance of REM sleep in solidifying memory for repetitive tasks because of the recurrence of 1/f spectrum-like states that occur during sleep.

> The reiteration of 1/f neural activity patterns on a nightly basis during REM sleep in adults may provide a connection to the initial conditions under which key structures of the brain formed . . . or a kind of reference state useful in the long-term consolidation of new information, as well as a means of maintaining cognitive and attentional flexibility. (Anderson & Mandell, 1996, p. 96)

Brain wave states similar to REM sleep are generated during deep music listening experiences, which is explored at length in chapter 7, and may also function to solidify memory.

Another midbrain structure, the amygdala, is an important part of memory formation because of its primary importance in generation of emotion. "The heightened (emotional) charge at the time of the event increases the strength of memory, as if our emotions are telling us what is important" (Ornstein, 1991, p. 89). High-frequency sound has been shown to "turn on" cells of the amygdala through subcortical pathways as part of this emotion generation (LeDoux, 1996). Strong emotion is also related to hormone secretion in the brain. LeDoux (1996) stresses the importance of hormone secretion, especially adrenaline, for memory solidification. Research by McGaugh (1994), Cahill et al. (1994), and others has demonstrated how increased levels of adrenaline increase memory of learning situations in rats.

Much attention has been focused on where memory is located. Early research focused on a location theory of memory—Where are memories stored in the brain? Are there different areas for different memories? Is there a "grandmother" neuron or neuron group responsible for storage of memories of our grandmothers? The popular conception of memory is that, like a videotape, we store billions of intact images and events somewhere in our brain waiting for the right cues to access and display those memories. Believing this, we are confused when two people experience the same event yet have vastly different memories of what happened. The conflicting testimony of Anita Hill and Clarence Thomas during Judge Thomas's Supreme Court confirmation hearings is a good example.

Karl Pribram (1982, 1991) challenged this location storage model of memory. According to Pribram, memory is not recorded in a particular cell or structure of the brain. Rather, information is enfolded over the whole brain. He postulated that the brain works like a "hologram" storing vast amounts of information in all brain areas and neurons simultaneously. A hologram is a photographic record of the interference pattern of light waves that have emanated from the object (Bohm, 1980). In a hologram, every part of the pattern contains information about the whole object. According to David Bohm (1980),

> The form and structure of the entire object may be said to be *enfolded* within each region of the photographic record. When one shines light on any region, this form and structure are then *unfolded* to give a recognizable image of the whole object once again. (p. 177)

Using the hologram as an analogy, Pribram theorized that the brain converts sensory input into waveforms that are stored as energetic resonance. Memory is retrieved if a waveform similar to the one stored holographically passes through the brain. In this process, one small part of the memory with similarity to the whole can retrieve the whole memory (Briggs & Peat, 1989).

> Pribram has given evidence backing up his suggestion that memories are generally recorded all over the brain in such a way that information concerning a given object or quality is not stored in a particular cell or localized part of the brain but rather that all information is enfolded over the whole. This storage resembles a hologram in its function, but its actual structure is much more complex. (Bohm, 1980, p. 198)

As an extension of this theory, it would make sense that these waveforms could be stored throughout all the neurons of the central nervous system. There is no reason why this energy would be cut off at the neck. Potentially, memory, and in fact all aspects of mind, may not be limited to the brain but, rather, may be generated from the whole body.

If memory is not physiological changes per se, what, then, is it? Memory, like all naturally occurring systems, is not a simple, one-step process. Memory is composed of multiple separate processes involving various brain systems (Squire, 1998). To remember something, you first have to *encode* the information, going through a process of translating the material into information usable by the brain. Then there has to be a *storage* process for that new information. Finally, to have an effective memory, there must be a system for *retrieving* the information when it is needed.

To add to the complexity of this system, there are three kinds of memory: short-term (lasting a few seconds), active working memory (where multiple components of a task are held long enough to complete an activity), and long-term memory (lasting from a minute to a lifetime [Levine, 2002]). We use short-term and working memory to remember the phone number we just looked up or the tune of a song we just heard on the radio. This memory does not last long. Working memory resides in the frontal lobe and has a limited capacity—about seven separate items or bits of information. This memory is an immediate memory. It holds the contents of our present awareness. Long-term memory, in contrast, is durable memory. Short-term/working memory and long-term memory are really different processes mediated by distinct brain systems.

There are also two contrasting types of memory (Squire, 1987). The first is *declarative* memory. This cognitive process is where memories of a specific nature are stored and can be brought to conscious awareness as images. This form of memory is probably encoded by the temporal lobe. It is this memory that is so devastated by Alzheimer's disease as the upper cortex is destroyed.

This is what we typically think of as memory. The second form of memory is *procedural* or *nondeclarative* memory. Procedural memory is acquired over time through rehearsing a skill or task. "It is developed and maintained through the specific network created in the formation of that skill. Procedural memory includes motor skill, cognitive skills, and simple classical conditioning" (Tomaino, 1998, p. 22). The motor skills involved in musical performance are a good example of procedural memory.

To further add to the complexity, the brain system involved in forming *new* long-term memories is different from the one that stores *old* long-term memories. LeDoux (1996) notes, "Long-term memory involves at least two stages, an initial one requiring the temporal lobe regions . . . and a later stage involving some other brain region, most likely areas of the neocortex. The temporal lobe is needed for forming long-term memories, but gradually, over years, memories become independent of this brain system" (pp. 185–186).

From the perspective of complexity science, memory is an emergent property of a complex brain structure and complex interaction among its component parts. Memory is a dynamic process and a system property that is not equivalent to the sum of the synaptic changes and neural processes that underlie it. It is a dynamic property of populations of neuronal groups (Edelman, 1992). Memories arise as relationships within and between entire neural networks. Memories, then, are distributed in the central nervous system through a shifting network of relations. "A memory . . . is not an isolated bit; it is a pattern of relationships. . . . The memory floats in an undulating sea of relationships that are continually, if subtly, changing" (Briggs & Peat, 1989, p. 173). It is this richness of information, the complexity of chaos, that constitutes a vigorous memory. Recalling a memory is not a matter of searching for a bit of stored information.

> The random character of the chaotic attractor places the system into a nonbiased state ready for the next [sensory stimulation] with instantaneous access to all possible non-strange attractors. . . . [T]here is therefore no "search" through a memory store, only a subtle shift in dynamics which settles the system into an appropriate recognition limit cycle. . . . The rich dynamics at the edge-or-chaos are crucial to the attainment of the final recognition attractor [which is the memory]. (Alexander & Globus, 1996, pp. 42–43)

To retrieve or store a specific bit of information, the entire network of connections must be activated.

Based on the principles of complexity science, memory, therefore, is an ongoing dynamic *process*. To think of memory as an exact snapshot of "what happened" would be a mistake. Memories are actually reconstituted from scratch every time we remember something. Memories are actually "made up" as the need arises, and, in keeping with the world we inhabit, our minds adapt to fit the complexity and changing nature of the world around us. We remember the semblance of things. Each time a memory is recalled, it alters the component parts of the memory. The brain never remembers an event in exactly the same way twice. Errors occur easily and readily. "Since perceptual categories are not immutable and are altered by the ongoing behavior of the animal, memory, in this view, results from a process of continual *recategoriza-tion*. . . . Unlike computer-based memory, brain-based memory is inexact, but it is also capable of great degrees of generalization" (Edelman, 1992, p. 102).

The relationships that constitute memory are sharply altered by a number of factors: current attitudes and social norms, strong emotion, and unconscious values and desires. Current attitudes are created by current emotions and by societal values as to what is appropriate now. An ex-criminal may not remember the viciousness of an attack twenty years after the fact because his or her current self-image does not allow for cruelty to others. Strong emotion at the time of memory formation and at each recall shifts the patterns of memory. Emotion focuses attention on certain aspects of a memory, and that is what is remembered. Events that occur between the storage of memory and the recall also influence what is remembered (Ornstein, 1991). The environment we find ourselves in also affects memory. The context surrounding both storage and recall has a powerful impact on memory. Where we are, whom we are with, and what is happening around us play a powerful role in memory.

Music and Memory

We have all experienced the various ways music affects memory. Music helps us encode, store, and retrieve information from memory. I learned to spell *encyclopedia* by hearing Jiminy Cricket sing the "Encyclopedia" song on *The Mickey Mouse Club*. I still recall how to spell that word by singing that little tune. *Sesame Street* songs and countless other children's songs are used to help children remember numbers, letters, simple arithmetic equations, and safety information. These are excellent examples of how music helps to encode information as a mnemonic device.

Music is also a powerful trigger for memory recall. Who hasn't had the experience of hearing a song or melody and being suddenly flooded with a whole, intense memory? I experienced this while listening to an "oldies" station when a song came on from the late 1960s. I immediately had an intense, almost hallucinogenic memory of my freshman dorm room. I saw it, smelled it, felt the smallness, and vividly recalled my roommate's face and voice. Clearly, this was a song I heard while studying in that room in the Old Main Dormitory. The song and all the details of that place were linked in my memory. Hearing the song retrieved all aspects of that memory in a vivid, complete way.

We can speculate as to the reason music influences all aspects of memory. First, we know that the auditory nerve has an effect on the midbrain structures that mediate long-term memory processing, including the hippocampus and amygdala (Tomaino, 1998). The role of the amygdala in memory, especially the role of high frequencies and timing on activating this structure, was previously noted. The high-frequency overtones of complex sound and the timing elements of music may be acting directly on this important amygdala function. Because of this neural innervation, music/sound may also be increasing the general brain arousal needed for a memory to be formed. Morton, Kershner, and Siegel (1990) found that prior exposure to music increased memory capacity and reduced distractibility on a monosyllabic memory task. The researchers postulated that this effect might occur because the music provided bilateral cerebral arousal levels through the action of midbrain structures and the right hemisphere needed for memory formation. However, this arousal effect relates to general sound input. There must be something specific about the unique impact of the organized sound of music that also affects memory.

The first unique aspect of music is the presence of the 1/f spectrum fractal time. Research on the involvement of REM sleep in solidifying memory demonstrates the ongoing importance of 1/f spectrum input to brain function like memory. "REM sleep may involve one particular type of stimulation of brain circuits that helps consolidate and strengthen the new learning and memory which the day's experience has half-crocheted into your brain" (Robertson, 1999, p. 47). Since music also has the 1/f patterns inherent in melodies and harmonic shifts, it has a potential to provide this needed input. There is, in fact, a similarity between REM sleep and sound-induced altered states of consciousness. Music and music-based altered states of consciousness can also be used therapeutically to solidify memory.

Another unique aspect of music, its emotional nature, may also be very important in memory formation. As discussed previously, music is an emotional art. It expresses emotion in ways language never can, and it directly evokes emotion through connections to the limbic system. The importance of emotion in memory is now supported by considerable research (Squire, 1987). Music may stimulate the hormone secretion associated with emotion and needed for memory storage (LeDoux, 1996). As music therapist Connie Tomaino (1998) notes, "To stimulate recognition memory, the more emotionally charged the song is, the more likely a person will respond" (p. 26).

Emotion plays another role in memory because memory recall is state dependent. Pert (1997) notes that positive emotional experiences are more likely to be remembered when we are in a positive mood and, conversely, negative emotional experiences are recalled more easily when we are in a negative mood. Music may influence this type of memory recall by establishing a mood that is conducive to the recall of this state-dependent memory. Could music put us in the same "frame of mind" that existed when the memory was formed so that it can be retrieved more easily? This is discussed more fully in chapter 6.

As previously noted, memory is not an exact recall of events as happened. Memory is altered each time we recall it. Our memories are changed by the context in which they are formed and recalled. Context, in fact, is extremely important in formulating memories. "The main function of context is to provide a way of organizing information beforehand, therefore making it more memorable" (Ornstein, 1991, p. 187). Music acts as a form of context for memory. Information imbedded in music, like songs, makes that information more memorable. Levine (2002) believes the best way to remember something is to change the information in some way. Music linked with information as in a song may facilitate memory in this way also.

Edelman (1992) postulates that memory relies on a temporal succession of events and patterns of movement. "Remember that categorization depends on smooth gestures and postures as much as it does on sensory sheets. The cerebellum and motor cortex together undergo the synaptic changes yielding the smooth movements that underlie both categorization and recategorization" (Edelman, 1992, p. 105). Music may affect memory because it is a sensory event that is a succession of patterns of movement. If, as Edelman postulates, memory relies on temporal succession of events expressed through movement, then music would be a natural enhancer of memory process.

Finally, when memory is viewed from a holonomic, dynamic perspective, music influences memory because it is in itself a shifting network of relations just as memory is from this perspective. In Pribram's model discussed previously, the brain converts sensory input into waveforms, which are stored throughout the central nervous system. Memory is retrieved if a waveform similar to the one stored holographically passes through the brain. Music, then, as a similar waveform, first helps set the memory and can also serve to trigger the memory retrieval later (Briggs & Peat, 1989).

Intelligence

There is a great deal of attention currently focused on the question, "Does music make you smart?" Contradictory research information has made this a very controversial subject. Much of this research focuses on increased test scores—IQ tests, math and verbal scores on SAT tests, and so on—because of participation in music. But the impact of music on intelligence really depends on your definition of intelligence. If intelligence is defined as a high IQ score or an isolated ability like mathematical calculations, then there is no conclusive research that verifies that exposure to or participation in music increases intelligence defined in this way. But this is only one of many ways to define intelligence. In fact, there is little to no agreement as to what intelligence is. The word *intelligence* has many meanings and serves many purposes (Richardson, 2000).

What is intelligence? The current popular conception of intelligence is based on the intelligence quotient model, which views an IQ test as a basic index of potential mental activity by educators, psychologists, politicians, and parents alike. In this definition " . . . intelligence is something that can be described and measured as a single variable on which people can be ranked, as with physical strength" (Richardson, 2000, p. 24). Intelligence becomes a set of fixed properties of the mind, each adapted to different problem areas encountered in interaction with the environment and specified by our genetic code (Richardson, 2000). The computational model of brain functioning supports this definition of intelligence as a collection of "rules" residing in simple mental units (computational symbols), each doing a simple task as a reflex. These simple units respond in a fixed and logically defined manner to specific inputs (Richardson, 2000).

IQ tests and other standardized tests of intellectual achievement have come under a great deal of criticism in past decades. They are accused of being culturally biased, racist, and overly dependent on verbal skills. Though these criticisms are serious, perhaps the most serious accusation is that these tests are completely invalid in the first place. As already noted, there is very little agreement as to what actually constitutes intelligence. IQ test designers declare they can test intelligence, but do they really know what they are testing? If a test is not measuring what it says it is measuring, it is by definition invalid. IQ testing began with little more than a guess about what was being tested and with a completely unsubstantiated idea that IQ scores correlated with other tests and measurements, such as school performance (Richardson, 2000). Recent research also shows that IQ score is not correlated to advanced cognitive ability of any kind. Ceci and Liker (1986) found that performance on cognitively complex tasks, having dynamic, nonlinear characteristics, is unrelated to IQ scores. Whatever an IQ test measures, it does not measure the ability to do a cognitively complex form of reasoning. Richardson (2000) concludes that IQ and other standardized achievement tests do not measure innate intellectual potential, do not really know what they are measuring, do not tell us much about people, are not long-term predictors of ability or social worth, and have no connection with complex cognitive tasks needed in interaction with the outside world. A definition of intelligence based on IQ score and computational units is seriously flawed.

With the intense research being conducted on the human genome, emphasis has been placed on finding the seat of intelligence in genetic programming. This research is endeavoring to determine what genes "program" the development of areas of the cerebral cortex to take on specified functions. Yet, as Richardson (2000) reports, "all we know for sure [about genes and intelligence] is that rare changes, or mutations, in certain single genes can drastically disrupt intelligence, by virtue of the fact that they disrupt the system as a whole" (p. 62). This is seen in conditions like Down syndrome, where general intellectual functioning is impaired, and William's syndrome, where some specific abilities (like music and social skills) are enhanced and others (mathematics) are impaired.

Many theorists postulate that intelligence comprises many separate factors. These theories came to culmination in 1983 when Howard Gardner proposed a theory of intelligence he called "multiple intelligences." Gardner defines intelligence as a set of skills for problem solving that entail the potential for finding or creating solutions to problems, which lays the groundwork for knowledge acquisition. He initially theorized seven "intelligences" and currently theorizes nine. These include verbal–linguistic, logical–mathematical, visual–spatial, bodily–kinesthetic, musical–rhythmic, naturalistic, interpersonal, intrapersonal, and spiritual–existential intelligence. Gardner believes these intelligences are biologically specified modules that differ in strength or prominence from person to person. Each has a differing computational mechanism, which defines the function of the intelligence. He believes each one is based on a distinct neural structure, set by the genetic code irregardless of varying circumstances or experiences with the environment (Richardson, 2000). Though on first appearance these seem to be separate capacities, Gardner believes these intelligences are linked together in complex ways. As Armstrong (1993) notes, "Although you may strongly identify with one or more of the . . . descriptions [of intelligences], you actually possess all seven intelligences. Moreover, virtually any normal person can develop every one of the seven kinds of minds to a reasonable level of mastery" (pp. 11–12).

However, in contrast to this idea that development is preset, such as is postulated by gene theory, computation models, or Gardner's multiple intelligences, a theory of divergent development has emerged from complexity science. A system of divergent development has no controlling codes, recipes, programs, or blueprints, only internal interactions and their reactivity to external conditions (Richardson, 2000). Intelligence could not come from a set map or collection of abilities because it is a complex and infinitely variable quality. Rather than a set of abilities, features, or symbolic representations of the world, intelligence is the ability to predict outcomes based on deeply structured interactions among a whole set of variables. It is knowing (not necessarily consciously) and using the deeper and more complex relations experienced in the natural world to predict and cope with novel situations (Richardson, 2000). Our brain does not register features, images, or other coded symbols. Instead it experiences patterns of redundancy, known as covariations, through our sensory experiences of the world. "Indeed, much of sensory behavior . . . has the purpose of collecting sample covariations . . . rather than preformed images" (Richardson, 2000, p. 182). The brain is interested in deep covariation structures in experience. We recognize and store these patterns of redundancy (like the 1/f spectrum) on many levels of brain organization.

Intelligence constitutes the integrated, interacting levels of organization and regulation (Richardson, 2000, p. 180). "In this nested system, interactions between levels, rather than the constitution of the levels themselves, is what is important: all intelligence emerges from them" (Richardson, 2000, p. 193). What this complex interaction does is allow intelligence to ". . . arise as emergent properties from the interactions between levels [of genesis and regulation], creating a final level of regulation incorporating all those evolved before . . ." (Richardson, 2000, p. 167). *Emerges* is the key word here. It seems that intelligence, as so much else in our complex world, is about the interaction of many levels of our recursively organized brains, with new and greater properties emerging from the interaction. Intelligence emerges out of this interaction as an attractor. Intelligence is the complex web of interactions and the reactivity to the ever-changing external conditions. In this view of intelligence, an individual is an active adapter to a constantly changing environment. Intelligence is the ability to anticipate and cope with new situations. This is fluid intelligence where individuals have the ability to solve new or novel problems when no previous experience with the situation exists. This is raw problem solving (Robertson, 1999). This adaptive ability has historically been one of the most prominent features of human intelligence (Richardson, 2000).

So how do we gather these pattern interactions so necessary to the emergence of intelligence? Quite simply, we interact with our environment. We have multiple and varied experiences with our complex world. To interact, we use our senses and, in particular, our bodies. We move, bump into things, touch, taste, hear, smell, and experience our world. The body is certainly implicated in intelligence, and again, so are emotions because they put value on experiences, focus our attention, and enhance experiences. Since there is no thinking without emotion, intelligence could not develop without it (Bennett Reimer, personal communication, February 18, 2000).

In general, intelligence evolved because animals interacted with a complex environment. But human intelligence developed far beyond the behavioral responses to environmental cues characteristic of animal intelligence. There is a communal dimension to human intelligence, which depends on interactions with others. Many theorists now believe human intelligence arose because of the rise of culture and patterns of affiliation among early humans. Human intelligence initially develops within a two-way interpersonal interaction between parent and child as the first social relationship (Bunt, 1994). Engagement in social cooperation led to both the relative increase of human intelligence and the numerous forms it takes (Richardson, 2000).

Intelligence is always manifested within a cultural context. "The origins of specifically human intelligence in cognition–culture interactions means it will develop fully only when keyed into or hooked up to external cultural tools" (Richardson, 2000, p. 193). According to Bennett Reimer, intelligence is the ability to make increasingly fine distinctions as related to increasingly wide connections in contexts provided by culturally devised role expectations (personal communication, February 18, 2000). Human interaction and the large forms of that interaction—culture—shape intelligence.

Music and Intelligence

Music is the quintessential cultural tool that mirrors the complex relationships and interactions of our world. This is one way that music ultimately influences intelligence. It is first a two-way interpersonal process with early tonal and rhythmic interplay between child and parent. It is a primal social discourse. Further, as explored in chapter 3, music uses and implies the deeper covariations or patterns of redundancy on which intelligence is based, especially the 1/f spectrum. Music helps us achieve an explicitness about deeper relationships in nature not attainable by ordinary language, which is the basis of intelligence (Richardson, 2000). Involvement in music readily and easily provides ways to interact with the environment using our senses and our bodies. We use our vocal chords to sing, our hands to manipulate sound-making instruments, and our bodies to move rhythmically. It is these activities that lead to intelligence.

Another important factor in intelligence, emotional value, is also reflected in music. The emotion attached to musical expression may create the sense of value needed for learning and memory to occur. This may well be why imbedding knowledge in songs is such an effective means for remembering. Finally, being a cultural tool, music creates a communal dimension. Music is a shared experience. Ensemble playing is the ultimate expression of this sense of community (Ruud, 1998a), but all forms of music are meant to be shared with others. It is in these ways that music may affect intelligence.

Music Therapy Practice in Learning, Memory, and Intelligence

There is a large body of music therapy practice that relates to problems in learning, memory, and intelligence (Gfeller, 1983; Larson, 1978; Michel et al., 1982; Morton, Kershner, & Siegel, 1990; Prickett & Moore, 1991). From children with learning problems derived from the cognitive impairment of mental retardation or learning disabilities to older adults with Alzheimer's disease and other conditions that impair memory, music therapy interventions address the multiple difficulties clients encounter in this area of mind functioning. Music therapy practice for clients with mental retardation is used as an example.

Individuals diagnosed with mental retardation have below-average general intelligence as measured by an IQ test, impairment in adaptive behavior, and severe problems in learning and memory. Engaging these clients in active music making, such as singing a song or playing basic rhythm instruments, addresses their learning needs in many ways. The music provides increased general neural arousal and the attention needed for learning and memory storage to occur. The physical movement and sensory input stimulate the brain areas needed for memory to occur and utilize neural connections necessary for brain functioning. The same activities allow for development of perceptions and concepts through sensory integration. Such skills become the building blocks of learning. Academic learning, such as counting skills contained in teaching songs, provides the practice with feedback needed for this specific kind of learning to occur (Robertson, 1999). In general, music supports the motivation to engage in learning activities by giving those experiences affective value to undermotivated children.

Creativity

Creativity is a particular manner or style of being intelligent that helps us pursue a particular purpose. Until the mid-1950s, creativity was thought to be a rare human skill that was bestowed on only a few specially selected individuals. Creativity was measured by the uniqueness of the product produced by the creative individual—the painting, the composition, the novel.

With the work of Guilford (1968) and others, creativity came to be seen as one form or component of human intelligence.

Creativity may be the most obvious emergent property of brain functioning (Richardson, 2000). In a way, our brain is hardwired for creativity. It brings together the diverse functioning of the left and right hemispheres so that, as in any nonlinear reaction, the whole (creativity) is greater than the sum of its parts. The left hemisphere functions as a means of convergent production, while the right functions as divergent production (Gowan, 1978). Creativity occurs when both hemispheres coalesce. "The two streams of the brain meet in a tremendous outburst of creativity" (Diamond, 1985, p. 87). The ancients saw creativity as the tension between chaos (right hemisphere) and order (left hemisphere [Briggs & Peat, 1989]). That tension is the edge of chaos, the place of the most vigor in a system.

With the understanding that all people have varying degrees of the intellectual quality known as creativity, it can be studied and researched as a human ability that can be fostered, developed, and, perhaps, taught. Developing a person's creativity became a psychologically and educationally relevant activity (Crowe, 1987; Treffinger, 1983).

In examining creativity as a form of intelligence, researchers have identified both characteristics of the creative individual and a set of creative behaviors in individuals showing high creativity (Treffinger, 1983). Characteristics of the individual or, as identified by Treffinger, affective behaviors of creativity include self-assurance, independence, willingness to take risks, curiosity, positive reactions to new elements in the environment, seeking new experiences, persistence, and a capacity for wonder. Extensive study of creativity has identified creative behaviors or cognitive skills as delaying judgment, *divergent thinking* (discovering many alternatives to solving a problem), examining a problem from all angles, *synergy* (associating elements in a new way so the whole is greater than the sum of its parts), *serendipity* (unexpected discovery of something not actively sought), and exploratory means of expression.

Treffinger (1983) not only delineates both the cognitive and affective components of creativity but also looks at the development of these skills in a hierarchy of increasing complexity and difficulty. The affective and cognitive skills are broken down to their most basic expression in the first level of development, with the other levels of the hierarchy showing increasingly complex abilities. This makes the development of basic creative skills possible for very young children and individuals with varying cognitive disabilities, as demonstrated by research I conducted on developing creative behaviors in children with developmental delay (Crowe, 1987).

Music Therapy and Creativity

Music is universally recognized as a creative art. Composition, improvisation, and performance of previously composed works all involve affective and cognitive behaviors of creativity. Though performance is often considered a re-creative art, Reimer notes, ". . . the performing arts require a second level of creative involvement—exploring and discovering expressive potentials in the yet-to-be-finished work of art and bringing those potentials to fruition in the performance of it" (1989, p. 65). The basis for musical creativity may stem from music's direct stimulation of the right hemisphere in the Wernicke area without the left hemisphere intervening (Gowan, 1978). A number of music educators have identified characteristic creative behaviors in music expression (Gorder, 1980; Vaughan, 1971; Webster, 1983). Webster (1983, 2001) proposes a model of creative thinking in music that identifies both convergent and divergent thinking constituting musical intelligence. Convergent thinking skills include recognition of rhythm and tonal patterns and the ability to imagine sound. Divergent thinking involves fluency (free-flowing, uninhibited response), flexibility (ability to manipulate sound), originality (unusual musical responses), and memory. Webster (1983) conducted research to show these creative behaviors can be demonstrated in spontaneous musical performance and reflect the general skills of creativity in children.

Music is certainly a natural way to encourage and even teach both the affective and cognitive behaviors of creativity. Affectively, music is motivating and engenders curiosity. What small child is not curious about a sound-making instrument and is not willing to explore its sound-making potential? What parent hasn't experienced a toddler happily banging on pots and pans with a wooden spoon? Expressing creativity requires facility with the tools required for expression. There are numerous techniques and equipment used in music therapy that make creative expression possible with little or no skill development in playing music. Electronic instruments, computer applications, and particularly rhythm instruments allow for expression with no skill development. The drum circle movement (Hull, 1998) has capitalized on this ability, bringing together hundreds of people from diverse backgrounds and ages to creatively express themselves simultaneously on rhythm instruments.

Imagery

Creativity involves three separate levels of functioning: perception, feeling/intuition, and thinking/imagination (Kenyon, 1994, p. 144). The first two of these levels were discussed previously. Let's turn to imagination and the importance of mental imagery. Creativity is dependent on mental imagery, which is an attribute of the senses. Imagery is a sensory experience when no immediate sensory stimulus is present. It is mental "pictures" or "sounds." Jourdain (1997) calls imagery ". . . a sort of 'perception' in the absence of sensation" (p. 163). In fact, the brain areas responsible for a given sensory perception give rise to that form of image. The visual cortex is activated during visual imagery, while the auditory cortex is active during an auditory image (Damasio, 1999). According to Baars (1997), "There is a close overlap between the brain areas involved in perception and imagery. Images and inner speech are truly internally created sensations" (p. 62). Imagery and imagination are the way the senses have of throwing themselves beyond what is immediately given.

However, as in all cognitive functioning, generation of images cannot come from one area of the brain alone. Imagery is yet another emergent property of brain function. As Hunt (1995) notes, "Imagery is far too broad and fundamental a phenomenon to be restricted to but one of its forms or to one area of the cortex" (p. 162). Imagery and its other form, dreams, are too pervasive for a simple explanation. Images and imagination are essential to cognitive functioning. "Imagery seems to occur not as an independent mental faculty, but as an extension of the anticipations required for any cognitive act . . ." (Jourdain, 1997, p. 227). Images spring from the interaction of human experience and memory. Since images arise without immediate sensory input, they must arise from the *memory* of sensation and perception.

Hunt (1995) postulates that there are two types of images: sensory and autonomous. He sees the pluralistic nature of images and dreams emerging from the functioning of the cortex's two hemispheres. "It would make the most sense to postulate a right-hemisphere form of holistic, spontaneous imagery and a left-hemisphere imagery based more on volition, analysis, and propositional control" (Hunt, 1995, p. 169). The first type of imagery reflects gained sensory knowledge—awareness closely aligned to the original sensation and arising from sensory brain areas as discussed previously. This type of imagery can only express what the brain already knows and can never produce novel knowledge. It is needed to regain a skill, such as walking, after loss of the ability. Oliver Sacks (1985) gives an excellent example of using this type of imagery as he regained his ability to walk after an accident left him with impaired movement in one leg.

The second type of imagery postulated by Hunt is more like thinking where new insights and knowledge can emerge. In this type of imagery, individuals can learn new things from the actual images, which leads to new insights beyond previous learning. This second type of image is a natural expression of the psyche. It is the language of the inner self. "It establishes a bridge between body, mind, and spirit as well as forming a vital link with the inner self. The metaphoric content of images provides access to various levels and states of being" (Bush, 1995, p. 48).

Music and Imagery

Music is widely recognized as a stimulus to imagery (Bonny & Savary, 1990; Bush, 1995). This likely occurs for several reasons. Images arise from many areas of the mind interacting with each other. "Images emerge as a result of a purposeful interplay of mind, feeling, and imagination" (Bush, 1995, p. 47). Music does exactly this. It is an interplay of multiple faculties of mind, emotion, and imagination. Sound input directly affects the midbrain structures responsible for emotion generation. Also through lower and midbrain structures, sound input serves to activate and alert all areas of the brain responsible for the three types of imagery: intuitive (receiving impressions), sensate (bodily sensations), and visual (Bush, 1995). The sound input engages these other brain areas and evokes the imagery. Sound input engages not only the emotional brain structures but also the right hemisphere of the cerebral cortex. The right hemisphere is the metaphoric part of the brain. It is the part that visualizes, dreams, creates, and holistically solves problems. In a word, it images. Musical input to the right hemisphere provides a dynamic element with needed structure and direction for the production of images. "Its dynamic, ever-changing quality transforms and moves the psyche along" (Bush, 1995, p. 73). Music is ever growing and evolving, which evokes an evolving, growing quality to the inner imagery. "With music as the stimulus the imagery often emerges with clarity and feeling, providing a dramatic soundscape and fluid container for an experience with the inner self" (Bush, 1995, p. 48). Music is a multilayered, stimulating, and, of course, complex input to the brain that stimulates a multilevel complex response like imagery (Summer, 1988). Finally, music has culturally assigned meaning. Music communicates meaning because the musical element refers to the extramusical elements of concepts, actions, and emotional states. A musical element would then evoke an image that relates to that meaning (Bonny, 1978). For example, in Western music, minor mode is associated with sadness. Hearing music in minor mode evokes imagery of sadness. The impact of music-generated imagery on various aspects of emotional functioning is addressed in later chapters.

Music Therapy and Creativity and Imagery

Music therapy activity interventions to foster creativity and imagination usually involve the spontaneous music making of improvisation. From simple playing on rhythm instruments to the complex musical patterns involved in an improvisation form like jazz, improvisation involves self-expression. This ability to express the unique attributes of self is important for all clients from young children with mental retardation to adults dealing with depression. Children, in particular, need opportunities to use their imagination as one aspect of cognitive functioning. Involvement in music can provide both sensory and autonomous imagery. Neurologist Oliver Sacks (1990) used sensory images of movement evoked by familiar music with his patients frozen by Parkinson's disease. He found that rhythmic music that patients associated with movement was best in reestablishing movement in these individuals with severe disabilities. As explored extensively in chapter 6, music also evokes the deeply personal autonomous imagery that helps clients with mental illness uncover deep causes of their problems.

Language and Speech
The next faculty of mind to explore is language and speech. Language is an interaction between an internal capacity and the social regulations that extend and shape it. "Language translates deep structures of cognitive representation into linear, temporal patterns of sound and visual symbols [and gesture] interpretable by others" (Richardson, 2000, p. 164). The auditory expression of language is speech. Language and speech are both products of culture. Language is ". . . another cultural tool through which social regulations mediate the cognitions of participants in the culture" (Richardson, 2000, p. 166). However, speech is not the only expression of language. Many theorists believe gesture is a more basic expression of language. French author Maurice Merleau-Ponty (1973) believed speech is gesture made with our mouths. He theorized that language developed from gestures—the spontaneous expression of feeling. "Active, living speech is just such a gesture, a vocal gesticulation wherein the meaning is inseparable from the sound, the shape, and rhythm of the words. Communicative meaning is always, in its depths, affective . . ." (Abram, 1996, p. 74). The gesture is the feeling of delight or anguish in its tangible, visible form (Abram, 1996). A gesture does not make us think of an emotion; it *is* that emotion. The work of Manfred Clynes (1977), explored in chapter 3, linking specific emotional states with motor expression also supports this contention. The direct representational ability of gesture in terms of musical expression was also addressed in that chapter.

Increasing amounts of research over the last decade have shown that gesture is an important part of communication and speech acquisition. Jana Iverson's (2000) research with children with visual impairment and gesture found that individuals with visual impairment use gestures when speaking even to others with blindness. Another study (Johnston, 1999) showed that toddlers who are visually impaired used gesture to communicate even before they were able to talk. With no visual input to imitate, gesture remained a form of communication. These research results demonstrate the intrinsic nature and importance of gesture as a vehicle for expression. Goodwyn and Acredolo (2000) report on extensive research showing that babies by the age of one can and should use expressive gestures to increase their language abilities and, potentially, their overall intelligence (based on IQ scores).

Problems in this area involve language dysfunction, including aphasia seen in patients dealing with strokes (Baker, 2000) and problems with receptive language—the inability to understand verbal, spoken, or written communication. Speech difficulties involve problems with expressive language or the production of speech (Levine, 2002).

Music as It Relates to Language and Speech

Is music a language? This question has been debated for centuries. The old adage, "Music is the universal language," is repeated endlessly. It is likely that music and speech evolved together two million years ago. Both functions—speech and music—are based on abilities common to all vertebrates that evolved into human-specific abilities (Wallin, 1991). Both use the same auditory and vocal systems and the same sensory processing. They "time-share" many neurological underpinnings (Falk, 2000). There is a close and complex connection between speech and musical function. They both apparently consist of a multitude of subfunctions, many of which rely upon the same psychological mechanisms (Borchgrevink, 1982). Falk (2000) notes that results from brain-imaging studies show that music and language are part of one large, vastly complicated, distributed neurological system for processing sound in humans. Music and speech share more of the brain mediating structures than previously realized. It is commonly believed that speech and music, particularly singing, are processed in the two different hemispheres of the cerebral cortex: left processing speech and right processing music. To a large extent, this is true. However, as the newer forms of processing needed for speech evolved, the older form of expression—musical forms—was required for limbic control, basic social learning, and a holistic experience of space and time. These different processing needs led to a lateralized cerebral dominance (Wallin, Merker, & Brown, 2000). But a simple assignment of these complex behaviors to one hemisphere or another does not reflect the complexity of the processing involved. For example, musical rhythm and the overall act of singing are processed by the speech hemisphere (Borchgrevink, 1982). Processing of the shape of a melody is a right hemisphere function (Radocy & Boyle, 1997).

However, there are significant melodic elements to spoken speech. In fact, speech and music share many qualities known collectively as *prosody*. These include rhythm, tone, emphasis, inflection, and melodic contour (Taylor, 1997). Based on Merleau-Ponty's work, Edie (1973) notes that there is an "... affective tonality, a mode of conveying meaning beneath the level of the words themselves ... which is contained in the words *just insofar as they are patterned sounds* ... which are more like a melody—a 'singing of the world'— than fully translatable, conceptual thought" (p. xvii). Being a function of the right hemisphere and midbrain structures, prosody reflects the common neurological basis of this aspect of speech and music (Taylor, 1997). Prosody gives speech and music their affectual quality expressed through timbre and tone. "The emotional content of speech depends more upon the music of language, that is, the intonational, inflectional, and prosodic elements of speech than upon content, itself" (Isenberg-Grzeda, 1995, p. 147).

Premusical and prespeech vocalizations likely developed first based on two channels of auditory sensory-motor functioning. The first channel was for sustained distance calling and was rich with redundant vocal sounds. This vocal ability evolved into music. The second channel uses rapidly changing, nonrepetitive sounds like exclamations created by consonant sounds. Consonants are shaped by the actions of lips, teeth, tongue, palate, or throat. The movement of these body parts breaks the flow of breath and gives form to our words and phrases. Vowel sounds are made by unimpeded breath. Vowels are sounded breath (Abram, 1996). In fact, music, especially singing, may have evolved before speech. "There is no a priori way of excluding the possibility, for example, that our distant forebearers might have been singing hominids before they became talking humans ..." (Brown, Merker, & Wallin, 2000, p. 7). Our ear physiology supports this contention.

> The fact that a full two-thirds of the cilia in the inner ear ... resonate only at the higher "musical" frequencies (300 to 20,000 hertz) suggests that at one time human beings communicated primarily with song or tone. One hypothesis is that human communication evolved from singing to primate-like grunts, before finally arriving at what we recognize as modern speech. (Campbell, 2000, p. 10)

Some scientists are now even speculating that music, not language, development was the catalyst for the rapid development of the human brain. Brown, Merker, and Wallin (2000) contend, "There is an alternative candidate [compared to language] for a structurally complex, syntactically rich, acoustically varied, socially meaningful human function that might have driven this brain expansion, namely, music" (p. 9). Ruud (1998b) sees music as a protocommunication, a form of social interaction that actually precedes verbal speech. Because of the additional diversity and complexity of music, it may actually transcend language. It clearly crosses cultural lines and communicates with a basic repertoire of body language, gestures, and sound combinations (Clynes, 1977).

Music and speech share another commonality in that they require a temporal sequence pattern of complex sound occurring during a certain time period (Borchgrevenk, 1982). This temporal patterning proceeds from event perception, to motor control, to the planning of extended strategies of behavior (Jackendoff & Lerdahl, 1982). These behaviors are similar in music and speech because they are temporally structured cognitive capacities. Ornstein (1991) postulates that the sequential movement of swinging in trees in our primate forbearers became the neurological grammar of the development of language and "musical" communication. Music does differ from speech in that the temporal organization is more rigorous and it has an organizing pulse (Scartelli, 1991).

To return to the earlier question, "Is music the universal language?" the answer depends on the intention of the question. If this question implies that music is a universally recognized form of communication, the answer is yes. If it means that music conforms to the linguistic requirements of a language, the answer is no (Chomsky, 1980; Farnsworth, 1981). Though music does not meet the standard linguistic criteria for a language, there are many parallel and similar origins and functions of the two human behaviors

Music Therapy and Speech and Language

Though being involved in music, especially singing, does not automatically improve speech because of some of the differential neurological processing, music therapy interventions are quite effective in work with clients with speech and language dysfunction (Cohen, 1993; Michel & Jones, 1991; Walker, 1972). Music therapy practice with problems of speech and language encompasses work in helping children develop receptive and expressive language (Cartwright & Huckaby, 1972; Colwell, 1994), in supporting speech development for children who are deaf (Darrow, 1984; Staum, 1987), and in working to help patients who are poststroke to regain speech (Baker, 2000; Cohen, 1992, 1995).

Music therapy assists in the area of speech and language dysfunction in several ways. First, speech and music abilities occupy adjacent areas of the brain. Music may provide a related neurological channel for initial development of communication skills (Michel & Jones, 1991) or for remediation of speech/language problems. Music therapy interventions provide a form of neurological exercise that helps new brain areas take over for speech functions (Sekeles, 1996). PET scan research (Weiler, 1995) shows that after a stroke, neighboring areas of the brain become more active to assist in regaining speech ability. A specific technique, Melodic Intonation Therapy, uses the presence of these shared and parallel brain areas to systematically move a patient from singing expression to speaking (Baker, 2000; Galloway & Kraus, 1982). A second way music therapy interventions can affect speech/language is to have music, especially singing experiences, assist in developing prelinguistic abilities (Bunt, 1994; Hoskins, 1988; Loewy, 1995). Since music and aural language have a great deal in common, including the importance of gesture, affect, timbre, rhythm, and movement patterns, involvement in singing and other music production can have an effect on the skills needed for speech. For example, ". . . pitch is a basic element of both the sound and verbal memory systems and that specific pitch work has potential in helping sort out prosody, intonation and general comprehension of language and speech" (Bunt, 1994, p. 55). The gestural quality of both speech and music is also important. Gestures inherent in music and gestures that accompany music, like action songs, are important precursors in promoting speech (Aldridge, 1996; Madsen, 1991). Speech/language and music skills seem to follow a similar developmental pattern (Michel & Jones, 1991). Music therapy interventions move the client through these developmental stages, including prespeech sound making and babbling. Singing words also provides practice and exercise for articulation. Finally, music experiences support establishment and ongoing development of language and vocabulary (Schunk, 1999). Singing songs, songwriting, and memorizing songs with active listening methods (where the music therapist focuses attention on the lyrics and their meaning) all increase receptive language and promote effective use of words.

Consciousness
The final aspect of mind to be considered is consciousness. There is no other faculty of mind that has so many diverse definitions and so much argument as to what it is than consciousness. "Consciousness is a word with several meanings and it is used to describe a variety of mental phenomena, including being awake rather than asleep, having control of one's behavior, having a concept of one's self and of the world, and so on" (Scott, 1995, p. 139). There are about as many theories of consciousness as scientists and philosophers studying it. Such a profound mental event is almost undefinable. According to Hunt (1995), no one definition or system of consciousness can do justice to the full range and variability of the human mind. There is cer-

tainly no consensus on a definition of consciousness in the scientific community. This debate over what constitutes consciousness is centuries old. Aristotle (1958) wrote on the nature of consciousness. Descartes' theory of dualism, separation of sense of self from the physical self, came from his struggle to define and explain consciousness. William James (1890), the great pioneer in psychology, struggled with the question. A great deal of scientific attention has been focused on the subject in recent years (Baars, 1997; Chalmers, 1996; Damasio, 1999; Edelman, 1992; Hunt, 1995; Jackendoff, 1987; Jaynes, 1976; Penrose, 1989; Wade, 1996; Wilber, Engler, & Brown, 1986). The *Oxford University Dictionary* provides seven definitions for *consciousness* from a state of being awake to the dissociative consciousness of a person with multiple personalities (Hunt, 1995). For the purpose of this book, two general levels of consciousness—core or waking consciousness and self-referential consciousness—are delineated.

Core Consciousness

Core consciousness is the state of being awake, alive, and aware of the surrounding environment. It involves basic wakefulness or alertness. To be "unconscious" implies not being awake, to not be alert to our surroundings. Alertness comes from the nervous system's exposure to basic sensory input (Jourdain, 1997) and to action of specific nuclei in the brain stem (Purves et al., 1997). A change in awareness like this is a psychological bifurcation, when awareness abruptly changes from wakefulness to sleep, for example (Combs, 1995). Core consciousness is the simplest form of consciousness, providing a sense of self in the here and now separate from the "outside" world. It is not dependent on memory, reason, or language (Damasio, 1999). All living, moving creatures have this level of consciousness. Even a protozoa will move away when it bumps into an object, demonstrating some level of awareness of the difference between itself and the environment.

> In short, core consciousness is a simple, biological phenomenon; it has one single level of organization; it is stable across the lifetime of the organism; it is not exclusively human; and it is not dependent on conventional memory, working memory, reasoning, or language. (Damasio, 1999, p. 16)

It is our first and most basic awareness. Our more complex, multilayered extended consciousness develops from it.

Core or waking consciousness stems from the actions of the reticular formation and thalamus (Baars, 1997). This core consciousness develops early. Research by Verny and Kelly (1981) and Restak (1986) puts ". . . the start of consciousness in the third trimester, when fetal EEGs show cortical response to peripheral sensory stimulation, and distinct waking and sleeping patterns" (Wade, 1996, p. 32). PET scan studies show that infants' brains are first active in the brain stem and hypothalamus, the somatosensory cortices, and the cingulate.

> As you can see, the set of activated structures entirely matches those needed for the proto-self [core consciousness] and second-order maps. The functional maturity of these structures at birth is noteworthy. Given that other brain systems have also been in full swing, e.g., auditory, the activation suggests a considerable functional precedence. (Damasio, 1999, p. 266)

Through these connections, the rhythmic component of auditory stimuli, especially music, serves to alert the whole cerebral cortex and subcortical areas (Scartelli, 1991).

From a basic sense of being awake, core consciousness also involves a higher level of attention leading to focus and purposeful behavior. Core consciousness orients us to our environment. It propels intentional movement that establishes a relationship between the organism and the environment (Damasio, 1999). It is evoked by a higher level of arousal triggered by high-intensity, unexpected or important sensory events, like music. Because sensation is based on movement, sound/music input can have a significant effect on attention.

Because we are aware of sound before birth, sound and rhythmic movement make up our first awareness, our first model of our world. Since experience with the world shapes our mind, sound and rhythm profoundly shape who we are. "Indeed, some of the prenatal learning by the fetal source of consciousness (e.g., vocalization recognition) seems to be retained as a cognitive foundation of early experience accessible to the neonate" (Wade, 1996, p. 73). Our first interaction with the world is through sound before and immediately after birth. As Berendt (1983) notes,

> Our ears are open before we are born. Even in the womb our ears are more important than our other senses. Our consciousness begins with them. The child in the womb hears its mother's heartbeat—and, later, sounds from the outside world—which means that before we perceive the world with any other sense, we hear it. (p. 139)

The internal and external sounds experienced by the fetus in utero are the first interaction with the environment that differentiates between self and other (the world). Core consciousness and a sense of temporality or flow over time are two sides of the same phenomenon (Hunt, 1995). Early exposure to this sense of flow through music may be a large part of core consciousness. Additionally, Damasio (1999) contends that core consciousness is inexorably linked to emotion. Emotion and core consciousness require the same neural substrates. Auditory innervation also shares these neurological structures. Music, as a basic expression of emotion emanating from the same neurological roots, also becomes, then, a part of core consciousness. This early awareness can be considered *auditory consciousness*.

Auditory consciousness is a multidimensional awareness of time and space, a nonlinear reaction that is unitary in nature. The consciousness of listening is continuous, ever present, and unavoidable. It is an awareness of wholeness and, simultaneously, of the constantly changing and evolving moving relationships inherent in sound (Berendt, 1988). Auditory consciousness is the capacity to experience the world whole, to perceive events as they combine simultaneously (Burke & Ornstein, 1995). It reflects the primal human functioning of the midbrain and right cerebral hemisphere— functioning that precedes language and visual discrimination. Sound from the external environment certainly includes human vocalizations, but, as noted previously, it also includes the rhythmically regular, organized sounds of music.

Self-Referential Consciousness

Higher-order consciousness or *self-referential consciousness* involves recognition by a thinking subject of his or her own acts without the direct involvement of sensory input. Self-referential consciousness is being aware of being aware (Edelman, 1992). Unlike core consciousness, self-referential consciousness requires memory of what went before and a projection into the future. According to Edelman (1992), this higher-order consciousness ". . . involves the ability to construct a socially based selfhood [distinction between self and non-self], to model the world in terms of the past and the future, and to be directly aware. Without a symbolic memory, these abilities cannot develop" (p. 125). This higher-order, self-referential consciousness involves deliberate, intentional acts rather than automatic control. "Conscious processes occur one at a time, take effort, and are inefficient. They are more flexible than unconscious processes. At any moment the content of consciousness is what we are prepared to act on next" (Ornstein, 1991, p. 230).

Self-referential consciousness is widely believed to be a biological imperative in that it is a major factor in adapting to change (Baars, 1997). It is an evolutionary survival mechanism with multiple functions, allowing the brain to interpret, learn about, interact with, and act on the world around us. Consciousness is the framework for processing information that guides behavior in adaptive and meaningful ways (Winkelman, 2000). All the faculties of mind are intercorrelated and lead to consciousness. Baars (1997) sees consciousness as the basis of the synthesizing, directing, and volitional abilities of the mind. Consciousness is a system of functions, including physical, mental, emotional, and extrasomatic, which interact to make an individual self-aware and environmentally responsive. "The properties of consciousness are not just the properties provided by brain structures; they are derived from inter-relationships of systemic properties of the brain with symbolic information and meanings provided by learning and culture" (Winkelman, 2000, p. 24). As the label "self-referential consciousness" implies, this level functions to create an elaborate sense of self. Jackendoff (1987) sees consciousness as the building of an internal model of the world containing the sense of self, reflecting back on one's own mode of understanding.

Self-referential consciousness begins with sensory input and a process of mapping the outside world and the "self" that is experiencing it. How does this representation or map occur? It happens through human interactions with the environment. "Consciousness and world are inseparable" (Hunt, 1995, p. 12). Self-referential, symbolic consciousness is based on a primary flow of perception. As Damasio (1999) states, "Consciousness begins as the feeling of what happens when we see or hear or touch. Phrased in slightly more precise words, it is a feeling that accompanies the making of any kind of image—visual, auditory, tactile, visceral—within our living organisms" (p. 26). Our perceptions are based on movement—our bodies moving and encountering the world and the movement in the form of vibration of light and sound impacting our bodies through the sensory channels. This movement occurs over time. Hunt (1995) believes consciousness and time are the inner and outer versions of the same flow. "To notice consciousness is to notice time, and vice versa" (Hunt, 1995, p. 246).

However, this higher-order, self-referential consciousness arises not just from this basic experience of sensation but from the human capacity for cross-modal translation and transformation. This occurs among multiple perceptual modalities, specifically vision, audition/vocalization, and touch/movement (haptic sense). Norman Geschwind (1965) first developed this cross-modal theory of consciousness, which states that all these sensory inputs have different rates and forms of brain processing. There are, therefore, innumerable ways in which these three sensory channels will flow into and transform the patterns of the others. These cycles of reciprocal transformations will reorganize the patterns of basic perception in an open-ended and emergent fashion as a higher rearrangement of perception. This becomes the genesis for self-referential symbolic consciousness (Hunt, 1995). Hunt states that ". . . a cross-modal *translation* capacity, as exemplified in language, the arts, and complex synthesis, is basic to the emergent symbolic capacity" (1995, p. 149). The multiplicities of connections in the human neocortex from these three sensory areas converge on the angular gyrus of the inferior parietal area. Singer (1998) has shown that damage to these neocortical zones of convergence affects various forms of symbolic cognition and, in the right hemisphere, self-referential awareness, supporting the assumptions of this theory. As Hunt (1995) observes, "Geschwind's insight that a neocortical cross-modal translation is the basis for self-referential symbolic cognition and consciousness has been broadly supported . . ." (p. 86).

Since interaction with the environment is essential to development of self-referential consciousness, it can be thought of as *consciousness-with*, an inherently social activity. Consciousness-with is a social "world" (Hunt, 1995), because it is socially shared knowledge (Winkelman, 2000). Scott (1995) believes that ". . . consciousness is the highest level of organization in the brain, and it is an atom at the level of human culture" (p. 186). Since social mirroring and cross-modal translations are the core of symbolic capacity, the separation of consciousness and the world postulated in so many theories of consciousness is eliminated. Consciousness is, therefore, not private but validated through shared experiences in a particular "world." These basic forms of perceptual awareness are organized in terms of the common dimensions shared within a culture with the culture producing many "worlds." Because self-referential consciousness involves a socially based self-hood, it is significantly influenced by culture, unlike core consciousness, which is not influenced by culture at all. The word *consciousness* comes from the Latin *scire*, meaning "to know," and the word *com*, meaning "with." Consciousness is the "with" by which we know the world (Winkelman, 2000). Self-referential consciousness is an event, not a thing. In fact, we should consider the word *consciousness* to be a verb, not a noun (Combs, 1995).

The first social world of self-referential consciousness is infant–mother mirroring—social mirroring with emotional content. "Social mirroring . . . and cross-modal translations—as the core of the symbolic capacity—are co-emergent and inseparable. Human cognition is, from the beginning, structured in the form of a dialogue" (Hunt, 1995, p. 88). This dialogue does not have to be linguistic but is often based on visual, kinesthetic, and auditory imagery and on awareness of movement over time. In fact, early mother–infant mirroring is a cross-modal interaction primarily involving haptic communication (touch with movement) and the mirroring of vocal sounds and timbres rather than visual mirroring of facial expressions. The touching, stroking, and cooing we do so instinctually with babies is the first social dialogue experienced by a newborn. During development, consciousness is further structured ". . . through internal conversation based on the contents of social life and the presumed perspectives of others" (Winkelman, 2000, p. 20). These "others" can include internal, personal images as the others, often seen in children as projected images of imaginary friends, and in later life, as a form of internal conversation (McNiff, 1992).

Consciousness as an Emergent Property

Consciousness involves highly complex interactions within most of our brain structures and, likely, our body. The event of consciousness is an emergent property of this highly complex interaction, created when many discrete events fuse together as a single experience. Emergence is central to understanding consciousness (Lewin, 1992). Consciousness then becomes a bottom-up emergent phenomenon where a series of brain systems, each producing some kind of global property, interact with each other to generate another level of emergent properties (Lewin, 1992). Van Eenwyk (1996) notes that

> . . . consciousness is a dynamic that replicates itself on many different levels. Increases in awareness occur when aggregations of fractal attractors become subsumed under yet more fractal attractors. . . . Consciousness is never "set." It is an ongoing process of fractal cascades, the result of which is a continual increase in the capacity of its attractors to metabolize life experiences. (pp. 324–325)

Reflecting its complex, emergent nature, consciousness is an ever-evolving, fluid process. Hunt (1995) notes that ". . . much of what consciousness 'does' is open-ended, unpredictable, and not rule-specifiable" (p. 60). In fact, noting the fluid property of consciousness, many people now see it as a form of energy. Pribram (1991) theorizes that consciousness is part of a unified field of energy. Tiller (1997) believes consciousness is converted to various forms of subtle energy. This brings us to a possible physics of consciousness. Consciousness could have a physical radiance.

> If consciousness itself, as opposed to its temporally antecedent neural substrates, is a physical field of some kind, then it would be emergent from the molecular level of processing in the nervous system. Consciousness . . . becomes part of a "unified field" of subatomic composition linking all levels of physical and psychic reality. Accordingly, consciousness would quite literally be a kind of rarified substance that flows and pulses. (Hunt, 1995, p. 260)

The topic of subtle energy and consciousness as a subtle energy is addressed in the next chapter.

Music and Consciousness

Many aspects of consciousness and its origins have been explored. It is now time to explore how music factors into these. There are many fundamental parallels between music and the various explanations of consciousness. In fact, many writers on consciousness use music and musicians as metaphors for consciousness. Baars (1997) explains, "Mozart was a master of consciousness" (p. 12) because of his ability to combine extreme and incompatible elements into a sparkling conscious unity.

First, consciousness is associated with motion, with flow. Historically ". . . the empirical terms for mind in Greek and Sanskrit originally referred to an embodied vitality, heart, flowing of blood, and breath. All these usages had in common a streaming based on metaphors derived from the qualities of water, air, and fire" (Hunt, 1995, p. 118). As explored previously, music is the motion of vibration and the sense of forward motion of melody and rhythm. It has the same streaming quality as consciousness. More important, this motion happens over time. As Edelman (1992) notes, "The sense of time is first and foremost a conscious event" (p. 168). Music is organization of sound and silence *over time*. To experience time is to experience consciousness, making the flow of music over time an experience of consciousness. As Baars (1997) notes, consciousness has a great preference for predictable structure over time. "Evidently the *structure and cohesion* of the conscious stream is also an important factor" (Baars, 1997, p. 24). By definition, music involves the structure and cohesion of auditory events organized over time. Even the most basic form of consciousness, the development of core consciousness, is based on a ". . . *coherent collection of neural patterns which map, moment by moment, the state of the physical structure of the organism in its many dimensions*" (Damasio, 1999, p. 154). The moment-to-moment physical response to music may even contribute to development of the core awareness. This is a more basic response than even the perception of hearing, which is not believed to be involved in proto-self-development per se.

The very basis of mind and core consciousness is about expression of life and the life urge within a boundary (Damasio, 1999). As explored in chapter 7, music is an expression of the life urge. It may very well be an external sonic representation of the internal processes of life, especially neural activity. Consciousness is

> . . . the possibility of bringing the system of life regulation—which is housed in the depths of the brain in regions such as the brain stem and hypothalamus—to bear on the processing of the images which represent the things and events which exist inside and outside the organism. (Damasio, 1999, p. 24)

Sound is the basic link between these deep brain regions and the outside world.

Music also factors into the development of self-referential consciousness. Music is certainly made possible by consciousness, but could it also be possible that experiences with music's flow, time, complex structure, and cross-modal dialogue help develop self-referential consciousness? Music is cross-modal because it involves audition in its most varied and complex forms and frequently involves vocalization. The earliest music was vocal, and the earliest forms of vocal interchange between mother and infant involve the same elongation of vowel sounds and the modulation of timbre variables as forms of emotional expression. This first mirroring of mother and infant is this form of sound production—the precursors of music—followed by the sung lullaby, which is a universal expression. As humans develop, music adds to the cross-modal experience since performing music uses vision (to a lesser extent) and, especially, the haptic sense. This sense of touch with movement is required for playing or manipulating objects to create music. Listening to music is even a cross-modal activity involving audition but also the movement sense of gesture. Music is a highly complex, culturally determined organization of numerous parameters of sound. It is a cross-modal world of dialogic mirroring with emotional content and, by the criteria of this model of consciousness, potentially a fundamental activity in the development of self-referential consciousness. Music continues to be a culturally based dialogue long after the initial mother–infant interactions. Within a culture, music is a dialogue between performer and listener, between composer and performer, and between performer and one's inner self. As the cross-modal theory of self-referential consciousness requires, music has emotional content.

Music is one of the "worlds" from which self-referential consciousness springs. It is a unique experience, a world of its own within the cultural matrix. As noted in chapter 1, philosophers and theorists have speculated as to why all human cultures have had music. Perhaps it is because music is a primary, fundamental activity in the development of self-referential, symbolic consciousness deriving from the prominence of auditory consciousness early in human development. Perhaps humans have engaged in the activity of music simply because they must as the genesis of the consciousness that makes them human. As Wallin (1991) notes, "Intense attention to a tonal flow-becoming-music . . . means to experience, observe, to read-off the evolving process of mind-becoming-consciousness" (p. 1). It is this lifelong process of "mind-becoming-consciousness" that is the essential element of soulmaking.

Music Therapy and Problems of Consciousness

Music therapy interventions are used with problems of both core and self-referential consciousness. Clients with problems of core consciousness have difficulties with alertness and wakefulness, such as a patient in coma or suffering from Alzheimer's disease. Music therapy interventions are used with such clients (Boyle, 1989) because a conscious state does not have to be present for the brain to respond to auditory input (Taylor, 1997). Music affects basic alertness because it requires the brain to maintain a constantly changing auditory sensory field, which keeps arousal level high (Taylor, 1997). A great deal of response to music is subcortical and available to clients who have upper cortex damage. "But the response to music, it would seem, is widespread and probably not only cortical but subcortical, so that even in diffuse cortical disease like Alzheimer's, music can still be perceived, enjoyed, and responded to" (Tomaino, 1998, p. 13). This makes music therapy interventions an important part of treatment for clients with severe impairments to core consciousness.

Clients with other forms of attention difficulties including children with attention deficit hyperactivity disorder (ADHD) can benefit from music therapy interventions related to consciousness. These children are unable to focus their attention and engage in meaningful educational activities. Music therapy is used extensively with these clients (Overy, 2000; Steele, 1984). Music has the ability to grab and focus attention. This occurs first because of the alerting nature of sound through subcortical structures. It has also been found that individuals with ADHD generally do not generate beta brain wave patterns. Beta is the brain wave associated with active alertness (Kenyon, 1994). When beta production is increased, attending behavior increases. Because of the high information stimulus of music, it may positively influence beta brain wave production. Music includes both orderly elements and novelty to keep attention high. "Human music shows an unusual combination of order and chaos, with some elements highly ritualized and stereotyped, such as tonality, rhythm, pitch transitions, song structure, and musical styles, and others highly variable and innovative, such as specific melodies, improvisation, and lyric content" (Miller, 2000, p. 344). This may be why learning tasks linked to music are useful in teaching children with learning disabilities.

Music therapy interventions also work with problems of self-referential consciousness. This appears in issues of self, ego, psychological development, and self-image. These music therapy interventions are addressed in chapter 6.

Altered States of Consciousness

Since consciousness is a continuum of states and not a specific or discrete value, an altered state of consciousness is the recognition of a describable difference in the state of consciousness. "Our normal waking consciousness builds us a model of the world, based on sense and body information, expectations, fantasy and crazy hopes, and other cognitive processes. If any of these factors is radically altered, an altered state of consciousness may result" (Ornstein, 1991, p. 228). As music therapy pioneer Helen Bonny (1978) states,

> Consciousness emerges from one's total capacity for sensory perception and the inventive-creative activity of their cognitive processes. Consciousness also involves dimensions of awareness not subject to the usual scientific measurements. So, while consciousness is not totally outside the scope of science, it is not limited by scientific judgements, for consciousness serves as the personal faculty which integrates one's varied perceptions of reality. (p. 4)

Consciousness and especially altered states of consciousness as "varied perceptions of reality" are addressed in later chapters. Altered states of consciousness, their therapeutic value, and the role of music in producing an altered state of consciousness are explored as problems of emotion and feeling. Altered states of consciousness as a therapeutic intervention for problems of the human spirit are addressed in chapter 7.

Specific Applications of Music Therapy for Problems of Brain and Mind

Many client groups can benefit from music therapy interventions designed to remediate problems of the brain and mind. A good illustration of music therapy interventions that address these basic cognitive functions is work with clients who have suffered a traumatic brain injury. A traumatic brain injury, whether caused by a severe blow to the head or an internal vascular accident like a stroke, causes a wide range of problems, including impairment to cognitive functioning. Therapy to restore this cognitive functioning is known as cognitive rehabilitation. Music therapy interventions can affect cognitive rehabilitation in all its stages. The first stage is sensory input and sensory stimulation. As noted previously, music, especially participation in a music activity, provides an enormous amount of sensory input and opportunities for sensory integration. From this, basic perception is relearned. The second stage of cognitive rehabilitation is attending to sensory input. This occurs because music is attention grabbing and provides alertness through neural arousal. With increased attention, cognitive skills of attending to, recognizing, and responding to sensory input can begin. The third step in cognitive rehabilitation is memory work. As discussed earlier in the chapter, music can influence memory on many levels. The fourth step in cognitive rehabilitation is relearning the HBFs, which, as previously explored, can be supported by music therapy interventions.

The human brain is a vastly complex structure that gives rise to the many functions of mind. Music, being a product of the human mind, affects brain functioning and the processes of mind on every level. Music therapy is used in remediating a wide range of problems associated with the brain and mind. The problems of the body—physical diseases and disorders—and the use of music therapy in dealing with them can now be addressed.

~

CHAPTER FIVE

Music Therapy and Problems of the Body

A professional musician and I are providing music for patients on a general medical/surgical unit of a local hospital. We approach a room where a sixty-year-old woman with respiratory problems is resting in bed. Her breathing is shallow, and her face shows tension and fear. I approach her and ask if we could play some music for her. She agrees, and my colleague wheels in his electronic keyboard and begins to slowly improvise using rich, full harmonies and gentle, underlying rhythms. After about thirty seconds, the woman's breathing slows down and deepens. Her face muscles relax, and she closes her eyes. When the music stops after twenty minutes, she and I discuss her reaction to the music. She reports that she is feeling much calmer and that the fear has subsided. She also tells me her breathing is easier and she has less pain in her chest. As we are leaving, she says, "Thank you for bringing me the music. I was feeling so alone and without hope. The music made me feel embraced and loved."

Having explored music therapy and problems of brain and mind, music therapy in the treatment of disorders and problems of the physical body is now addressed. Physical functioning is another aspect of soulmaking. In this chapter, the principles of biology and how music and music therapy interventions affect this biological functioning are delineated.

According to Maranto (1991), medical music therapy is the functional use of music in medical specialties. However, even here it is clearly impossible to separate out the body from issues of the mind. In this chapter, the case is made that the mind and emotions have a direct and important impact on physical functioning, disease processing, and overall health and wellness. In reality, mind and body cannot be separated. This is the basic premise of a newly emerging approach to medical practice, holistic medicine. Holistic medicine recognizes a constant and reciprocal action and communication between mind and body (Scartelli, 1992). As Benor (1992) states, "Holistic medicine views the person as a unity of body, mind, and emotions and spirit" (p. 89).

In this chapter, the issues of bodily functioning, which have many layers of processing, are investigated. First, the *content* of medical interventions— defined as some agent or action that alleviates or remediates the dysfunction— is addressed. The content of healing, thought of as curing, provided by traditional Western medicine addresses the physical body primarily from a chemistry perspective. Until now, it is chemical and, to some extent, structural interventions that have been the focus for treatment of the body. These interventions include surgery, chemotherapy, medication, and now gene therapy. However, there are other processes occurring in the body that have been recognized by non-Western medicine for centuries and are now increasingly recognized by Western medical practice. These include energetic systems in the body and energy medicine, the mind–body connection, the link of emotion and immune system functioning, and, of course, the nonlinear, edge-of-chaos dynamics typical of optimum vigor. Later in the chapter, the *context* of healing—the external and internal environment conducive to recovery and health—is explored. Medical music therapy is addressed by overviewing the use of music therapy in the content of healing—impact on physical aspects, interface with essential rhythmicity of physical functioning, vibrotactile stimulation, nonlinear dynamics, human energy systems, and the mind/body interface.

Music Therapy and the Content of Healing

Music therapy interventions may affect physical functioning in a number of ways. Though some of these effects are verified by research, further investigation needs to be done in this area in order for these techniques to gain widespread acceptance.

DNA and Human Cells

The investigation of music therapy's contribution to content of healing begins with a basic level of physical human organization, *deoxyribonucleic acid* (DNA). DNA makes up the building blocks of the body. DNA, and all matter, is composed of atoms. Because atoms are in a constant state of vibration, Frohlich (1986) theorizes, based on the principles of quantum (atomic) physics, that the living matrix must vibrate and produce coherent or laser-like oscillations. This theory is verified by laboratory experiments. Each layer of organization that constitutes the body, starting with atoms, has its own mode of vibration so that individual molecules, assemblies of molecules like DNA, have vibrating characteristics. The living cells that DNA creates also have these characteristics. Research has verified that DNA and human cells have certain modes of vibration (Eyster & Prokofsky, 1977; Frohlich, 1977). Anything that vibrates has a specific resonance frequency. As discussed in chapter 3, anything that can vibrate with a certain frequency can be acted on from outside if that frequency is matched. This is how sound vibrations may potentially influence functioning at the level of DNA and cells. Vibrational modes of DNA and cells may, in fact, form the basis for the interaction of electromagnetic radiation and sound waves with living tissue. Such waves could influence humans both physically and psychologically (Hado Music Corporation, 1996).

Another way in which sound may affect DNA is through the arrangement of the molecules. The DNA molecule exists in the form of a double spiral or helix. Each helix is made up of tiny molecular building blocks known as nucleotides. "Now what is important about these nucleotides is their order, or the way they are laid out on the helix, the form, if you will" (Kenyon, 1994, p. 10). Research by Dr. Susumu Ohno (1988) has found that the form or sequence the nucleotides take is not random but, rather, much like the organization of a melody. Dr. Ohno used a computer to ascribe musical notation to DNA sequences. Not only did the resulting arrangements of notes come out as melodies; they consisted of particular melodies depending on the DNA used. "While working with a gene for a kind of cancer, Dr. Ohno recognized the basic melody. It was from Chopin's Funeral March" (Kenyon, 1994, p. 186). Researcher Joel Sternheimer (1983) says, "The masses of particles behave and maneuver among themselves as if they were musical notes on the chromatic tempered scale" (quoted in Maman, 1997, p. 61). Richard Voss (personal communication, April 2000) verifies that DNA has the same characteristics as music. These include patterns of redundancy and predictability where boundaries lie between the random and the predictable and power law behaviors based on the 1/f spectrum discussed in chapter 2.

French musician and researcher Fabien Maman (1997) conducted experiments with biologist Helene Grimal that explored the potential effects of sound on DNA and human cells. In this research, they observed that sound has an impact on the cell nucleus and the electromagnetic fields of the cells. As Maman notes, "With a specific frequency (different with each type of blood cell and each person) I observed a stimulation of the cells, as if they were energized" (1997, p. 65). He also observed that the frequency of sound altered the color of the magnetic field surrounding the cell. Maman found that the shape of the cells varied with the timbre of sound—the same note would affect the cells differently when played on metal, wood, or wind or nylon string instruments. Additionally, physicist Joel Sternheimer (1983) discovered that each molecule in the body has a corresponding melody and, therefore, each of these molecules can be reactivated through external resonance when that particular melody is presented. Maman believes that all individuals have a tone or fundamental sound that resonates with them in their entirety.

> Perhaps one day, when the technology will be available to enter more deeply the vibrational world, it might be discovered that the fundamental sound is the particular resonance of the individual's DNA. . . . Fundamental sound can be very helpful for the physical body through its harmonizing and regenerating effect at the cellular level. (Maman, 1997, p. 20)

Music Therapy and DNA

Though there are no specific music therapy techniques currently working to influence this level of physical functioning, certain sound healing techniques do claim impact at this level (Hado Music Corporation, 1996). Maman (1997) predicts that specific combinations of frequency patterns could positively or negatively influence the form of DNA and the physical and energetic makeup of the cells of our body. Traditional forms of sound healing have postulated and utilized frequency, melody, and timbre differences to affect changes at this basic level of functioning (Goldman, 1992; Leeds, 2001; McClellan, 1988; Rael, 1993). This is an area that needs further investigation.

Brain Chemistry

There has been a great deal of research interest in the last two decades on the effects of sound/music on another level of human organization—brain chemistry. Much of this research explored whether music promotes the production of certain biochemical and neuroendocrine levels in the body. Bartlett, Kaufman, and Smeltekop (1993) and VanderArk and Ely (1992) found short-term decreases in cortisol levels in healthy individuals after music listening, an indication of immune system functioning. Other studies, some with the added element of mental imagery, have found similar results (McKinney et al., 1997a; McKinney et al., 1997b; Miluk-Kolassa et al., 1994). Rider, Achterberg, Lawlis, Goven, Toledo, and Butler (1990) and Rider and Weldin (1990) found that secretory IgA shows a greater increase when using music and imagery than for music alone, also an indication of healthy immune functioning. In an extensive research project on well older adults, Koga and Tims (2001) found significant increases in human growth hormones following active music making, in this case keyboard instruction. The ability of music to stimulate bodily chemicals associated with increased immune system functioning and music therapy practice in this area are addressed later in this chapter.

Autonomic Nervous System

Physiological responses to music were explored in chapter 3. These physiological responses are created by the input of sound on the structures of the autonomic nervous system. Research by Harrer and Harrer (1977) indicated that active music performance creates strong autonomic reactions that cannot be suppressed by deliberate intent. Of particular interest to medical music therapy are the effects of music on heart rate, blood pressure, and respiration rate. White (1997, 1999) found that music listening significantly decreased heart rate pressure in individuals compared to that of subjects in non-music-listening groups. Augustin and Hains (1996) report a decrease in heart rates for patients waiting for surgery when music listening was added to preoperative instructions. Miluk-Kolassa et al. (1994) found a significant decrease in autonomic nervous system markers of stress response (arterial pressure, heart rate, cardiac output, skin temperature, and glucose level) for presurgical patients who had one hour of music listening.

Research on physiological changes associated with music, however, shows that these changes are inconsistent and unpredictable (Radocy & Boyle, 1997). As Thaut (1990b) notes, "Experimental investigations have shown that (1) physiological changes are reflected in a highly idiosyncratic manner, and (2) music stimuli, within the concept of response stereotypes, can markedly affect these changes" (p. 34). In other words, music does elicit physiological changes but in a highly personal manner for each individual. This occurs because of differing experiences with the musical elements, such as tempo and rhythm, and because of the many variables specific to the particular individual. These variables include current mood, general attitude and preferences toward music, the person's level of alertness, and general autonomic and emotional reactivity. "This means each individual has his own biological response pattern to a given stimulus. He responds in an idiosyncratic manner that shows a consistent relationship among stimulus characteristics, physiological response, and psychological experience" (Thaut, 1990b, p. 34).

Music Therapy and Autonomic Nervous System

The individual physiological response to music has several implications for music therapy practice. First, if effects on physiological functioning are to occur, the music therapist needs to assess and account for as many of the variables involved as possible. The music therapist's training allows this to happen. Furthermore, because the physiological reaction is clearly a highly complex, interactive effect, it is difficult to predict results. These physiologic effects of music are used in various areas of music therapy practice. However, they are not prescriptive as to a particular sound, melody, instrument timbre, or genre of music affecting a physiologic response, like heart rate, in a specific way each time it is used.

A number of music therapy applications utilize these physiologic responses to music. For example, music therapists use music listening with and without vibrotactile stimulation for people in coma or who have a traumatic head injury (Boyle, 1989; Claeys et al., 1989). Because the autonomic responses are mediated in the brain stem, individuals with cortical damage can and do react to music, since the auditory nerve affects these structures (Radocy & Boyle, 1997). Music therapists who use the physiological impact of music as part of the strategies to manage symptoms treat patients with high blood pressure and heart disease. Similarly, music therapists use these physiologic responses in general programs of stress reduction and management to be discussed later in this chapter.

Nerve Stimulation
Direct physical effects of sound/music may also occur because of stimulation of peripheral and cranial nerves. Much evidence for this effect comes from acupuncture research. Shi-Jing, Hui-Ju, Guo, and Maranto (1991) conducted research using music transduced into electrical impulses and fed into acupuncture needles. The research found that music electroacupuncture enhanced muscle strength and use in patients with hemiplegia in contrast to traditional acupuncture or electroacupuncture without music. This effect is likely due to the shared spectral power densities in voltage fluctuations in music, natural sounds (babbling brooks), and the action of myelinated nerve fibers (Voss, 1989). This shared spectrum of fluctuations is the previously discussed 1/f spectrum. The significance of electrical current in the body is discussed in a later section of this chapter on the human energy systems.

Other musical elements that stimulate nerve conduction pathways involve the cranial nerves. The auditory nerve interfaces with all of the cranial nerves. Research by Dr. Alfred Tomatis found that all cranial nerves lead to the ear. "Furthermore, the 10th cranial, or vagus, nerve had an origination point on the outer surface of the eardrum. . . . The vagus nerve is involved in many psychosomatic diseases as it connects from the ear [to] the lungs, heart, and stomach" (Rider, 1997, p. 103). For example, vocal toning (elongated vowel sounds with varying pitches) provides a continuous high-frequency stimulation (Campbell, 1990), an increased immune response (sIgA production), and decreased heart rate as compared to singing familiar songs (Rider et al., 1991).

Rhythm and Entrainment

Another layer of processing that occurs in music therapy interventions in physical medicine is the use of rhythm and the mechanisms of entrainment. Rhythm, as the sense of measured recurrence, is pervasive in nature. Periodicity, the rhythm of the regular recurrence of things, is expressed in the phases of the moon, the ebb and flow of the tides, the earth's rotation, and the orbit of an electron around a nucleus (Hughes, 1948). "The world of living organisms originates from this rhythmic universe and represents one part of it. Therefore, the organism is part of the rhythmic order and life is a rhythmically organized process, again with frequencies extending over a huge range . . ." (Koepchen et al., 1992, p. 39). In fact, rhythm is fundamental to life and our very existence. The heartbeat, neurons firing, and movements of our digestive tracts all occur in a regular, though complex, rhythm (Clynes & Walker, 1982). "Everywhere in nature we experience rhythm. . . . For living organisms rhythm is an essential feature. As soon as it disappears, so does the possibility of living. There is no living organism which exists without rhythm" (Wilkes, 1993, p. 72).

The human body has a complex biological rhythmicity on many different layers and ranges of functioning. "The rhythms within the different ranges of this scale have different characteristic properties and interdependencies" (Koepchen et al., 1992, p. 41). Rhythms recorded in milliseconds include molecular rhythms, the action potentials of muscle fibers, and brain cell activity. Activity recorded in seconds is the next layer of this complex rhythmicity. Activities such as brain waves, heart rate, voluntary movement, and respiration are on this level. Our bodies also work in macrorhythms such as circadian rhythms that are measured over days (Scartelli, 1991).

> Every one of us is a multiplicity of internal clocks. Our cells have their own individual timekeepers that switch on and off various biochemical processes. Cells organize into individual organs whose internal clocks instruct them to secrete hormones and chemicals. These chemical messengers cause the time rhythms of various organs to couple together in the larger, self-organized system of the body. Some of the subsystem clocks operate on limit-cycle repetitions. . . . Other of our internal clocks—such as the many rhythms of consciousness—are more open to environmental influence. (Briggs & Peat, 1999, pp. 133–134)

All these bodily rhythms have harmonic relations to one another (Moses, 2000).

The bodily rhythms that are particularly important to music are found in the medium range. Within this medium range of human rhythmicity is found music and other outer world rhythms like dancing and walking, rhythmic movements of the body controlled by motor control system, and the internal rhythmicity controlled by the autonomic nervous system.

> The middle of this medium range between 10 Hz and 10^{-2} Hz is the proper domain of musical rhythms in the usual sense of the word. It is here that we find the inner rhythms of the heart-beat with all its variations, those of the respiratory system, and the frequencies of most of our normal movements. (Koepchen et al., 1992, p. 41)

In considering the impact of musical rhythm on human functioning, it is important to realize that these external rhythms are not acting on a passive or inert organism but on one that is a moving, dynamical system of complex, interacting rhythms.

One particular mode of interaction between biological rhythms in this medium range and external musical rhythms is the mechanism of entrainment. Entrainment or mutual phase locking occurs when two oscillators vibrating in the same field in close rhythms will tend to "lock in" or synchronize. "Entrainment is universal in nature. . . . It is a physical phenomenon, but it is more than that, because it informs us about the tendency of the universe to share rhythm, that is, to vibrate in harmony" (Berendt, 1983, pp. 116–117). Entrainment is seen in electronics, making it possible for radio receivers to lock onto signals even when there are small fluctuations in their frequencies. It is also seen in biological systems, allowing multiple heart or nerve cells to work in synchronization to phase (Gleick, 1987). This tendency toward phase locking is due to the nonlinear nature of these complex vibratory systems. When the vibratory ratio between two oscillating bodies is close to a whole number, nonlinearity tends to lock those vibrations in (Gleick, 1987). The entrainment is not to a single frequency but to a range of frequencies that are "tied together" by nonlinear dynamics. A common example of entrainment is the synchronization of the inner circadian rhythm of the human body, which is naturally approximately twenty-six hours, with the twenty-four-hour day–night cycle.

Music Therapy Practice and Rhythm and Entrainment

A lack of rhythmicity is characteristic of many pathological states. An arrhythmic heartbeat is associated with a diseased heart, and constipation is the result of the loss of normal rhythm in the small intestines. In music, both the musical rhythms and the frequency on tone (a rhythmic perception) can be mechanisms of entrainment. Music therapy practice utilizing the rhythmic nature of music is based on the idea that outer rhythmicity corresponds to the natural rhythms of our bodies and brains and, therefore, the external rhythms (as occur in music) can create synchrony between the two. There are many ways that entrainment mechanisms affect physical functioning. Research shows that music with a beat just below the pulse rate can entrain diaphragmatic breathing associated with a nonhyperventilating state (Fried, 1990). Rider (1985) demonstrated that music designed to entrain neural functioning significantly decreased pain and EMG tension. Flatischler (1992b) contends that drum rhythms act directly on the human heartbeat. Scartelli suggests that entrainment affects the medulla oblongata or brain stem area of the brain. He (1991) notes,

> Auditory input that has a strong, discernible, and organized rhythm or pulse (thus delineating the stimulus from non-musical sounds) would directly relate to or associate with the nature of the medulla oblongata's rhythmic commands that sustain heart and respiration rates. In other words, rhythmically formatted input creates a sympathetic reciprocity with certain areas of the brainstem by virtue of the natural, innate, pulsative function of these areas, *automatically*. (p. 33)

According to medical doctor Deepak Chopra (1990), any form of music that engenders entrainment is healing.

Motor Rehabilitation

The most prominent bodily response to rhythm is gross motor movement. Highly rhythmic music stimulates us to move, usually unconsciously. We find ourselves tapping our toes or drumming our fingers to a strong, complex rhythm with an obvious underlying pulse. As Dick Clark said for many years on *American Bandstand*, "The song has a good beat, you can dance to it." The ability of music to stimulate gross motor movement is known as the *thalamic response* and occurs due to the presence of neurons in the thalamus, which respond to specific tempi (Rider, 1997). As Koepchen et al. (1992) note, there is a common rhythmicity shared by the somatomotor and autonomic functioning.

In addition, rhythmic auditory stimuli (RAS) influence the initiation and timing of motor response. The effect of RAS on motor behavior was noted by neurologist Oliver Sacks (1990), when he and the hospital's music therapist used familiar music to "unfreeze" patients with Parkinson's disease and allow them to initiate movement. He notes that Parkinson's disease and other disorders of the basal ganglia are disorders of time, particularly disorders in the temporal organization of movement. Music acts ". . . as a sort of temporary substitute, a 'prosthesis,' for the basal ganglia, in particular of its functions as a temporal organizer and sequencer of movement" (Sacks, 1998, p. 7). Thaut (1997) theorizes this phenomenon is based on an oscillation-entrainment model where rhythmic processes in neural gait networks in the brain become entrained to rhythmic timekeeper networks in the auditory system. There are many links between the auditory system and motor system that make sound/music's impact on motor functioning possible.

A number of research studies (Pal'tsev & El'ner, 1967; Rossignol, 1971; Rossignol & Melville-Jones, 1976) show that auditory stimulation physiologically primes and entrains subcortical motor structures. Thaut reports on extensive research verifying that

> . . . nerve pulses induced by sound signals—in particular, musical sound patterns—travel from the cochlear nuclei not only along the pathways ascending to the cerebral cortex, but simultaneously spread to the spinal cord via the alternate auditory pathway, where they raise the excitability of the motor nuclei. (1990b, pp. 38–39)

The research by Rossignol and Melville-Jones (1976) further shows that this activation of motor potential neurologically by auditory input results in synchronization between the neural activity and the repetitive auditory input, thus facilitating timed muscular response patterns. This rhythmic auditory stimulation has more than a pacemaker role. It is, in fact, the primary coordinator of the control structure in the generation of complex movement sequences (Thaut, 1997). The potential effect of auditory rhythmic stimuli on temporal accuracy in motor movement is auditory–motor coordination (Thaut, 1990b). This auditory–motor coordination produces motor rhythmic responses that are less variable than other sensory modalities. Research verifies that ". . . auditory presentation mode produces consistently faster reaction times and better response qualities than the visual, tactile, or combined auditory/visual presentation" (Thaut, 1990b, p. 41). In fact, rhythmic auditory stimulation serves as a predictable timing cue that facilitates the anticipation of the motor response.

As Sacks (1998) notes, the effect of music on initiation of movement is instantaneous and therefore cannot be due to chemical changes in the basal ganglia. In rhythmic movement, the response is synchronized with the presentation of the stimulus. "This sets apart a synchronized musical experience from other forms of activity, as generally reactions succeed the stimulus. Anticipation of the ensuing event is crucial in synchronizing a movement with a specific sound . . ." (Bunt, 1994, pp. 62–63). Though any rhythmic, auditory input can create these effects, music in particular is effective in overall motor rehabilitation. Sacks (1998) observes,

> It is not just a matter of motion and time, but of inner force and energy of intention and impulse. And it is these inner characteristics which make it wholly different from a mere pacemaker or metronome—it is the inner life, the "will," of rhythm that has such power and that calls to the "will" of the performer. (p. 8)

Music Therapy Practice and Motor Rehabilitation

Music therapy for motor rehabilitation developed using auditory rhythm as a sensory stimulus to facilitate gait patterns. In rhythmic auditory stimulation, music provides a template or pattern around which the movements of walking can be reorganized and centered. "It helped to reorganize, or re-create, motor programs or engrams (or allow access to them) necessary for the recovery or reconstruction of what one might call motor identity" (Sacks, 1998, p. 6). Dr. Michael Thaut and his colleagues at the Center for Biomedical Research in Music have conducted extensive research on the use of RAS for patients with various diseases affecting gait. Thaut, McIntosh, Rice, and Prassas (1993) and Thaut, Miller, and Schauer (1997) found RAS improved general gait patterns and specifically gait velocity and stride length. Prassas, Thaut, McIntosh, and Rice (1997) demonstrated that RAS produced smoother forward gait trajectory. McIntosh, Brown, Rice, and Thaut (1997) showed that RAS improved velocity and stride length for patients with Parkinson's disease even when basal ganglia dysfunction existed. Additionally, Hunt (1996) found patients with head injury increased their gait velocity using RAS stimulation. Dr. Thaut (1997) believes RAS provides for a more efficient recruitment of motor units needed in skilled movement, leading to a quicker recovery of motor control and skill, a greater exercise benefit to enhance strengthening of weak muscles, and increased duration of muscle activity and co-contraction between antagonist muscle groups to add stability around the joint during therapeutic exercise.

In RAS, music synchronizes internal processes, not just motor events. This is accomplished without cognitive involvement. The sensory input rhythmically drives the motor response, but the actual process occurs below the sensory threshold. A whole movement pattern is rhythmically reprogrammed. The rhythmic stimulus drives the motor synchronicity by approximating the auditory signal. This approximation is scattered around the set signal in a fractal pattern, making the rhythm an organizational effect through time but not as a timekeeper. Musically based rhythmic input is best for this process because, with music, there is better carryover. "Although rhythm is enough to cue gait, the more one can internalize the music the more likely there will be a carry-over outside of the therapy session" (Tomaino, 1998, p. 25).

Music therapy is also used in other aspects of physical rehabilitation. Music is used to motivate exercise. The increased time of participation that comes when music is paired with movement helps to increase physical endurance, increase coordination and muscle control, and improve joint mobility and range of motion. Playing musical instruments also supports specific physical rehabilitation goals by improving grip, muscle strength, and fine motor coordination. There is a large body of research that supports this contention (Cofrancesco, 1985; Thaut, 1990b; Zelazny, 2001).

Music also motivates participation in physical rehabilitation by reducing the perception of pain or discomfort. There are several possible reasons for music's ability to reduce pain perception. First, music may be a distraction from pain (Clark, McCorkle, & Williams, 1981; Hanser, Larson, & O'Connell, 1983; Mandell, 1988). Research by Spintge (1989) showed an increase in pain threshold, an increase in pain tolerance, and a 50 percent reduction in the dosage of pain medications using music. Marteniuk (1976) believes music accomplishes this pain distraction because of a selective attention process. This involves the person's perception of a pleasant auditory stimulus predominating over attention to the less pleasant stimuli of the physical exertion. Additionally, Hernandez-Peon (1961) demonstrated that a pleasant sensory input like music could facilitate electrical activity in one sensory channel while blocking the transmission of other pathways, such as physical discomfort. Taylor (1997) believes sound input may block pain reception in the brain through activation of neurons in the medulla. The axons of these neurons activate the anterior horn to inhibit the activity neurons that bring pain sensation into the central nervous system for transmission to the brain. Pain sensations are carried by slow nerve fibers so that pain perception can be blocked or decreased by rapid, powerful stimuli such as strong rhythmic music (Sekeles, 1996). As Taylor (1997) notes, "Music should be effective as an environmental stimulus in decreasing the ability of the CNS to carry pain stimuli to the brain for conscious awareness" (pp. 60–61).

Another way music decreases pain perception is the ability of music to stimulate brain production of endorphins, which are natural painkilling substances. Substantial research supports this effect (Prince, 1982; Scarantino, 1987). Music produces a "high" similar to a runner's high through this stimulation of endorphins.

Third, music likely decreases pain perception due to exposure to 1/f spectrum fractal time. Complexity science research has shown that exposure to 1/f stimulation decreases pain perception (Takakura et al., 1987). In this study, two sources of 1/f stimulation, white noise and the extracted long period changes present in classical music, were used on subjects. Results showed the 1/f stimulation from classical music was significantly more effective than white noise in reducing pain. Anderson and Mandell (1996) believe this occurs because ". . . 1/f patterns of stimulation interact directly with the sub-cellular and cellular processes involved in creating the pain. Thus, unlike pharmacological approaches that involve blocking receptors, 1/f stimulation may resonantly support the endogenous 1/f processes that are affected by the pathology" (p. 113). Takakura et al. (1987) also found that the positive effects of 1/f-spectrum fluctuations in music were most effective when the subjects enjoyed the music.

The Takakura et al. (1987) research brings us to the final way in which music affects pain perception—the positive influence of the patient's general mental attitude and emotional state. Taylor (1997) notes there is substantial music therapy research showing music influences pain perception when it is ". . . selected by, preferred by, or meaningful to the patient" (p. 61). The impact of music on pain perception is important in physical rehabilitation and many other areas of medical music therapy.

An additional way in which music therapy techniques support rehabilitation goals is in aiding respiratory rehabilitation. It first contributes to this physical goal by helping to time breathing rhythm. Music activity causes the brain

> . . . to exert conscious control over the otherwise automatic rhythmic discharge emanating from the respiratory center in the medulla. . . . During controlled breathing such as that used to play a wind instrument, the cortex takes over direct control of these muscles by imposing its own timing priorities on the pace and strength of their contractions. (Taylor, 1997, p. 91)

Music can also be used for breathing training (Fried, 1990). Involvement in singing and blowing a wind instrument like a recorder provides a means for individuals with shallow or shortened breath capacity to improve their ability to take a long, deep breath. The music provides the motivation to take deeper breaths and extend the breath capacity. It is musically more satisfying to sing an entire phrase than just a few notes. I used this technique myself after recent surgery. Great emphasis is placed on doing breathing exercises and taking deep breaths after surgery to avoid pneumonia. I sang songs with long phrases as a means to deepen my breaths. It also gave me motivation to take deeper breaths and sustain them longer.

Vibroacoustic Stimulation and Resonance

Another way music influences physical functioning is vibroacoustic effects and resonance of bodily structures through the entrainment process. Resonance, as discussed in chapter 3, is the tendency of a body that can vibrate with a certain frequency (resonance frequency) to be set into vibration when an outside vibratory force is oscillating at the resonance frequency. Resonance occurs throughout nature—from the movement of electrons moving from one energy level to another to the shattering of glass when exposed to a tone of a specific frequency and amplitude (Gerber, 1988). Vibroacoustic music therapy utilizes the vibrations of musical sound occurring at specific frequencies to set the entire human body or particular organs into vibration through resonance. Eagle (1996) reports that research in radionics (a specific application of vibration to the body) shows that humans are sensitive to sound not only through hearing but through our whole bodies. Music becomes the means to shift the vibratory frequencies that are out of resonance, giving rise to disease (Parker, 1998).

Based on this idea, Wigram and Dileo (1997) define vibroacoustic therapy as ". . . the use of music and sound (as auditory and vibratory stimuli) transmitted to the body to achieve physical and psychological therapeutic goals" (p. 7). In this theory, illness is the energetic imbalance of the human organism as a whole. Sound/music is used to shift the vibratory frequencies that are out of resonance and causing illness. According to Fernandez (1997),

> A complex tone stimulates whole and partial vibration of a body, causing an effect in the human being of a perception of vibration in specific locations, and also general vibration in the body, experienced as a whole body vibration. Mechano-receptors sensitive to vibration are responsive in specific frequency bands, and therefore the sensation of vibration will vary depending on the frequency and upon the overtones above the fundamental tone. (p. 35)

Music therapy research on vibroacoustic effect shows promising results. Standley (1991) found positive reports of vibroacoustic stimulation, while Darrow and Goll (1989) found that deaf children identified rhythmic changes better with vibroacoustic stimulation versus vibration alone.

Skille (1992) has developed a specific form of vibroacoustic therapy where sinusoidal, low-frequency (30–120 Hz) rhythmical sound pressure waves are mixed with music as the therapeutic agent. Extensive research shows that this technique relaxes muscles, increases blood circulation, and affects the autonomic reactions (Skille, 1992).

Based on the principles of homeopathy, another application of sound resonance involves matching the vibratory signatures of chemical substances, including dietary nutrients, through sound vibration (Parkhurst, 1998). Sherry Edwards has developed a similar therapeutic intervention (Crowe & Scovel, 1996). Many of these techniques are currently not in the mainstream of music therapy practice but do give us an initial introduction to the use of sound and music to positively influence our highly complex human energetic system.

Nonlinear Dynamics of Health and Disease

Chapter 2 explored nonlinear dynamics in human anatomy and physiology. The human body is a dynamical system. Processes in human functioning from blood pressure regulation to neural firing patterns follow the principles for nonlinear dynamical systems. Let's turn now to look at disease processes from the perspective of deterministic chaos and processes in dynamical systems.

As researchers investigate the nonlinear dynamics of our physical functioning, they find that health is associated with intricately complex patterns of functioning. To be healthy is to be composed of shimmering cycles of fractal time (Briggs & Peat, 1989). Stability of the body is a limited range of states in the constant flux of complexity, moving back and forth across the edge of chaos (Damasio, 1999). Disease occurs when a system in question loses the complexity needed to maintain vigor (health). To be healthy, the organism must move around the edge of chaos. "The complex type of variability generated by healthy systems may be due in part to deterministic chaos. A reduction in this apparent chaos characterizes certain diseases. . . . This phenomenon represents an example of the principle of decomplexification of disease" (Goldberger, 1992, p. 321). A broad variety of disease processes, drug toxicity, and even aging may decrease the amount of deterministic chaos and complexity in physiologic systems. For example, researchers (Goldberger, Kobalter, & Bhargava, 1986; Mackey & Glass, 1977) found that normal blood displays chaotic fluctuation in white blood cell counts from one day to the next. However, for patients with leukemia, highly *periodic*, linear oscillations of white cell count may occur. The leukemia patients had *nonfractal* changes and showed a marked decrease in complex rhythms of blood cell fluctuation. The implication is that these normally complex processes became too regular. *Decomplexification* occurred.

Decomplexification occurs as a generic physiological response to multiple influences (stress, drug effects, repeated injury, etc.) on the body as a whole or particular systems, which ultimately leads to a pathological state by reducing the ability of the system to function in a complex manner. Nonlinear dynamics are seen in most systems in the body. Edge-of-chaos dynamics are seen in immune system function, respiration, digestion, and most other systems (Briggs & Peat, 1999). Let's use heart functioning as an example of this process. We think of a healthy heartbeat as a clocklike, regular pulsing. This is the "rhythm" we feel as our pulse or see on EKG (electrocardiogram) markings, but, in reality, the heartbeat is never quite the same each time. There are definite yet subtle variations of that pulse each time our hearts beat. These slight variations show nonlinear complex vibrational patterns (Briggs & Peat, 1989). The heart rhythm is actually the superimposition of numerous rhythms into a complex dynamical system (Koepchen et al., 1992). As Goldberger (1992) notes, "When one analyzes the interbeat interval variations in healthy individuals more carefully, it is apparent that the normal heart rate fluctuates in a highly erratic fashion . . . the type of variability that one sees under healthy conditions is consistent with nonlinear chaos" (p. 322).

The type of nonlinear variability seen in healthy heart functioning is consistent with nonlinear chaos in several ways. This includes the fact that phase space pictures of healthy heart rate variability show complex movement consistent with a strange or chaotic attractor mechanism (Goldberger, 1992). The chaotic variability of the heart rate is due to a complex interaction of the sympathetic and parasympathetic nervous systems when these two systems entrain for maximum efficiency (Childre, 1991). There is now substantial evidence that heart disease is characterized by a disruption of these chaotic movement patterns in the heart. If the heartbeat is too regular (nonchaotic), congestive heart failure results. If the heart rhythm is completely aperiodic, defibrillation occurs. Something like heart fibrillation is clearly a disorder of a complex system (Gleick, 1987). Healthy heart functioning must dynamically rest between these two extremes. "The heart that has locked itself into a limit cycle is on its way to heart failure, but the heart that is open and fluctuating with fractal variance is vibrant" (Briggs & Peat, 1999, p. 135). A healthy heart beats in a complex nonlinear fashion holding at the edge of chaos, thus ensuring vigor and viability. When this complex dance between impulses of the sympathetic and parasympathetic nervous systems is disrupted, heart "disease" ensues.

Numerous factors could potentially disrupt and diminish this complex movement dynamic in the heart. These include the buildup of plaque in arteries and veins, inflammation of the artery walls, high blood pressure, and the aging process itself. "Another candidate in which there is apparent loss of physiologic chaos is the aging process. As we grow older, the complexity of our cardiovascular dynamics appears to decrease . . ." (Goldberger, 1992, p. 326). Both natural aging and the buildup of plaque contribute to decreased flexibility in the arteries that inhibits the movement patterns needed for the heart to generate nonlinear chaotic movement patterns.

As explored next, emotions and feelings are also a factor in complex heart rates. Rider (1997) notes that ". . . individuals who disclose more feelings and achieve more emotional closure in psychotherapy have been found to display a more variable and chaotic heartrate than those who exhibit more emotional repression" (p. 18). Heart rate changes are influenced by any stimulus the brain processes—thoughts, sounds, light, and emotions (Childre, 1991).

To be healthy, an organism must have dynamic flexibility in all its systems and tissues (Hunt, 1996). Two general approaches address the loss of the complex functioning needed for physical health. First, address and eliminate the factors impinging on complex functioning (such as inflammation or artery plaque buildup), or second, directly affect the system as a whole by adding complexity. Most Western interventions for physical disorders address the former. It has been difficult to envision how music therapy might contribute to that form of content of healing. However, Eastern medical traditions have addressed the energetic systems of the body as a whole. Many interventions, including music therapy, may appear to introduce complexity into the energetic system. In general, chaotic, open systems and the input that keeps these open systems at the edge of chaos constitute our bodies. This allows the body to be responsive to the environment and at optimum vigor.

However, complexity can also help the body maintain form and order by introducing small amounts of energy into the system.

> Just as small disturbances rapidly alter chaotic systems, so can minute adjustments stabilize behaviors. Physics has found that by periodically introducing energy into chaotic systems, they can be pulled back toward order. Because the human energy field is so resilient, manipulation techniques [such as massage and vibrotactile stimulation] . . . introducing subtle energies into the system can more effectively preserve health than those therapies using chemical or mechanical interventions. (Hunt, 1996, p. 56)

This introduction of energy into a complex system is known as proportional feedback—small "nudges" to keep a dynamical system near a fixed point and not breaking into chaotic movement. Ditto (1996) researched proportional feedback techniques and found they controlled chaotic cardiac arrhythmia and epileptic brain activity.

When considering music as an intervention on this level of healing, music is actually a fractal, complex dynamical system and can add complexity to the energetic system as a whole, keeping it in that state of edge of chaos. It may also serve to provide proportional feedback to maintain stability and form. Composer and researcher David Isom composed music with particular nonlinear time patterns that mirrored the respiration patterns of premature infants. In a controlled study, he found that his specifically composed music was more effective than other music in assisting the timing of infant's breathing (David Isom, personal communication, October 1995). Though Western verification of nonlinear dynamics in human functioning is ongoing and application of this knowledge in the content of healing is still in the early stages (Goldberger, 1992), an exploration of human energetic systems and the use of music as an intervention in this system will be useful in exploring the reasons why music can contribute to the content of healing.

Human Energetic System

Current models of intervention to treat physical illness are based on traditional Western medical models of human anatomy and chemistry. Looking at physical health from an energetic perspective is new to Western medicine. However, a human energy system has been postulated and used by non-Western medical traditions, such as Chinese medicine and Indian Ayurvedic medicine, for thousands of years (Gerber, 1988). Only recently has Western medicine begun to acknowledge the impact of the human energy system on health and healing. Since sound/music is a complex energetic system, its influence on the energetic system of the body is another way in which music therapy can interface with physical functioning.

Mechanical physics defines energy as the ability to do work. Energy is the ability of something to act on and influence something else (Laskow, 1992). In classical physics, this term includes an entropic dynamic—the amount of energy or power diminishes over time and space. In acoustics there is the phenomenon of diffusion—the loss of acoustic wave power over distance as an example of an entropic process. However, when referring to a human energy system or field, the term *energy* is also used to describe processes that act on something, have impact, but which may not lose power over time or distance. Much of this form of energy is generated at the atomic or quantum level, which does not follow the rules of mechanical physics. Though many theorists question whether these quantum fields affect the large or macroscopic world, there is much evidence that shows quantum mechanics apply in all physical situations regardless of scale (Wolf, 1989). Glenn Rein (n.d.) notes that

> . . . in addition to having real physical effects on inert matter, quantum fields have effects on living biological matter. . . . Since quantum fields exist at more

fundamental levels than traditional EM [electromagnetic] fields, it is proposed here that quantum fields regulate the action of the more dense EM fields. EM fields in turn regulate or effect biological processes. (p. 12)

Before exploring both electromagnetic and quantum energy fields, it is important to understand what an energy field is. Fields are nonmaterial regions of influence, of pattern information, and of action at a distance. Fields allow objects to affect one another even though they are not in physical contact (Whitmont, 1994b). It was Albert Einstein who first formed the Unified Field Theory in physics. There are five basic premises of this theory. He first postulated that matter is organized energy and, second, that fields—the underlying energetic patterns—are characteristic of the universe. In his third premise, he states that all matter is underlain with energy fields, which are the basis of substance itself. As a century of research in quantum physics has taught us, everything in our material world is made of energy, including the human body. "The earth is one enormous energy field—in fact, a field of fields. The human body is a microcosm of this—a constellation of many interacting and interpenetrating energy fields. . . . [W]e are beings of energy, living in a universe composed of energy" (Collinge, 1998, pp. 2, 4). Einstein's fourth premise states that there are no firm boundaries between these fields. Because there are no boundaries between energy fields, they become continuous mediums of transmission and information storage. This is especially true of the interaction of human energy fields and the fields that surround us. As Hunt (1996) observes, "The most important level from which to understand the world and human beings is the level of the field transaction. We know that living things have dynamic fields which constantly and selectively transact with all environmental fields" (pp. 47–48).

Finally, Einstein affirms that fields extend everywhere, evolve and grow, and are frequently in a state of disequilibrium (deterministic chaos), evolving into higher levels of complexity (Hunt, 1996). Energetic systems evolve and grow through the nonlinear dynamics of self-organizing systems. The human body is an energetic field that evolves and becomes more complex. The human energetic field interacts with the energy fields around it. Our cell membranes, existing at the edge of chaos, allow the information from surrounding fields to enter our bodies. "Theorists of complex systems believe that biological membranes, where the edge of chaos is found, serve as the space transition between field and tissue. This is the place where information gets in" (Hunt, 1996, p. 24). It is now believed that the human energy field is a complex, multilayered organization of energy from its densest form in physical structure, through the lighter energy of molecules and body tissues, to the electromagnetic energy of brain waves, to the subtle energy of consciousness.

Human Bioenergy Anatomy

We have an energetic anatomy as well as a physical one. There is an energetic communication network in addition to the chemical mechanism. The human bioenergy body is composed of ". . . multiple, interacting energy fields that envelop and penetrate our physical body, govern its functioning, and extend out into the world around us. This anatomy serves as a vehicle for the circulation of vital energies that enliven and animate our lives" (Collinge, 1998, p. 20). This energy body comprises a combination of physical and *subtle energies*—energy that is currently unmeasurable. According to energy researcher Glenn Rein (n.d.), "The bio-energy body is seen as a complex, nonlinear synergetic interaction between these forms of energy around the body. The new energies generated by such a non-linear interaction would be quantitatively and qualitatively different from the individual components" (p. 4).

Our physical bodies are encased in and penetrated by these energy fields, and this influences what happens to us physically (Collinge, 1998). According to Western medical approaches,

> . . . these energy fields [EKG, EMG, EEG] are usually considered by-products (almost waste products) of the biochemical reactions in the body and are not considered by most [Western] biomedical researchers to be involved with the basic functioning (or healing) of the body. The basic tenet of energy medicine is that these fields are not only involved with the functioning of the physical/chemical body but regulate these processes. (Rein, n.d., p. 7)

This theory contends that the energy body serves as a template or mould for the physical body. The energetic template preserves the shape, arrangement, and fundamental function of the material parts of our body.

> Molecules and cells are constantly being torn apart and rebuilt with fresh materials from the food we eat. But, thanks to the controlling L-field [life-field or energetic body], the new molecules and cells are rebuilt as before and arrange themselves in the same pattern as the old ones. (Burr, 1972, pp. 12–13)

The human energy field maintains the pattern in the midst of the physical, chemical flux over time, regulating and controlling living things. "It must be the mechanism, the outcome, of whose activity is wholeness, organization, and continuity" (Burr, 1972, p. 33). As energy researcher William Tiller (1997) notes,

As one digs deeper into the nature of living systems, one finds that they are very complex photoelectrochemical devices that emit a wide spectrum of photons, and that homeostasis at the chemical level requires a network of fields and currents flowing within the fabric of the body's cells and tissues. (p. 3)

The bioenergetic field creates and organizes the form and substance of the body. These energy fields are dynamical systems and are regulated by the principles of complexity science and nonlinear dynamics. Once the field is structured, it becomes self-organizing and able to perpetuate itself (Laskow, 1992).

Based on this human bioenergetic field theory, illness and disease have their genesis in disruptions or disharmony in the energetic body. As Hunt (1996) observes, "I believe that all diseases are caused by a break in the flow or a disturbance in the human energy field. Eventually, this disturbance is transferred to the organ system creating functional, and ultimately, destructive changes" (pp. 77–78). Several possible mechanisms are working here that could cause disruption in energetic systems to create disease states. First, there may be a disruption in the movement of energy.

The more complicated the structure [like in the human body], the more it requires energy transactions to maintain its integrity. Open systems have a dynamic and shifting balance, whereas more closed ones have a static balance and are more threatened by sudden, catastrophic field changes. When a system becomes closed and stagnant, structural mutations occur. Probably cancer is such a mutation. (Hunt, 1996, p. 48)

The lack of complex movement in the energy system causes the physical structure to become rigid, losing its ability to stay dynamically at the edge of chaos. "The healthy body is a flowing, interactive electrodynamic energy field. Motion is more natural to life than non-motion. . . . What interferes with flow will have detrimental effects" (Hunt, 1996, p. 48).

Another way in which the energetic system may cause disease in living cells occurs when some agent (virus, bacteria, toxin) creates a phase shift in the energetic resonance. If sufficient phase shift occurs, eventually biochemical changes occur in the cells, which precipitate disease (Hado Music Corporation, 1996). Each disease or functional disturbance would have its own energy field signature, which would need to be reversed before healing could occur.

In a bioenergetic theory of disease, healing requires the reharmonization and re-energization of the bioenergetic body. Healing involves the activation of the body's energies toward ". . . dynamic equilibrium, growth, and evolution. . . . [Health] should be viewed as the perfection and maintenance of a dynamic energy field which is flowing, coherent, and strong, giving it the capacity to vibrationally interact" (Hunt, 1996, pp. 244–245). A *coherent field* is one in which energies have a fixed relationship over time that allows the energies to "hold together." The energy is in phase (Lehrman, 1990). Frohlich (1986) theorizes that to maintain health, living systems must produce coherent or laser-like vibrations in all parts of the living matrix. He believes the living organism is very sensitive to information conveyed by coherent signals. Such signals integrate the system processes and the functioning of the organism as a whole. He further believes that each cell, tissue, and organ has a resonant frequency that coordinates its activities (Oshman, 1996). For healing to occur, the energy system has to be retuned and re-energized through resonance of these coherent signals. "In this case information is transmitted by external fields of similar frequency, with healing occurring through a 'tuning' effect" (Pecci, 1997, p. xvi). More complex energetic fields, such as those that occur in human functioning, require greater energy and more complexity in the energetic input to effect this retuning process. Music influences energetic healing on all levels of the bioenergetic field. Let's explore these levels, starting with the densest biological energy.

Levels of the Bioenergetic Body
The bioenergetic body is made up of energies ranging from dense or low frequency to subtle or immeasurably high frequency. Our energetic anatomy includes "octaves" of energies stacked one on top of the other from dense to subtle. The physical body is nested in this series of energy bodies. Each level has its own characteristics (Christie-Murray, 1988; Hutchinson, 1986; Pearson, 1957; Ten Dan, 1990). According to Hunt (1996),

> Human energy fields display a continuum. The extremely low frequencies (ELF) are directly involved with life's biological processes. The extremely high frequency (EHF) patterns ally with the mind-field and awareness. The general pattern of ELF is similar for all people, while the EHF reveals a personal signature of emotional patterning for each person. (pp. 110–111)

Each type of energy in the human energy field can and does influence functioning. There are three general types of energy involved in a healing process—dense energy, subtle energy (SE), and uncharacterized forms of SE or non-Hertzian energy (Rein, 1992). The human energy body is composed of these same energetic forms.

Dense Energy
  The first and most dense energetic level is *electromagnetic energy* (Collinge, 1998).

Electromagnetic energy (EM) is a physical energy that can be measured. Electromagnetic energy extends from low frequencies to radio, microwave, heat (infrared), visible light, ultraviolet to X and gamma rays. The lowest frequencies are indeed found in living systems. Thus heart activity and brain waves are in the extremely low frequency range of about 1 Hz to 100 Hz. (Srinivasan, 1997, p. 1)

Our bodies produce direct electrical current (DC). The electrical energy of the body is recorded in the range of 500 to 20,000 Hz (Hunt, 1996). Interestingly, this is the approximate hearing range of the human ear. This dense form of energy is electromagnetic because electricity and magnetic fields are related. As we know from basic physics, electric currents create magnetic fields, and changing magnetic fields create electricity (Brophy, 1999). The body itself generates this measurable EM energy. Every atom, molecule, cell, gland, or tissue of a living animal generates at least one EM energy band. EM energy radiates from the body as a result of electron orbit changes and the physical rotations and vibrations of the molecules, flexure of cell membranes, and pulsations of organs and body movement in general (Tiller, 1997). Candace Pert (1997) theorizes that the joining of the neuropeptide receptor and its ligand in the immune system generates this EM energy. Additionally, each substance in our bodies—chemical, protein—has a unique EM signature, which serves much like a fingerprint to identify specific material.

> The number and variety of electromagnetic fields in and around the human body are beyond our power to calculate. Still, it is reasonable to suppose there must be a subsuming, overall field that is ever changing yet unique—your own personal electromagnetic signature, as distinctive as your face, fingerprints, voiceprint, and DNA. Such a field would be weak in terms of energy output but extremely specific and highly organized in terms of information. And information theory tells us that the more precise and coherent the information, the less energy is needed to carry it. (Leonard, 1997, p. 14)

DC electricity specifically and EM fields generally have been investigated extensively as physical healing agents. Becker and Marino (1982) showed that manipulation of the body's electromagnetic field stimulated healing in ways not possible through mechanical or genetic means. Adey (1981) has shown that external EM fields directly affect a wide variety of tissues including the immune, cardiovascular, nervous, and muscular-skeletal systems. Rein (n.d.) points out that ". . . biological systems show nonlinear responses to weak EM fields—i.e. the cellular response is greater than and/or different from the energy which is put into the system" (p. 22). Extremely low EM fields can help or harm the body.

> The low frequency activity of the nervous system is both a problem and a blessing. These endogenous fields could couple easily with external fields; thus, the external fields could be used both for destabilizing the nervous system as well as for therapeutic purposes. (Srinivasan, 1997, p. 1)

Research using weak EM fields on cells showed that the flow of calcium to the cells exposed to EM radiation was significantly greater than in the controls, showing that weak EM fields can significantly affect living human cells (Leonard, 1997). This research found that it was the frequency of the EM energy and not just the amplitude that created the effects. Tyler (1975) found that application of weak EM fields had observed effects at the organism, cellular, and molecular levels. Through extensive research, Becker and Selden (1985) also found that small amounts of applied DC current creates changes in red blood cells that begin regenerative processes, including bone healing. They also found that DC electricity induces sleep and decreases pain.

One of the most interesting potential applications of weak EM fields involves the electrical charge that emanates from an energy healer's hands. In research, healers generated large measurable voltage pulses ten to the fifth power times normal levels (Tiller, 1997). Large amplitudes of frequency change have been noted in healers who meditate or focus intention on healing (Fahrion, Wirkus, & Pooley, 1992; Schwartz, Russik, & Beltran, 1995). As Tiller (1997) notes, "One sees the large electrical voltage pulses as physical level correlates of the subtle level energy manifestations associated with the healer's intentionality to create a healing event . . ." (p. 17). This hints at where the dense EM energy may interact with subtle energy, which is explored next.

In addition to direct application of DC current to the body for healing either through external electrical current or biological current from a healer's hands, DC current is also generated within the body itself through a process of *transduction*. Transduction involves the conversion of one form of energy into electrical energy. Mechanical vibratory pressure on the body, especially the bones, generates an electric charge. This is due to the *piezoelectric* structure of the human body. Piezoelectric property involves the conversion of pressure or vibration into an electrical charge and vice versa. This attribute allows various bodily structures, including DNA, connective tissue, and cells, to readily convey information and transfer energy (Laskow, 1992). Hunt (1996) notes that connective tissue ". . . has piezoelectric capacities, which can act like an electrical system, where stretching enhances the electrical capacity. . . . Connective . . . tissue seemed to dictate the flow of electromagnetic energy throughout the body at the finest level" (p. 12). Once generated, this electrical energy and the magnetic fields it creates could propagate throughout the body, ". . . through the extracellular matrix (the space between cells), which is composed of a complex lattice network. . . . This network is composed of several highly structured protean molecules (like collagen) which are wound around each other into double and triple helixes. . . . [T]hese proteins are piezoelectric" (Rein, n.d., pp. 17–18). Because of this piezoelectric phenomenon, the vibrotactile impact of sound on the body may be a source of potentially healing DC electrical current.

Another form of dense energy is bodily acoustic energy. This also factors into the internal piezoelectric system of the body. Acoustic energy involves the sounds produced by bodily function, including digestion and muscle activation (Barry, 1991).

> Unlike intrinsic EM fields, which are generated in the body from moving ions and electrons, acoustic energy is produced from oscillations [of] large biomolecules or even whole tissues. . . . Of particular interest is the acoustic oscillations of DNA . . . due to the vibrating and undulating motion of the helix itself. (Rein, n.d., p. 9)

Bentov (1976) found a special system of tuned oscillations in the body driven by the rhythms of heart action. Through feedback, a 7-Hz acoustical standing wave is created that reverberates in the skull cavity via cerebrospinal fluid pulses. Our bodies are sensitive to this acoustic energy. These bodily sound waves produce corresponding electromagnetic waves, which are carried via piezoelectric effect through the crystal lattice system of the connective tissue. The sonic resonances for a particular body part occur in a significantly lower frequency range than its electromagnetic resonances. "Because collagen, tissue and bone are all piezoelectric materials, the small stresses produced by the sound wave patterns generate associated electric field patterns and thus emit EM wave patterns" (Tiller, 1997, pp. 106–107). Additionally, as discussed in chapter 3, the ear itself transduces the mechanical energy of sound waves into electrical impulses of neurons, providing yet another source of electrical current in the body.

The question then arises: Can external acoustic input from music create or add to the electrical current of the body? Rein (n.d.) states that the body is sensitive to EM and acoustic fields when applied externally. Vibrotactile impact of sound on the body may be a source of potentially healing DC electrical current because of this piezoelectric phenomenon. Additionally, if the music therapist is generating electrical pulses from his or her hands while playing in response to the intention to heal, a potentially high level of DC current may be generated. In a music therapy intervention, then, there is potential for generation of a large amount of electrical energy—through vibrotactile stimulation activating the piezoelectric transduction of mechanical energy, through the ear transducing sound waves into neurological electrical impulses, and through the therapist's hands as the music alters his or her state of consciousness and creates the healing intention.

The best-known healing system utilizing the generation of electrical current through piezoelectric processes is acupuncture. Eastern medical practices of China, India, and Japan theorize a system of energy transfer throughout the body. This involves *chakra* points—primary energy centers in the body—and *meridian lines*—routes of energy distribution in the body. The "geography" of these routes forms the basis of acupuncture treatment. Research by Hiroshi Motoyama (see Jackson, 1992) has now scientifically measured the location and energy flow in the human meridian lines hypothesized by Eastern medicine. These energy centers are located at points where external energy— dense and subtle—is transduced into subtle energies used by the body.

> This model allows the external EM and subtle environment to communicate with the internal physical and subtle substance of the body via a network of points on the surface of the body. . . . [W]e should think of the individual chakra–endocrine pairs as transducers of energy from the subtle levels to the physical level. (Tiller, 1997, p. 121)

Music is used to directly stimulate acupuncture needles (Jing et al., 1991). This research showed music electroacupuncture was more effective than traditional electroacupuncture, acupuncture, or ultrasonic therapy in treatment for muscle tone loss. According to Diamond (1981), the body receives sound in two ways: through the ear and through the acupuncture points. Since acupuncture circumvents brain activity tapping directly into the energy field (Hunt, 1996), music may influence the energy system in the same fashion.

Our bodies produce EM fields, but, based on acupuncture theory, they also receive EM energy from the outside environment through these energy centers (Schwartz et al., 1996). Tiller (1997) notes that the material of the body both emits EM energy in some pattern and also absorbs it: "Thus, each system is in communication with the outside world (transmitting and receiving) via its resonant frequency spectrum" (p. 106). The human body can be thought of as both a receiving and a transmitting antenna. The energy field surrounding our body ". . . is both an information center and a highly sensitive perceptual system. We are constantly 'in communication' with everything around us through this system, which is a kind of conscious electricity that transmits and receives messages to and from other people's bodies" (Myss, 1996, pp. 33–34).

How the transfer of energy from the outside environment to the interior of the body occurs is open to much speculation and research. One prominent theory postulates the use of *soliton waves* moving through the body as the mechanism of transfer. Soliton waves are coherent, highly ordered, nonlinear waves that are capable of loss-free energy transport. They move through space, including the human body, without changing shape and without breaking apart even if they interact with other nonlinear waves (Campbell, 1996). Soliton waves consist of individual sine waves of both EM and subtle energy bound by nonlinear interactions and coupled by feedback (Briggs & Peat, 1989). They carry the memory of this energetic nonlinear coupling. In contrast to linear waves, soliton waves remain localized and self-stabilizing. However, a weak external field of the appropriate frequency can break the soliton, releasing a large amount of energy. In a characteristic nonlinear reaction, a weak external force can produce a strong effect. Solitons are macroworld phenomena. Tidal waves and tsunami are soliton waves that can travel over great distances without dissipating. Soliton waves carry information from one point to another.

Soliton waves are present in the human body and serve this information-carrying function. Nerve signals are known to be soliton waves since nerve impulses move at a constant speed and do not dissipate. "Some theoreticians have called the nerve soliton the 'elementary particle of thought'" (Briggs & Peat, 1989, p. 129). In the human body, energy brought into the body from the energy centers is transduced at the receptor points through piezoelectric processing, and soliton waves are generated. These waves are then propagated throughout the body along the collagen network of the body. Collagen constitutes the connective tissue in the body and may be the anatomical, electromagnetic circulating system. Collagen is the main structural material of the body and consists of a metastable biopolymer—chain-like molecules marked by a slight margin of stability. Because it can become changed or unstable, collagen can serve as a conductor of EM energy (Becker & Selden, 1985). Solitons propagate along the backbone of these biomolecules.

The theory proposes that glycoproteins on the surface of the cell membrane interact cooperatively in response to weak EM fields and communicate this information to the inside of the cell via solitons that propagate through the cell membrane along the backbone of helical proteins. (Rein, 1992, p. 291)

The soliton wave traps the EM energy and carries it along as the wave moves through the body. When a weak force finally breaks the soliton at a certain place in the body, the undissipated EM energy is released. This is an amplification effect that allows very weak fields to influence cellular activities. If an external force of a particular frequency due to piezoelectric phenomenon triggers this whole process, it has potentially important implications for the impact of music on physical healing. Could the complex interactions of certain sound combinations be the force that instigates the soliton wave in the body? Could music at a particular frequency break the soliton so that the EM energy is released?

It is also possible that the large acoustic waves of sound serve as carrier waves for EM energy. A carrier wave is a wave of low frequency that transports vibrations of higher frequency, such as EM energy. The acoustic wave would then instigate a piezoelectric reaction and generate a soliton wave. Additionally, the acoustic wave, and particularly the frequencies of the higher harmonics of a complex tone, may serve to break the soliton and release the EM energy. This potential impact of music on the human energetic system needs further study in order for music therapy interventions of this type to be appropriately used to influence physical functioning.

Subtle Energy

In addition to EM energy, solitons can also carry another type of energy found in the human energy system—*subtle energy*. EM energy serves as a carrier wave for subtle energy, delivering it to bodily structures. Subtle energy is the next layer of the human energy body. Dense, measurable energy (EM and acoustic) has a mirror relationship with subtle energy. These energies interact in complex ways. Albert Einstein was the first physicist to use the term *subtle energy* (Rein, 1992). He defined subtle energy as the "energy" or force remaining in the absence of all known forces. Subtle energy is a nonphysical yet active field. It is an information field, not a force field (Rein, n.d.). Numerous researchers, healers, and scientists have been developing a theory of subtle energy and its underlying mechanisms (Gerber, 1988; Hunt, 1996; Rein, 1992; Rubik, 1992; Tiller, 1997). Many terms have been used to identify this level of energy. These include quantum potential, scalar energy, zero point energy, longitudinal waves, vital energy, and time-reversed waves (Rein, n.d.). All these terms are used to describe subtle energy because this type of energy does not obey the laws of classical electromagnetic field theory. Subtle energy is nonphysical causality interacting with the physical.

As an information potential, many believe that subtle energy is initially generated at the quantum level. For a long time, it was believed quantum dynamics had no relevance to biological processing. However, the emergence of a new discipline, quantum bioenergetics, has changed that with its descriptions of the anomalous energetic properties of biological systems. "The quantum processes described in this discipline are postulated to be the fundamental energetic phenomenon behind the natural self organizing and self healing capabilities of all biological systems" (Rein, n.d., p. 6). According to this theory, subtle energy mediates the communication network between all cells in the body. Based on research by Olariu and Popescu (1985), Rein postulates two additional components to the energetic system. "These two extra components, which are referred to as quantum potentials can be viewed as subtle forms of the electric and magnetic components" (Rein, n.d., p. 10.). He further contends that these quantum fields in the body will resonate with external fields (like music) when applied to the body.

Subtle energy cannot currently be directly felt or measured, but its effects have been demonstrated apart from other energetic influences. Subtle energy fields have been generated experimentally (Abrams & Lind, 1978; Pepper, 1982; Smith, 1964; Wells, 1970). Extensive research demonstrated various effects of subtle energy, including an impact on biological systems (Gagnon & Rein, 1990; Puharich, 1984; Reid, 1989; Rein, 1989). Reid (1989) demonstrated subtle energy effects on salt crystallization at a distance, while Rein (1989) and Gagnon and Rein (1990) found a 76 percent increase on immune system lymphocytes (in vitro) exposed only to subtle energy. Tiller (1997) has shown that subtle energy mechanisms can affect DNA. Rein (1989) showed that subtle energy can have even more profound effects on the nervous system than conventional EM fields.

Because subtle energy is not physical in the sense that the dense energies of EM and acoustic waves are, scientists have been unable to measure subtle energy with scientific instruments that have no parts above the physical. We just do not have the instruments with the parts needed to extend into the realm of subtle energy. Currently, the human body/mind is the only instrument that can perceive subtle energy.

We all have a remarkable capability to sense energies that may not be detectable by technological means. Each of us has, in effect, a subtle perceptual system that we often rely upon without even being aware of it. . . . [I]t appears that our ability to detect and work with subtle energies is based on a transduction system that involves our endocrine glands, our nervous system, and our own biofield—*to which these systems are coupled.* (Collinge, 1998, pp. 15, 17)

The collagen that makes up our bodies comprises liquid, crystal-like receptors sensitive to subtle energy, and ". . . our right brains, freed from the limitations of the left brain, are capable of quantifying the reception of subtle energies from other dimensions" (Tiller, 1997, p. xiii).

Non-Hertzian Energy

A higher dimension of subtle energy, known as *non-Hertzian energy,* has also been proposed. Non-Hertzian energy fields do not reside in our ordinary four-dimensional space/time as the previously mentioned quantum potentials do. Non-Hertzian energy is a fundamental quantum energy field underlying the quantum potential fields and the dense EM field. It is these layers of the energy body that ultimately manifest as matter (Rein, n.d.).

The non-Hertzian fields have a number of interesting properties, including *nonlocality.* Nonlocality is information or influence transfer without local signals such as electromagnetic or physical means of influence (Haaland, 1999). The effects from them can occur at a distance since, according to quantum theory, all matter in the universe is related by nonlocal forces or implicate order out of which the explicate order (energy and matter) unfolds (Bohm, 1980). The studies on distance healing, including prayer, are examples of the nonlocal effect of non-Hertzian energy (Aston, Harkness, & Ernst, 2000). In this way, non-Hertzian energy is information as distinguished from classical forms of energy. This energy exerts influence not through an agent of force but, rather, as information transfer agents. These fields have a subnuclear origin, generated ". . . in the monopoles and anti-monopoles located within protons [of the atom]. . . . [P]rotons and neutrons in the nucleus . . . absorb scalar [non-Hertzian] energy when it interacts with matter" (Rein, 1992, p. 294). Like quantum coherent states, non-Hertzian energy implies a sense of oneness, where instant knowing occurs. Haaland (1999) writes, "The quantum-wave properties of the very small are shown in some degree with the complexity of information patterns inherent in *living systems.* It is postulated that the metabolic energy and dielectric properties of biological systems are sufficient to result in large-scale *quantum coherence*" (p. 15). This non-Hertzian energy can interact directly with the nucleus, which implies that this energy can interact with matter at a fundamental subnuclear level. It is, therefore, nonlinear in nature. Because of this, non-Hertzian fields do not diminish with distance and are not easily shielded by conventional four-dimensional means.

There is a field of subtle energy information above non-Hertzian energy that has also been theorized. This level of subtle energy underlies all other forms of energy. This energetic state was first postulated by ancient Eastern traditions of India, China, and other highly developed civilizations. Scientists are now also postulating this level of energetic information based on the principles of quantum physics and complexity science (Brophy, 1999; Hunt, 1996; Rein, 1992; Tiller, 1997). Rein (n.d.) refers to this form of subtle energy as "spiritual," acknowledging the ancient philosophical and spiritual interest in this field of energy underlying all other energetic forms. This level of subtle energy constitutes energies,

> . . . often referred to as spiritual due to their association with the non-physical world and higher states of consciousness that exist at a level even more subtle than the non-Hertzian level of the super-quantum potential. Thus, non-Hertzian energy is particularly important as a bridge between the higher dimensional levels of consciousness and the more dense levels of 4D space/time. . . . [C]onsciousness would be considered the most fundamental level of all [subtle energy]. This is the energy source from which all other forms of energy are derived. (Rein, n.d., p. 14)

In this view, higher-order awareness or states of consciousness, and perhaps, a universal consciousness, and the products of consciousness—thoughts, intention, imagery, and emotion—become the fundamental field that gives rise to and informs subtle energy. Consciousness itself becomes a form of energy and is equivalent to quantum information (Matzke, 2001).

> It is the highest form of energy and is integrally involved with the life process. If we consider consciousness as a fundamental quality and expression of life energy, we come closer to understanding how spirit interacts with and manifests through many forms of physical matter. (Gerber, 1988, p. 418)

This "spiritual" energy directly influences subtle energy, which, in turn, shapes electromagnetic energy. All these energetic levels then create and influence matter—in this case, our physical body. Intuition and consciousness operate interdependently with matter, and matter transforms them (Hunt, 1996). In other words, it is recursively organized.

Current research has begun to verify this connection of consciousness as the highest-order energy field and physical matter. Rein (1992) conducted a series of experiments using tumor cells in a petri dish. An experienced subtle energy worker with extensive practice in altering his state of consciousness was asked to instigate a particular mental state and imagery pattern or intent in an attempt to inhibit the growth rate of the tumor. Experimental results showed that different biological effects were seen when the intent or imagery of the healer was changed.

> When we included the intention for the cells to return to the natural order of the normal cell line together with the imagery of reduced growth, the inhibitory effect was doubled to 40 percent. These results suggest that imagery and intent each contributed equally in influencing the psychoenergetic inhibition of tumor cells in culture. (Rein, 1992, p. 306)

Rauscher and Rubik (1983) found the volitional intention of a healer significantly influenced bacteria growth compared to a control that held no intention. The implications of these findings are immense. Thoughts, including emotions, should be conceived of as specific subtle energy patterns. "Through the energetic patterns that we shape with our thoughts and emotions, we can support the natural healing processes in ourselves and others" (Laskow, 1992, p. 31).

Based on decades of research, Hunt (1996) theorizes that human emotion is the key subtle-energy element of consciousness that affects healing: "I strongly believe that the internal dynamics of the most complex biofield, the human energy field, are based on its emotional organization. . . . Emotion provides a force which flows and fluxes; it captains a field organization to maintain its integrity" (pp. 109–110). One particular human emotion, love, and its effects on heart functioning have been extensively studied at the HeartMath Institute (Childre, 1994; McCraty, Atkinson, & Rein, 1993; McCraty, Atkinson, & Tiller, 1993; Rein & McCraty, 1993a, 1993b). Love, defined as a benevolent intent focused toward the well-being of others, affects the heart energetically (Collinge, 1998). The heart creates the body's strongest electromagnetic field, and, ". . . with deep feelings of love, compassion, and caring this field actually expands and strengthens" (Collinge, 1998, p. 35). This supports the importance of EM energy in the human bioenergy field.

The significance of this research to music therapy practice acknowledges music as an overt energetic manifestation of unconditional love. Music embodies the wholeness and unity factor of universal love and is a concrete reminder of this state.

> [Music] activates the power of love for ourselves and for our fellow men. It alone of all the art forms can do this with such immediacy and facility. It does this whether the listener "likes" the music or not, whether he understands the music or not, whether it is part of his culture or not. This is its power. (Diamond, 1981, p. 31)

In the HeartMath research, the heart focus feelings needed for the development of strong coherent EM fields generated from the heart were enhanced when a conscious state of love occurred while simultaneously listening to music specially designed to facilitate mental and emotional balance (Childre, 1991).

The energetic significance of consciousness, emotion, and thought points out the fundamental importance of the therapist in this energetic healing. The therapist is an open energetic system exchanging energy, including thought, with the environment and with the energy fields of other individuals. The client is also an energetic system. "So, therapist and client are each a whole and complete, vibrating, rich energy form, full of potential. This form or field is experienced on the intuitive level by both therapist and client before the onset of 'therapy' . . ." (Kenny, 1989, p. 78). Healing includes interactions between the minds of the healer and the healee. "It proposes that contents of consciousness other than nonfocused thoughts, i.e., intentions and images are critical components necessary for psychoenergetic healing" (Rein, 1992, p. 311). Intention is directing attention toward a goal or outcome (Gallo, 1999). It refers to vigorous action based on vigilant observation (Wolf, 1999). Aharonov and Vardi (1980) experimentally verified the effects of intention.

The optimal mental state of the therapist conducive to healing is a high-performance mind or awakened mind state plus the ability to use that state (Wise, 2002). This state is first achieved by altering the therapist's normal state of consciousness (Laskow, 1992; Wade, 1996). The awakened mind state produces compassion, detachment, nonjudgment, clarity, equanimity, service, and unconditional love and regard in the therapist (Wise, 2002).

As explored in chapter 7, music is traditionally a means for creating an alteration in consciousness (Eliade, 1964; Harner, 1982). Through potential mechanisms of entrainment and hemispheric synchronization (Russell, 1993), music serves to create the needed consciousness state. A music therapist likely enters this state of consciousness, usually quite unknowingly, through the presence of the music and, in particular, through the act of creating music. Once in the mental state, the intention and imagery held by the therapist alter energetic patterns and become this higher-dimension energy field. This form of subtle energy is then carried to the client and amplified by the acoustical energy of music acting as a carrier wave. Rein (n.d.) believes that intention can be carried by sound waves. In music therapy practice, these intentions and imagery are formed by the knowledge of human functioning, a part of training in music therapy, and by the goals and objectives set for the client. Music creates the state of consciousness that allows for the generation of the subtle energy needed for energetic healing. While in this state, our knowledge of what needs to happen for normalization of functioning and the goals we set become the intention for healing needed for energetic impact. Gerber (1988) notes that the energetic or "spiritual" healer ". . . works as a power source of multiple-frequency output to allow energy shifts at several levels simultaneously. . . . [S]piritual healers usually work with the many levels of mind and spirit as well" (p. 319). Having explored these many levels of potential energetic healing, let's summarize how music and music therapy processing may affect the energy healing of the body.

Music Therapy and Energetic Healing

The complex, living human energy field responds more readily to elaborate, information-laden fields than to simple, isolated ones. The intricate patterns of vibration in music provide this information. Music is an external energy field that produces frequencies of vibration matching or close to bioenergetic frequencies. Complex sound organized in the complex forms of music creates the greatest amount of information and has the greatest potential for impact. This complexity of information comes not just from the harmonic structure and the vibration of the fundamental and overtones but also from the changes in rhythm, dynamics, timbre, and the regularly recurring patterns in melody and musical forms (Hunt, 1996). This exquisitely complex vibratory energy provides the human bioenergetic system with enough "information" to create the edge-of-chaos dynamics needed for it to come into resonance and coherence. The complex energy involved in music generally nourishes the dynamical system of the energy field. Disease is anticoherence in the energy field, and music acts to return this field to coherence.

For this process to occur, exposure to music must include the whole body, not just our ears, since the energetic system is a physical presence throughout and around the physical body. Since live music provides the biggest range of frequencies and dynamics, as compared to recorded music, this may be why researchers like music therapist Jayne Standley (1986) have found that live music, used by a trained music therapist, has the greatest effect in medical procedures. She found that of fifty-five dependent variables analyzed, fifty-four benefited more from the music therapy condition than from nonmusic conditions. Even if music does not exactly match the energetic vibration of the human energy field, it may still have an effect. "If, however, exact relations cannot be produced, approximate relations have a power if not of creation, at least of evocation . . ." (Daniélou, 1995, p. 4). The principles of complexity science support the idea of the "evocation" or approximation of the resonance needed to affect the bioenergetic system.

Music may affect the energetic system in other ways. Because of the piezo-electric properties of the body, the vibrotactile impact of sound may generate electromagnetic energy. A specific frequency or the harmonics of complex sound may create and/or release energetic information at the point needed in the body or energy field. If not the fundamental frequencies, then certainly the harmonic overtones in complex sound will have an impact. "Each physical body, composed of interacting, pulsating energy fields, has its own set of vibrating patterns, like musical notes, that are natural to it and with which it resonates. Since all notes have higher harmonics, we can assume the body does as well" (Laskow, 1992, p. 40).

Acoustic waves can also serve as carrier waves for both this vital electromagnetic energy and the subtle energy in the bioenergetic body. Music may very well serve to amplify and carry the subtle energy generated by the therapist's thoughts and emotions to the patient's energy field. Music embodies and creates the most beneficial of these healing states of consciousness: love. Music is, in fact, an overt manifestation of unconditional love, that state that derives from wholeness and unity. In addition, music creates the altered state of consciousness that must be present for this form of subtle energy healing to exist. It also evokes the imagery that contributes to these effects. This is explored in greater detail in chapter 6.

Mind/Body Interface

Having explored the impact of music on direct content of healing, let's now turn to the body/mind interface and the role music plays in this important area for physical functioning. Beginning with Descartes' theoretical split of mind and body (Damasio, 1994), Western medicine has assumed that aspects of mind do not influence physical functioning, health, or healing. This assumption has been challenged by non-Western medical traditions and by recent research that shows that there are anatomical connections between the nervous system and the immune system. Ader and Cohen (1975) found a bidirectional neurological link between the brain and the immune system, while Pert et al. (1985) identified and isolated identical chemical messengers in the brain and immune system. Other research documented the affect of emotional states on immune system functioning. Irwin et al. (1987) found that depression weakens the immune system. "Vulnerability to illness may arise in part because feelings of powerlessness depress the immune system and disrupt the cardiovascular system" (Robertson, 1999, p. 204). As will be explored in greater detail next, chemical discharges in the brain associated with improved immune functioning are triggered by various events or states, including environmental factors such as music, state of mind, and social and spiritual changes (Bartlett, Kaufman, & Smeltekop, 1993; Rider et al., 1990; Tsao et al., 1991). There is ever-increasing evidence that states of mind do affect physical functioning and health. These discoveries led to the science of *psychoneuroimmunology* (PNI), the scientific study of the mind/body connection.

Music and PNI

PNI acknowledges the connections among the body, its functioning, and states of mind. Such states of mind include emotions and feelings, events and experiences, sense of control, hope, beliefs, memories, attitudes, thought patterns, and motivations and behavior. Lloyd (1987) states that PNI focuses on reactive patterns of emotion and behavior that may predispose an individual to disease. More researchers are finding that the mind has *physical* effects on the body. Functions of mind have downward effects on the physical level (Winkelman, 2000). In fact, they are finding that aspects of mind affect biology in specific ways because there are numerous ways in which the central nervous system (CNS) and the immune system communicate. Our immune system defends the body against invasions from bacteria, viruses, toxins, and foreign bodies. The biological pathways that make up the mind, the emotions, and the body are not separate but, rather, intimately entwined (Goleman, 1995).

Early research by Rossi (1986) found that there were several messenger systems in the body: neurotransmitters of the autonomic nervous system (ANS), hormones of the endocrine system, and the immunotransmitters of the immune system. These three messengers target organs, tissues, and glands of the body (Maranto & Scartelli, 1992). The first evidence that the CNS and immune system communicate is in the anatomical similarity of the two systems. There is anatomical commonality between these two basic functions. Thought, emotion, and immune response are processed in the same areas of the brain and body (Rider, 1992). The nervous system and immune system are found at identical places throughout the body. "These nervous/immune system connections are extremely comprehensive. Both branches of the autonomic nervous system, the sympathetic ('fight or flight') system, and parasympathetic ('relaxation') trunks innervate immune tissues. . . . This means that both stress and eustress have direct involvement in the immune response" (Rider, 1997, p. 24).

A number of these common structures and their importance in sound and music were explored in previous chapters. For example, the reticular activating system (RAS) plays an important role in information transduction within the mind/body connection (Scartelli, 1992). Rossi (1986) noted that a state of alertness, derived from novel stimulus, is needed to be present in order for new learning to occur. The reticular formation is the brain structure that creates that alertness and receptivity to new information. As explored previously, auditory nerve input has an effect on the reticular activating system and allows sound to provide a high level of novel information through its complexity.

The hypothalamus, another brain structure influenced by sound/music, mediates all the functions of the immune system and has a large role in emotional response. "The hypothalamus, in effect, receives messages from all portions of the nervous system, therefore providing a connection between behavior and the generally automatic functions of the autonomic, endocrine, and immune complex" (Maranto & Scartelli, 1992, p. 143). This directly affects the neurotransmitters of these structures, the first messenger system in the body. The endocrine system regulates the secretion of chemical messages (hormones) that influence organs, tissues, and glands of the body. These chemicals, the second messenger system of the body, are another important part of immune system functioning.

The presence of certain hormones in the body shows improvement in immune system functioning. Extensive research on the secretion of one such hormone, IgA, has been conducted.

> IgA in the saliva is the body's first line of defense against germs entering through the mouth and nose that produce, among other illnesses, respiratory tract infections. . . . People with higher concentrations of IgA show a more rapid increase in antibodies to germs, making them less likely to become ill than people with lower levels of it. (Collinge, 1998, p. 154)

Increasing IgA levels has positive effects on health. Numerous studies have shown that music, especially music therapy interventions, through its impact on ANS, can help increase secretions of IgA (Rider et al., 1990; Tsao et al., 1991). Bittman, Berk, Felten, Westengard, Simonton, Pappas, and Ninehouser (2001) found that group drumming increased dehydroepiandrosterone-to-cortisol ratios and increased lymphokine-activated natural killer cell activity, indications of increased immune system activity. Music does affect the release of certain hormones, which, in turn, creates a chain reaction of immune system functioning. Other research found that music, music and imagery, and healing imagery in general affect the levels of other hormones like adrenal cortico-steroids (Rider, Floyd, & Kirkpatrick, 1985) as well as interleukin-1 and cortisol (Bartlett, Kaufman, & Smeltekop, 1993). In physical healing, a mental image was shown to activate the brain area responsible for sensing the corresponding actual input. So when a mental image of the sound of the ocean occurs, appropriate auditory areas of the brain are activated. As in other aspects of physical healing, health seems to require the dynamic stimulation of many portions of the brain. Music produces this stimulation and the rhythmic stimulation needed for the health effect (Rider, 1997). The importance of rhythmic shifting is explored later in the chapter.

The third messenger system in the body involves the immunotransmitters of the immune system or neuropeptides. Pert's (1997; Pert et al., 1985) research on neuropeptides and their receptors identified the mechanisms involved in the action of cells of the immune system and underscores the connection and, in fact, inseparability of mind and body. The immune system comprises the spleen, bone marrow, lymph nodes, and a variety of white blood cells—some circulating in the body and others residing in bodily tissue like skin. The immune system defends against invading pathogens and repairs damage various external agents might inflict. "To do this, the immune system must define the boundaries of the organism, distinguishing between what is self and what is not self . . ." (Pert, 1997, p. 181). To communicate this distinction, Pert identified a system of receptors and their corresponding ligands, which constitute this complex and comprehensive chemical communication system in our bodies.

The ligand-receptor information network links all our systems and organs—the brain, the glands, the immune system—through the coordinated actions of the discrete and specific messenger molecules (Pert, 1997). The neuropeptides ". . . serve to weave the body's organs and systems into a single web that reacts to both internal and external environmental changes with complex, subtly orchestrated responses" (Pert, 1997, p. 148). One of the most important internal environmental changes affecting immune functioning is emotion. Pert, in fact, concluded from her research that no state of mind exists that is not reflected by a state of the immune system.

Because of this extensive connection of emotions and the immune system, our emotional states have a strong impact on our physical health. According to Bittman (2000), PNI research has shown that general mental attitude makes a medical difference and interacts with the other factors primarily responsible for health: genetic susceptibility and lifestyle. Our general mental attitude or mood is deeply affected by music. As explored in the next chapter, music affects our overall mood and general emotional state, stimulates production of natural endorphins (A. Goldstein, 1990), and engenders a sense of community and belonging. Tiller (1997) reports extensive research demonstrating the immuno-enhancing effects of positive emotional state and the immuno-suppressive effects of long-term negative emotion.

Individual, specific emotional states also have a direct impact on health.

> Viruses use the same receptors as neuropeptides to enter a cell, and depending on how much of the natural peptide for a particular receptor is around and available to bind, the virus that fits that receptor will have an easier or harder time getting into the cell. Because the molecules of emotion are involved in the process of a virus entering a cell, it seems logical to assume that the state of our emotions will affect whether or not we succumb to viral infection. (Pert, 1997, p. 190)

Emotional states, especially long-term states like heightened stress, can diminish immune system functioning (Selye, 1978). Much of the PNI work focusing on the impact of emotions on the immune system involves long-term stress management and reduction.

Stress

Any emotion or behavior creates *stress*—a physical reaction of alertness and preparation to act. Stress becomes a problem only when it is prolonged or unmanageable and becomes a stress reaction or *distress*. Stress is a physiological reaction to the perception of threatening situations. "The perception of such threats generates a sustained stress reaction in which the adrenal glands secrete epinephrine which affects glucose metabolism, norepinephrine that increases heart output and blood pressure, and steroid stress hormones such as cortisol" (Taylor, 1997, p. 105). Distress causes increased wear and tear on the body and ultimately suppresses the immune system. The actions of the amygdala contribute physiologically to the stress reaction. The amygdala sends projection to parts of the brain that react to adverse stimuli. These include the lower brain stem, which controls ANS functions, and an area in the hypothalamus that stimulates secretion of stress-related hormones. The amygdala also organizes behavioral responses to emotions, especially fear and anger (Taylor, 1997). Prolonged stress contributes to many serious physical diseases, including coronary artery disease, hypertension, stroke, irritable bowel syndrome, and migraine headaches. These are often referred to as "time diseases" because they are caused or aggravated by concern with deadlines, worries, apprehension about the future, and obsession with past events. "In general, any illness in which anxiety and excessive time awareness have been shown to play a role belong in this growing category of human maladies" (Dossey, 1989, p. 39).

Music has been used throughout history to combat stress, induce relaxation, and promote health (McClellan, 1988). The biblical story of David soothing King Saul's depression and anxiety is a good example. More current music therapy practice and research (Mandell, 1996; Robb et al., 1995; Scartelli, 1984; Scartelli & Borling, 1986; Stratton & Zalanowski, 1984; Thaut, 1989) verified the effectiveness of music as a stress reducer. The mechanisms that produce this effect are not completely known, however. There are likely a number of factors contributing to music's relaxation effects.

The first possible factor relates to the idea of stress as a time sickness. A very effective intervention for this type of stress is to retrain the time sense. As noted previously, music is an event that occurs over time and has the capability of altering time perception. As with biofeedback training and meditation techniques, music can slow the perception of time passage and allow attention to be focused on the present moment. Cultivation of this focus is a known stress reducer (Green & Green, 1989).

A second way in which music may reduce the stress reaction is the various direct physiological effects of music on the body. Such effects may first be based on the shared or closely allied areas of the brain that mediate both sound perception and stress reaction. The initial stations of auditory processing, the cochlear and olivary nuclei, are in the medulla oblongata and are in close proximity to specific nuclei that control heart and respiration rates (Scartelli, 1991). Heart and respiration rates are often indicators of stress and anxiety levels. "Music has a direct effect on specific physiological processes whose functional variations are indicators of anxiety, tension, or stress" (Taylor, 1997, p. 103).

These physiological changes associated with relaxation may also be the result of direct stimulation of the parasympathetic nervous system. Stress involves long-term activation of the sympathetic nervous system (Winkelman, 2000). To counter this, the parasympathetic nervous system must be activated. The parasympathetic nervous system slows down all bodily processes including heart rate, respiration, blood pressure, and oxygen consumption (Collinge, 1998). Sound input activates both the sympathetic (arousing) and parasympathetic nervous systems (Taylor, 1997). Relaxation effects may be due to a particular sound input's direct stimulation of the parasympathetic nervous system. "Rhythmic music allows one to both arouse and relax, perhaps due to differential information outputs at different times" (Scartelli, 1991, p. 37).

Repetitive rhythm has been shown to be particularly effective in promoting the relaxation response (Neher, 1962). One area of the brain, the locus coeruleus, changes novel sensory input into heightened psychobiological states. However, dull, monotonous, or repetitive input, such as repeated steady drumming, decreases the activity of this brain area leading to relaxation, drowsiness, and even sleep (Scartelli, 1991). Koepchen, Droh,

Spintge, Abel, Klussendorf, and Koralewski (1992) elaborate on the effects of music on these physiological reactions, which they refer to as neurovegetative processes. Their research found that relaxation promotion did not occur because music created consistently slow or unchanging measurements of heart rate, blood pressure, and respiration but, rather, produced a regular shift between tension and relaxation. This regular rhythm of shifting in music matched that of the neurovegetative processes.

> It cannot be pure coincidence that the harmony of mind induced by many pieces of classical music is not based on constant low levels of tension . . . but on the organic change of strain and relaxation around a medium level very similar to the natural time course of our neurovegetative parameters. (Koepchen et al., 1992, p. 58)

This finding points again to the 1/f spectrum shift that occurs in nature, human functioning, and music.

A third potential physiological effect of music on the stress reaction is postulated by Taylor (1997), who theorizes that the complex input of music occupies the neural pathways that might otherwise be carrying increased arousal associated with stress.

> With musically stimulated impulses occupying neural pathways throughout the brain, the orbitofrontal cortex is less able to focus on self-concerns in determining emotional responses. The positive responses are sustained and replicated as the individual's brain stores conditioned emotional responses resulting from the effects of music on the medial division of the medial geniculate nucleus in the thalamus. (Taylor, 1997, p. 76)

Music-induced stress reduction has also been postulated to occur because of changes in brain wave speed. Chemical means of stress reduction, such as alcohol or barbiturates, do slow brain wave activity with resulting decreases in anxiety. Though a shift to a slower brain wave state cannot be assumed to *create* relaxation, the slower brain waves are associated with a relaxed state. Research, though not conclusive, has indicated that sedative music can produce an alpha brain wave state (Benson, 1975; Borling, 1981; Kenyon, 1994). This slower brain wave pattern is associated with meditative states, drowsiness, and daydreaming, which are all states of increased relaxation. A similar approach to relaxation involves the synchronization of neural discharge patterns between the two hemispheres of the brain (Russell, 1993). This synchronization is said to promote a sense of calmness and mental focus. Widely developed by the Monroe Institute of Virginia, hemispheric synchronization strives to ". . . produce in the listener whole-brain coherence, a state of consciousness defined when the electroencephalograph (EEG) patterns of both hemispheres are simultaneously equal in amplitude and frequency" (Russell, 1993, p. 15). Brain synchronization occurs because of a frequency following response—entrainment—and binaural beat stimulation. "When you listen closely to sounds of specific frequencies, you tend to reproduce those frequencies in your own physiology. Furthermore, you can become entrained to the state of awareness (such as relaxation) engendered by those frequencies . . ." (Russell, 1993, p. 15). Though the Monroe Institute techniques use specific beat frequencies created through binaural hearing to produce this effect, the potential for music and certain forms of musical production—use of gongs and metal bowls—has the potential to also create this effect (Leeds, 2001). Music and brain wave production and brain synchronization are addressed more fully in chapter 7.

As reviewed in chapter 3, the research on physiological reactions to music as it relates to stress reduction and relaxation has been largely inconclusive and inconsistent (Radocy & Boyle, 1997). Though music does influence human physiological processes, what these effects are, how extensive they are, and what will trigger the reactions vary greatly from individual to individual. There is likely a process of complexity working here where numerous factors in addition to the sound input are at work. As Koepchen et al. (1992) note,

> The reaction to these exogenic [outside] signals is different in different subjects. Music is a special kind of exogenic signal mediated by the auditory sense. Thus, it has to be expected that *the action of music will be quite different in different people.* Their constitution, education, and life history have a part of play. We can assume that this will likewise apply to the widely unknown action of music on neurovegetative rhythmicity. (p. 59)

As explored, music can potentially have a number of physiological effects that could engender a state of relaxation.

Another way in which music may affect the stress response is in the direct action of emotions. Koepchen et al. (1992) attribute changes in the neurovegetative rhythmicity to emotions and speculate that music's generation of emotion is faster in its impact on rates of respiration and heartbeat than on other physiological interactions. Positive emotions can support the relaxation response by offering a release of negative emotion. The link of music and emotion can have another important effect on our physical health. The overwhelming negative emotions of physical and emotional trauma can damage our health. It is not the experience of an emotion per se that is the problem. In fact, as Rider (1997) points out, ". . . a wide variety of emotions may provide the best balance for the optimum dose of chemicals associated with health" (p. 88). However, the repression of strong emotion has serious effects on our health. In a study of women with breast cancer, Greer and Morris (1975) found that the suppression or expression of anger was the key factor in whether a woman developed cancer or not. Other studies (Scherg, 1987; Temoshok, 1987) showed that repression as a coping skill directly affected physical health. Pert (1997) relates this suppression of emotion to the activity of the neuropeptides of the immune system. She sees disease-related stress in terms of an information overload,

> . . . a condition in which the mind–body network is so taxed by unprocessed sensory input in the form of suppressed trauma or undigested emotions that it has become bogged down and cannot flow freely. . . . When stress prevents the molecules of emotion from flowing freely where needed, the largely autonomic processes that are regulated by peptide flow . . . collapse down to a few simple feedback loops and upset the normal healing response. (1997, pp. 242–243)

The important emphasis here is simple flow versus the normal state of complex flow. Based on the activity of the neuropeptide network, repressed traumas caused by overwhelming emotion can be stored in a body part, affecting it directly. In this case, health is promoted by an honest expression of emotion. "All honest emotions are positive emotions. Health is not just a matter of thinking 'happy thoughts.' Sometimes the biggest impetus to healing can come from jump-starting the immune system with a burst of long-suppressed anger" (Pert, 1997, p. 193). The "jump-start" of emotional expression is known psychologically as *catharsis*, a deep, intense expression of emotion. An increasing body of evidence (Ikemi et al., 1975; LaShan & Gassman, 1958; Pennebaker, Keicolt-Glaser, & Glaser, 1988; Spiegel et al., 1989; Weinstock, 1977) shows that the expression of repressed emotion has positive effects on physical health and disease states.

Music is known to evoke and support cathartic expression. The link of music and emotion and the powerful effects of sound input on emotional centers of the brain give music the ability to evoke repressed emotional states. Music also then allows for the intense expression of those emotions (Bonny, 1978). Additionally, certain emotional states can positively influence the immune system. The emotional centers in general need regular use and activity just as our muscle and cognitive functions do. Specific emotional states, like having a sense of control, seem to positively counter stress and provide needed support to immune functioning (Scartelli, 1992). As previously discussed, music is an important stimulus to a wide range of emotions, with sound directly affecting the limbic system. Participation in music making also engenders the sense of control so important to immune system functioning. As we make music, especially with music therapy techniques like improvisation, we make the decisions about what sounds will be heard, when the music will begin and end, what emotions will be portrayed, and how others will respond. Such techniques give clients a true sense of autonomy and control.

PNI and the Importance of Rhythmic Shifting

Music therapist Mark Rider (1997) has proposed an expanded theory of psychoneuroimmunology he terms homeodynamism. Homeodynamic theory states that ". . . every atom, molecule, and cell in our body speaks the same language (homeo), and we just need to shift (dynamic) to the different mental frequencies to perceive this elegant symphony" (Rider, 1997, p. 33). Homeodynamism is based on the rhythmic and harmonic nature of our body/ mind functioning. In this theory, mind, brain, and body are organized harmonically with neuropeptides that promote quick and precise communication between the nervous and immune systems (Rider, 1997).

There are many examples of the rhythmic/harmonic organization of body functions and their relations to disease/health. Multiple frequency oscillations exist in the nervous, cardiovascular, endocrine, and immune systems. "It turns out that these multiple rhythms within any one system are integral multiples of each other, making any one rhythm the harmonic of another" (Rider, 1997, p. 34). As Rider points out, we are, in effect, musical instruments.

> Our acoustic spectrum in this case is the waveform of the EEG. And, if we play out of beat with the cosmic drummer (nonharmonically), we steer further from health. The fact that harmonic organization is more prevalent in health than in disease has important things to say about the communication between the nervous and immune systems, and the mind and body. (Rider, 1997, pp. 38–39)

For example, DNA patterns that vary from the harmonic models normal to our body/mind create proteins that are harmful to us. Optimal muscle health depends on rhythmic shifting between normal contraction limits and relaxation to baseline levels (Rider, 1997). As Pert (1997) points out, the T-cells of the immune system (attack cells) recognize a body as "not foreign" because of its harmonic relationship to the receptors on the T-cells. The relationship between the nervous and immune systems is rhythmic and harmonic. Individuals with suppressed immune systems have a deficient conductor function to time the sequence of immune reactions in an orderly

fashion (Rider, 1997). Another example of the rhythmic/harmonic functioning of the body/mind is production of brain waves (measured by EEG).
Brain waves are harmonically organized with alpha being twice theta and
beta being twice alpha. Nonhealthy individuals show nonharmonic EEG
patterns. These abnormal EEG patterns either cause disease or reflect a disease state. In fact, certain EEG (brain wave) frequencies are also directly involved in proper immune functioning. Delta brain waves foster the production of many immune chemicals (Rider, 1997). As just explored, alpha waves
may also play a role in immune system function.

Homeodynamic theory uses both the electrical properties of the CNS to
explain the immediate and direct PNI effects and the neuroendocrine
mechanism to explain the slower and less direct PNI phenomena utilizing
rhythmic shifting as the common element in these processes (Rider, 1992).
This theory assumes that the most adaptive and healthiest environment for
living systems is not homeostasis (maintenance of stability) but, rather, a
state of continual movement and flux of changes between levels of organization. This "state of flux" corresponds to the edge-of-chaos dynamics discussed in this chapter. Rider sees this flux as having predictable rhythmic
shifting that likely corresponds to the 1/f spectrum variations noted
throughout nature. It is this constant and complex state of shifting that is
essential to health.

The second basic principle of homeodynamism is based on the idea of dy-
namism, which includes the belief that all phenomena can be characterized
by interactions between forces. The healthy body is normally in periodic
(regularly recurring) flux. Stress and disease are produced when these regular
variations are *prevented* from occurring (Rider, 1997). Homeodynamic theory
states that living systems are constantly reorganized and reintegrated through
rhythmic activity (Rider, 1992). This rhythmic activity monitors and tunes
the body/mind to ensure adaptive functioning and constitutes regularly recurring periodic shifts that enable us to cope with environmental change and
life stressors. These rhythmic fluctuations are important to the body because
". . . information can be transmitted by variations in any oscillating signal.
When these variations are frequency-based. . . . the information can be transmitted more efficiently. Secondly, energy can be saved and even created
through an oscillating system" (Rider, 1997, p. 32).

Health and healing, then, depend on this constant, regular movement or
shifting. Mental shifts of some kind, an imagery or belief shift, are necessary
for physical healing because ". . . the more dynamic activity that occurred in
the brain, the more the immune system was boosted" (Rider, 1997, p. 7). The
connection of mind and body is absolute.

Thus, the EDR (electrodermal response) modulation by the baseline component of the EEG can be thought of as the mechanism for mind–body interactions. In other words, this electrical field is both our mind and our body, simultaneously. A physical shift cannot occur without a mental shift. (Rider, 1992, pp. 153–154)

Shifting is also essential for changes of psychological state, like depression and multiple personality, as will be explored in the next chapter (Putnam, 1989).

Music and Homeodynamism

For these necessary shifts to occur, the brain must respond to incoming stimulation without habituation. The brain responds to novelty, to the edges and changes in an input. As Rider (1997) notes, "Hearing is the one behavior that the least amount of habituation and adaptation occurs by an organism. . . . In other words, no matter how often they are repeated, sounds create more profound psychophysiological shifts than most other stimuli" (p. 93). Because of this, sound, and particularly music, can be very important in creating this shifting dynamic. Both the overt musical rhythm and the rhythmic input our ear translates as frequency create such shifts.

Increasingly, research has demonstrated the ability of music to produce several different types of brain shifts. These include shifts both in brain wave frequency and in hemispheric activity. The importance of music's ability to shift brain wave speed to promote PNI effects is in the shifting itself not in the promotion of any one brain wave state (Rider, 1992). Normal immune system functioning seems to require the brain's ability to shift dynamically and easily into a wide range of electrical brain wave activity.

Rider (1997) identifies several ways in which music creates the shifts in brain waves (the speed of electrical activity) needed. First is the impact of tonal and rhythmic elements of music on shifts in brain wave speed. From the use of Tibetan bowls, to chanting practices of medieval monks, to the relaxing "New Age" music of today, music has been used to alter our state of alertness by changing brain waves (Goldman, 1992; Halpern, 1985). A number of studies (Borling, 1981; Kabuto, Kageyama, & Netta, 1993; Neher, 1961; Nicosia, 1994; Wagner & Menzel, 1977) show that sound/music can produce shifts in brain waves. Interestingly, the shifts to slower brain wave states may not be due to particular characteristics of the music but, rather, to the listener's familiarity with it and the pleasure derived from it. Bruga and Severtsen (1984) found that the subject's determination of music as "relaxing" was the important factor in alpha brain wave production and EEG slowing. Stratton and Zalanowski (1984) found that self-reports of relaxation were significantly increased when the listener liked the music. Finally, Rider (1997) notes that there is a shift to slower brain waves during creative activity. This may be why no cultures have ever been discovered that did not have the creative arts, especially music. Creativity may be an adapting survival-linked behavior for two reasons: (1) it is a healthy expression of emotions harmful to the body, and (2) it promotes brain wave shifts so necessary to immune system functioning.

Changes in brain wave speed are often associated with alteration of states of awareness or consciousness, a subject addressed more extensively in chapter 7. Music may also produce brain shifting through alternating left–right motor patterns such as occur when performing music, which create shifts in brain wave activity (Nicosia, 1994). These alternating rhythmic movements produce a general increase in alpha activity and coherence between the left and right cerebral hemispheres in the brain wave range of theta and delta (Rider, 1997).

From this extensive discussion of the body/mind interface, it can be concluded that mind can and does affect immune system functioning and thus our overall health. Rider (1997) notes that there are ". . . many unexplored similarities between the nervous and immune systems, which will all point to the conclusion that total communication between the two is inevitable" (p. 23). In fact, one might go so far as to say that mind and body are actually one and the same. As explored previously, music affects mind and thus it influences the body, especially immune system functioning. A number of ways that music may directly affect the body as possible content of healing were explored. However, there is a second factor in healing on which music has an impact: this is the context of healing.

Music Therapy and the Context of Healing

The *context of healing* is the external and internal "environment" of the patient that is conducive to recovery and health. The context of healing influences the effectiveness of the medical interventions, the content of healing, and the overall success of the total healing process.

The external environment conducive to healing includes things like room colors, smells, lighting, visual aspects in the environment, and the auditory environment—what sounds are heard or not heard. This is the first aspect of context that can be addressed by music therapy. Music provides a humanizing aspect to an environment. Doctors implicitly recognize this by playing music in their waiting rooms. Music makes a sterile, impersonal environment inviting and gives us a link to our fellow human beings. Familiar music provides us with comforting familiarity and perceptual predictability to decrease anxiety. Music can also mask the disturbing sounds of a medical environment. I experienced this firsthand recently when I was admitted to a hospital emergency room. In this acute medical setting in close proximity to other patients, I found the sounds of various heart monitors, breathing machines, patients' cries, and doctors' and nurses' tense voice tones very disturbing. When I was able to listen to music through headphones, the sounds were masked, and I was able to relax.

Music therapists working in hospital settings contribute to this aspect of healing context in a number of ways. The hospital-based music therapist may make music—both live and recorded—available for patient rooms, in the hospital lobby, and in procedure areas. After a personal experience in a cardiac catheterization lab, I supplied the hospital with tapes of music to be played while patients undergo this procedure in this very cold and sterile environment.

The other aspect of context of healing—the internal environment of the patient—refers to the patient's psychosocial functioning and reactions. This area involves the patient's subconscious and conscious mental state. Pert (1997) affirms that our conscious mind plays a deliberate role in immune system functioning. Research reported in Rubik (1992) shows that an active role of conscious participation in the material world, including the functioning of our body, is vital. Though these effects are small, complexity science tells us that small things can make a large impact. The various factors contributing to an internal context of healing may be seemingly small factors but can have a large impact on health.

The first aspect of the internal context for healing is a person's general psychological state, including one's general mood. A positive, optimistic mood is far more conducive to health than sadness, fear, or anxiety. There is much support for the impact of music on mood (Radocy & Boyle, 1997). This is particularly noted in the use of music to reduce preoperative and other medical procedure anxiety. The music therapist prepares music programs for use in pre- and postsurgery areas. As mentioned earlier, having music playing while waiting for surgery significantly decreases anxiety. Music played through headphones is also used during surgical procedures and in the recovery room (D. Cowan, 1991; Miluk-Kolassa, Matejek, & Stupnicki, 1996; Robb et al., 1995). Music played to the patient during surgery decreases pain and nausea and promotes a faster recovery with fewer complications. It is also used to mask the voices of the surgical team and eliminate the possibility of "posthypnotic suggestions." "Studies show that language understanding continues during anesthesia, though explicit recall of what is said does not. But the understanding is enough to allow patients to recognize meanings of what is said to them" (Russell, 1993, p. 28). Music is further used to distract patients, especially children, from medical procedures (Malone, 1996; Turry, 1997).

Emotional awareness and expression make up the second aspect of the internal context of healing. As Goleman (1995) writes, "There is a margin of *medical* effectiveness, both in prevention and treatment, that can be gained by treating people's emotional state along with their medical condition" (p. 165). As previously noted, verbally and nonverbally expressing strong emotion has medical benefits. As explored at length in the next chapter, music is a powerful tool for evoking, recognizing, and expressing emotional states.

Context of healing also involves the patient's social ties and sense of affiliation to a group. Spiegel, Bloom, Kraemer, and Gottheil (1989) found that the survival rate of patients with breast cancer doubled because of their participation in a support group. They felt an affiliation with a group of women who had experienced the same disease and treatment they had experienced. This gave the patients a significant survival advantage. Childre (1991) reports that people with a strong sense of affiliation have decreased levels of stress hormone and higher IgA levels. As explored in chapter 7, music is a powerful tool for creating group experiences, feelings of affiliation, and social support. "Musical experiences also have the power to reduce physical symptomatology through group support, or sociospiritual, mechanisms" (Rider, 1997, p. 104). Music therapy experiences can help create patient groups, provide for family support groups, and offer social outlets when hospitals and medical facilities isolate people from each other.

Finally, the internal context of healing involves the overall state of mind including the general belief system of the patient. Hunt (1996) notes, "Healing and belief systems work together—the healing system being the way the body mobilizes all of its resources. The belief system is often the activator of the healing system" (pp. 253–254). A general belief system involves our outlook on life. Is the patient generally pessimistic or optimistic? Does he or she handle change by taking it in stride, or does it add to stress? It also involves a belief in the ability to get better, a will to live, a trust in the treatment modalities, and a hope for recovery (Schlitz, Taylor, & Lewis, 1998). These are deep-seated and often unconscious beliefs. For this aspect of context to influence healing, a person must have the ability to change the fundamental belief about the self from one who is sick to one who is well. This vital change of belief takes place nonverbally in the deepest parts of the brain (Achterberg, 1985). These brain parts include the limbic structures and our nonverbal right hemispheric processing. Both areas are critical in processing and appreciating music. In the next two chapters, the ability of music to reach and transform the fundamental beliefs we carry is explored in depth. Of course, our fundamental beliefs also involve spirituality and religious expression. There is increasing evidence that religious observance and general spirituality—the beliefs and values a person holds relating to one's place in the universe and to one's connection to a power greater than self and physical reality—are in and of themselves beneficial to health. Benor (1990) reviewed over 300 studies documenting the positive effects of "spiritual" healing and spiritual beliefs on health. As explored in chapter 3, music and religion have been intricately related since earliest human history (Gaston, 1968a). Music can link us to our beliefs about the Divine and remind us of the tenants of our religious faith. It fosters hope and brings us into a reality greater than ourselves alone. Through transcendent or peak experiences, music can also support all aspects of the human spirit and our spirituality, which is examined extensively in chapter 7.

Wellness

Before moving to the next two chapters to explore music therapy and emotions and music therapy and the human spirit, one additional topic related to music therapy and body—wellness and prevention—is addressed. The use of music therapy techniques to promote wellness and prevent physical problems from developing is a newer area of practice for the field. Health is a state of optimal well-being, not just the absence of disease. A state of wellness indicates the best possible individual condition. On the physical level it involves a correlation or resonance among all cells in the body (Wolf, 1986). As explored at length in chapter 8, it also involves a resonance with all parts of human functioning. Music therapy for wellness is the use of music therapy processes in the prevention of illness and promotion of continued health. Clearly, the discussion of music therapy and immune system functioning is relevant here. Music therapist Dr. Frederick Tims (Koga & Tims, 2001; Kumar et al., 1999) conducted extensive research with well older adults and found that active music making decreases anxiety, depression, and loneliness while increasing the growth hormone hGh by 92 percent. The production of this hormone indicates a state of health and wellness. Specific music therapy practice with older adults to foster wellness has been developed in recent years (Clair, 1996). These techniques are based on active music making. They emphasize enjoyable, social activities that engender fun and recreation. There is an emphasis on group bonding and attentional focus. Activity interventions include instrument playing, group singing, active music listening, and movement and dance.

This chapter explored the vast and complex biological theories as they relate to the music therapy theory of music and soulmaking. To understand this complex theory of health and healing completely, yet another layer of complexity—psychological functioning and theories of human psychology—must be added. Just as physics theories are insufficient to explain human functioning, so are biological theories. Understanding the biology of human functioning is necessary but not a complete or sufficient explanation for what is happening in a music therapy intervention. The next chapter turns to human psychology, and then we explore in chapter 7 the role of human spirit in this process of soulmaking.

~

CHAPTER SIX

Music Therapy and Problems of Emotion and Feeling

This case study comes from my personal experience as a music therapy client. I am taking the first training workshop in "Guided Imagery and Music," a depth psychology technique using music to evoke personal imagery and emotions. It is the first time I will experience this process as the client. After getting comfortable and relaxed, the preselected classical music begins. Prompted by my music therapist, images form in my mind. I'm in the house of my infancy. I see the living room and the hallway into the kitchen. Suddenly my Aunt Jessie appears. A close family friend, Aunt Jessie always had an important place in my life. Her image appears to me as she looked in her late eighties, just as she looked when she died in 1990. I feel great sadness. My therapist prompts me to ask this image why she came. "Because you have something to say to me," she replies. And I realize I need to tell her how sorry I am she died alone, how guilty I feel I wasn't with her. Huge waves of grief well up from deep in my stomach. I am sobbing, my body racked with the physical expression of this grief, this guilt. The music playing supports this emotional expression and shapes the images throughout the experience. I tell her out loud all I need to say and cry with deep heaving sobs. After thirty minutes the music and experience ends. I feel a great release. A sense of physical and emotional lightness grows, and I realize what has happened. This was a profound catharsis of long repressed emotions. The healing of an old wound has occurred.

Having addressed music therapy for problems of the mind and problems of the body, it is time to turn to problems of emotion and feeling, ego and identity, psychological development, and mental illness. These are the issues of human psychology—the study of human nature. Psychology deals with the mental structure of a person, especially as a motivating force. This study goes beyond the properties and faculties of mind addressed previously. It delves into the human psyche's relationship not only to biology and the environment generally but to the particularly human interactions of culture and society. Also addressed here are the problems that can arise in this area, referred to as mental illness. This area of practice in music therapy is known as psychiatric music therapy—the uses of music therapy techniques and interventions in treating mental illness. The current chapter addresses general psychological growth; problems of feeling, mood, and temperament; and the problems of mental illness. Chapter 7 addresses another psychological manifestation—issues of spirit or our reconnection to our essential wholeness as a state of being. As a physics theory alone could not explain human biology, we now find that a biological theory alone cannot explain human psychology. Psychological, anthropological, and cultural theories are now added to the overall complexity of the music therapy theory of music and soulmaking.

Stages of Psychological Development

Many theorists of psychology—from Freud, to Jung, to, Piaget, to Wilber—believe that human development unfolds in specific stages or levels. By moving successfully through each developmental stage, a healthy sense of individuality is established and ultimately a mature identity emerges that both transcends and includes the personal self (Schwartz, 1996). McCarthy (1978) defined a developmental stage model of human psychology that theorizes a set sequence of specific and increasingly complex developmental stages. The belief is that no developmental stage can be skipped and that each higher stage incorporates, transforms, and then reintegrates the previous one. The stage model requires a hierarchy of structural wholes where later stages are more complex and encompassing and are built on previous stages (Wilber, Engler, & Brown, 1986). This psychological theory mirrors the theories of recursive development in complex, biological systems explored previously. Psychological development can thus be seen as a self-organizing system. Wilber, Engler, and Brown (1986) postulate that this approach leads to two great areas of human development—one leading up to the personal, individual sense of self or ego development and one leading beyond it. The current chapter addresses the first area of human development and the problems that can occur as individuals move through the stages, while the next chapter addresses human development moving beyond the personal ego.

Stage theories of human psychological development began with the earliest theorists. Sigmund Freud (1920) did pioneering work in psychoanalytic developmental theory or the stages of psychological development (Bruscia, 1998c). According to Freud, this development involves psychosexual stages and culminates in the development of the individual ego. Erickson (1959) proposed a stage theory based on life cycle, while Mahler (1968) based her developmental theory on formation of object relations.

Jean Piaget (1977) postulated cognitive developmental markers in the mental skills of developing children. Each level in his hierarchy denotes certain cognitive skills that underlie knowledge and consciousness. This development proceeds through fixed stages that represent different degrees of adaptation to the environment (Winkelman, 2000). In Piaget's theory, each stage must be met in order for cognitive development to occur and is achieved only when a child matures to a particular stage. Rider (1977, 1981) theorized that various music skills correspond to the cognitive tasks at each of Piaget's developmental levels and found, in particular, that auditory conservation of sound concepts does occur as theorized by Piaget for visual conservation. As discussed in chapter 4, music therapy techniques can be used to help children develop these various cognitive skills and to promote movement through the developmental sequence.

Various non-Western traditions have postulated levels of human development beyond the personal or ego level. Ken Wilber (1977, 1986) proposed a theory of development he calls the spectrum of consciousness, which encompasses all these levels and theories. "Consciousness" was explored in chapter 4, using the word to refer to either core consciousness or basic alertness and self-referential consciousness, or being aware of being aware. In psychological theory, the full spectrum of growth and development from self-concept and identity and beyond is referred to as a "development of consciousness." Hunt (1995) states, "It would appear that the proper metaphor for becoming conscious is that of growth rather than of opening a door between separate areas . . ." (p. 39). As a psychological theory, the development of consciousness refers to ways or forms of seeing, acting, and interacting with the environment (Wade, 1996). Wilber envisions consciousness as having many dimensions composed of many levels. Each level ". . . contains a unique outlook on the world, in other words, each embodies its own form of perception. This has to do with dimensionality, the number of dimensions accessible to consciousness, and the form that they take" (Combs, 1995, p. 97). Each level has its own worldview and is shaped by its own neurological underpinnings and personal life experiences. Each level of consciousness involves and integrates increasingly more of the neurological system and, as Wade (1996) theorizes,

234 ~ Chapter Six

". . . perhaps other bioelectromagnetic fields" (p. 260). For individuals to grow, they must be able to access greater neurological capacity and thus shift their worldview—the form of awareness and the relations of self to the world. In Wilber's theory, psychological growth involves moving up step by step through these hierarchical levels. Consciousness evolves over the lifetime of a person, moving from identification with macroworld concerns to the more subtle or transpersonal aspects (Combs, 1995).

According to this theory, consciousness evolves when a crisis is faced that cannot be resolved by using the particular type of worldview currently available to the individual (Wade, 1996). Every stage of development has its own inherent limitations.

> The inherent limitations create a type of turmoil, even chaos, and the system either breaks down (self-dissolution) or escapes this chaos by evolving to a higher degree of order (self-transcendence)—so-called order out of chaos. This new and higher order escapes the limitations of its predecessor, but then introduces its own limitations and problems that cannot be solved on its own level. (Wilber, 1996, p. 50)

To grow and evolve through the levels of psychological development, individuals must be challenged and pushed through experiences to access more neurological capacity and shift the worldview of the level they currently utilize. Various music therapy techniques, such as improvisation and deep listening techniques like Guided Imagery and Music, can provide the intense, emotion-laden experiences needed to open consciousness to more neural capacity and shift the learned worldview.

Wilber (1996) identifies nine levels of consciousness. The first level is the *prepersonal* and includes reactive, naive, egocentric stages. The second level, *personal*, includes the conformist, achievement, and affiliative stages. The final level of consciousness is the *transpersonal*, which includes the authentic, transcendent, and unity stages. Each level of consciousness is linked to behavior characteristics and pathologies or mental illness, and each level responds to a different type of therapeutic approach. Most schools of psychology focus on one major level of this hierarchy of development. All are correct and useful at their level (Wilber, 1996). Music therapy techniques can and do fit into every level. As Bruscia (1995) observes, "Music is like consciousness in that it can be in one mode [level] fully, in transition to another mode, in several modes at once, or not in a mode at all" (p. 168). It is beyond the scope of this book to address in detail each of the nine specific levels of consciousness theorized by Wilber (1977), Wade (1996), and other writers. Music therapy practice as it relates to the three general stages of consciousness development is examined first. Subsequently, the issues of mental illness and treatment at each level are addressed. In Wilber's theory, the prepersonal stage includes core consciousness, the unconscious, and emotions and feelings. The second stage, the personal level, includes ego and identity development. The third stage is the transpersonal level, which involves awareness beyond the ego level and the human spirit (addressed in the next chapter). Let's begin with the prepersonal level. This level is important because it elucidates the issues of mental illness and its treatment utilizing music therapy techniques.

Prepersonal Level of Development

Prepersonal development involves early stages of consciousness development that lead up to and are necessary for the emergence of the personal self or ego. This level constitutes awareness before referential consciousness develops and involves subconscious processing and emotion and feeling.

Subconscious Processing

Much of psychological theory is based on the presence of two layers of psychic organization: the subconscious and the conscious.

> Depth psychology has attempted to model the adult human as two great psychic/somatic organizing systems: the unconscious one with many interconnected subsystems we share with all biological organisms, and the conscious ego-organizing system with abstract language capabilities that only humans seem to have developed. (Shulman, 1997, p. 129)

As previously explored, most of our cognitive functioning is subconscious, including our basic core consciousness and embedded unconscious structures, like grammatical rules that are unconscious to us yet govern speech patterns. In psychological theory, especially as it relates to mental health, unconscious material also implies submerged materials that are repressed, screened, or pushed to the background by the effects of the emerging ego structure (Washburn, 1995). Our unconscious processing influences our conscious activities, including memory, motivation, and especially behavior. As Jung noted, "Part of the unconscious consists of a multitude of temporarily obscured thought, impressions and images that—in spite of being lost—continue to influence our conscious minds" (quoted in Russell, 1993, p. 171). A large percentage of our unconscious material originates in childhood. "Adult consciousness has separated out from childhood integration and is unconscious of the continuing 'child'—integrating activities going on in the background of conscious life" (Shulman, 1997, p. 129).

Washburn (1995) identifies a number of ways in which childhood experiences become unconscious. The first way is through filtering. This involves predetermined ways in which the mental ego unknowingly organizes or interprets experience, such as habits, systems of condensed experiences (preconception of and response to experiences based on previous events), cultural assumptions and values, and biologically based patterns of response. When a new experience triggers a filtering mechanism, it is excluded from awareness because the unconscious filter responds below conscious level. A common example of the filtering process occurs when we are driving a familiar route out of habit. We can arrive at our destination without any conscious memory of the trip. Because we have a habit of making the drive, it is filtered from consciousness. Another form of filtering involves condensed experiences. An example of a system of condensed experience, known as a "COEX system" as theorized by Grof (1975), occurred with a roommate I once had. A COEX system is composed of highly emotional memories, meanings, and behaviors associated with a particular experience. These are formed when the first experience has a strong negative or positive impact, forming a preconceived and preprogrammed response to later similar experiences. In the case of my roommate, her first roommate had listened in on her phone conversations. The first time I inadvertently picked up the phone to make a call while she was on the extension, she reacted in an angry, aggressive manner. Her COEX system on this issue predisposed her to believe I was "snooping" and to react defensively even though my motivation and behavior were not the same as in her previous experience. A psychological "complex" that can affect mental health, like an inferiority complex, is an example of a COEX system (Washburn, 1995).

The second way in which experiences become unconscious is through ego identity. When an experience does not match our self-concept, our ego structure does not allow it to become conscious. If a person holds a self-concept as being a moral person, the conscious mind may not be aware of a behavior where the person committed an illegal or immoral act.

Finally, experiences can become unconscious through the action of psychological defense mechanisms. Psychological literature identifies these mechanisms as repression (rejecting unpleasant ideas, impulses, etc.), projection (attributing repressed aspects of the self to others), reaction formation (behavior formed in direct opposition to a repressed impulse), rationalization (attributing superficial but untrue motivations for behavior), intellectualization (ascribing rational motivations to emotional reactions), and denial (refusal to believe). These psychological processes can cause life experiences to be pushed into the unconscious as a means of defending the ego and self-concept. For example, highly stressful and emotionally charged events, especially in childhood, cause repression of experiences that can lead to serious problems, including mental illness.

> The most deeply buried materials of the personal submerged unconscious are those that have their origin in serious abuse or trauma during early childhood. . . . [These] cause grave psychic injury. To survive, the child must cover over the wound in its soul and attempt to deny the reality of its experience. (Washburn, 1995, p. 151)

This "repression" occurs in young children because of the biology of the brain and memory formation. The release of brain chemicals during a traumatic event can actually block memory formation (LeDoux, 1996). Goleman (1995) notes that these early memories are

> . . . stored in the amygdala as rough, wordless blueprints for emotional life. Since these earliest emotional memories are established at a time before infants have words for their experience, when these emotional memories are triggered in later life there is no matching set of articulated thoughts about the response that takes us over. (p. 22)

Additionally, the corpus callosum, the information channel between the left and right cerebral hemispheres, does not fully mature until age ten. "So a child has a wealth of experience available to the right brain that isn't transmitted to the left side; a good deal of unconsciousness exists before the age of ten simply because the information network isn't in full working order" (Janov, 1996, p. 202). The memories of early traumatic events are literally wordless. They exist only as emotional states and reactive behavior patterns. These suppressed, unconscious events and the wounds they cause affect consciousness development and mental health when they push into our conscious brains and, especially, into our behavior. It is emotion that carries these suppressed experiences into our current lives and functioning and is an important aspect of the prepersonal level of development.

Emotion

Previous chapters explored at length the importance of subconscious emotion for learning, memory, motivation, reasoning, and problem solving. Looking at psychological development and problems of mental health, it is important to examine the layers of emotional expression in humans. In psychological terms these are issues of *affect*. Affect is an organized pattern of changes comprising several physiological and psychological systems. These changes include arousal of systems (increased blood pressure), suppression of systems (decrease of gastrointestinal movement), or steering of the function of a system in a specific direction (imagination of anger such as fantasies of revenge). Specific affect is characterized by a typical configuration of such changes that can be identified (Noy, 1993). The word *affect* encompasses *emotion* and also *feelings, mood,* and *temperament*. The terms *emotion, feeling, mood,* and *temperament* are often used interchangeably, when, in fact, they are different properties of affective behavior. Each property can be thought of as a different nuance of our emotional lives. The entire process begins with emotion. Emotion is a collection of physiological changes occurring in the brain and the body (Damasio, 1994). As explored previously, these arise in various structures of the limbic system, especially the amygdala. Feelings or conscious emotional feelings are a secondary acquisition, a subjective learned response that occurs as a function of conscious awareness and memory. As LeDoux (1996) states, "A subjective emotional experience, like the feeling of being afraid, results when we become consciously aware that an emotion system of the brain, like the defense system, is active" (p. 268). In fact, emotion can overwhelm conscious processing.

> [While conscious control] over emotions is weak, emotions can flood consciousness. This is so because the wiring of the brain at this point in our evolutionary history is such that connections from the emotional systems to the cognitive systems are stronger than connections from the cognitive to the emotional systems. (LeDoux, 1996, p. 19)

We cannot stop emotion. We can and do, however, learn to prevent the external expression of the emotion as feelings.

The next level of emotional expression is mood. Moods are muted emotional states that last much longer than the core emotion to which they are related (Goleman, 1995). I may have an emotion of fright when I am cut off in traffic, which, in turn, creates a feeling of anger at that driver and a daylong mood of irritation. The final nuance of emotional life, temperament, is a mood state generalized over time. Temperament is the ". . . readiness to evoke a given emotion or mood that makes people melancholy, timid, or cheery" (Goleman, 1995, p. 290). Temperament is the emotional nuance that becomes part of our ongoing personality structure. Let's look at these four levels of our emotional life as they relate to music and music therapy.

Emotions and Music

There are a number of prominent theories of emotion and music, but only a few are discussed here. The first theory involves sound/music's direct input to the brain areas responsible for emotion. As previously noted, emotions are subconscious processes beyond the reach of language and cognition. Emotion begins with arousal of brain structures found in the loosely related limbic "system" of our brains. The neurological pathways of sound provide input to these structures—the hypothalamus and amygdala—providing needed arousal (Taylor, 1997). There are even more specific ways in which music influences the neural structures associated with emotion. Research using functional MRI (fMRI) conducted by Chen, Kato, Zhu, Adrian, and Ugurbil (1996) found that during musical cognition and processing of emotions, the hypothalamus and amygdala of the limbic system are activated differently in the right hemisphere. Since many properties of music are processed in the right hemisphere, this research points to potential arousal of emotions through musical input. Ornstein (1991) also notes that the left hemisphere controls small muscles of the hands and is the hemisphere that generates happiness. As a skilled motor behavior, music performance utilizes the small muscles of the hand and may contribute to a feeling of happiness while we play. As previously discussed, sound/music input also affects the areas of our brain that control hedonic reactions—experiences of intrinsic reward, value, and positive feedback—and arousal.

> Since these same centers play a major part in processing of music stimuli, it is reasonable to assume that music stimuli may have influence on those aspects of human behavior which are related to the function of those brain areas, i.e., emotionality, motivation, mood, alertness, etc. (Thaut, 1990a, p. 9)

A second theory of music and emotion involves the nonverbal nature of emotion and music. The mode of expression of emotion is nonverbal (Goleman, 1995). Because emotion is a subconscious process, we cannot willfully control emotions and usually do not know what triggers an emotional reaction. The cause of the emotional display is not conscious (Damasio, 1999). Music is a nonverbal expression of emotion. "Because pure music has no verbal referents, it can hurdle the left hemisphere finding itself in the right, speaking to us in the language of emotions" (Summer, 1988, p. 14). As philosopher Suzanne Langer (1942) notes, "The real power of music lies in the fact that it can be 'true' to the life of feeling in a way that language cannot; for its significant forms have that *ambivalence* of content which words cannot have" (p. 243). She also states that music is composed of the gestures, forms, and shapes that are the patterns of human emotion. All the primary or core emotions—anger, sadness, fear, enjoyment, surprise, disgust—are universal in terms of their facial expression and recognizability across cultures and are present in newborns and in children born deaf or blind (Goleman, 1995; Pinker, 1997). These core emotions are inborn, have their genesis in particular but differing brain regions, and are not conditioned by environment or culture (LeDoux, 1996). In fact, the Latin root word for *emotion* denotes movement.

> All emotions are, in essence, impulses to act, the instant plans for handling life that evolution has instilled in us. The very root of the word *emotion* is *motere* the Latin verb "to move," plus the prefix "e-" to connote "move away," suggesting that a tendency to act is implicit in every emotion. (Goleman, 1995, p. 6)

Fundamentally, music is about movement and particularly about movement in time. Music stems from movement of the body (Blacking, 1973). As Storr (1992) notes, "Only music affects our emotions [as opposed to feelings]. . . . Emotions involve the body, feelings do not" (p. 183).

Manfred Clynes, in his pioneering work on sentic states (identified as a specific emotion regardless of its intensity), found that, in addition to characteristic facial expressions, each emotion has a specific dynamic motor program (Clynes & Nettheim, 1982). Clynes found that an emotion and its expression form an integrated unit irregardless of the mode of expression—gesture, facial expression, tone of voice, motor movement, or musical phrase (Gabrielsson, 1995). These units are *essentic forms* and are the motoric expression of a specific emotion. They constitute a biologic principle of emotional expression. These forms have innate meanings that transcend cultural learning and conditioning and are, therefore, neurologically coded (Ornstein, 1986). Clynes and Nettheim (1982) identified a number of biologic principles of essentic forms as the means for emotional expression. Each of these relates to the possible way in which music conveys emotion.

The first biologic principle of emotional or sentic states is exclusivity. Only one emotion can be expressed at a time. The motor pattern for a given emotion is specific to it. Second, there is equivalence in expressing any one emotion. A sentic state can be expressed by any number of different motor output modalities but is identified by the characteristic movements of a given emotion. As Wallin (1991) notes, "For each emotion there was a characteristic form of expression with a beginning, middle, and end, and a particular duration as well . . ." (pp. 489–490). Each pattern is unique and characteristic of a particular emotion. Music also comprises patterns of form (beginning, middle, and end) and duration.

Another biological principle of sentic states is coherence. A brain program or algorithm specific to that state and governing all motor outputs governs the expression of a sentic state. Therefore, each motor expression of that emotion is coherent or unified with every other expression. As Clynes and Nettheim (1982) note, "There is increasing evidence that there appears to be a single common brain algorithm for the various sensory modes underlying the production and recognition of dynamic expression of specific qualities" (p. 51). The recent research of Joseph LeDoux (1996) substantiates this contention. Kenyon (1994) believes that essentic forms are distinct waveforms, so emotion can be conveyed purely through sound waveforms without the need for language. Emotional expression in music, therefore, is a neurologically programmed gesture, which animates and provides the emotional meaning (Hunt, 1995).

The fourth biologic principle governing sentic states is complementarity. Production and recognition of essentic forms are governed by inherent data-processing programs of the central nervous system so that the forms produced can be recognized by others and will create the same sentic state in the perceiver. In other words, when we communicate an emotional state through movement, not only can other people "read" and understand the emotion conveyed but the same state is generated in them. I recently saw a videotape of artificial intelligence research involving programming a robot with the facial expressions and movement patterns of different emotions. When an individual was asked to speak in an angry manner, the robot reacted with "sad" facial expression and eye movement. What was interesting was that the human subjects immediately also looked sad and unhappy because they had made the robot "unhappy." The principle of complementarity was clearly at work. Complementarity explains the ability of music to communicate emotion to others and to produce that emotion in the listener.

The fifth biologic principle of essentic forms is self-generation. Clynes found that the intensity of the sentic state was increased by repeated, arrhythmic generation of the essentic form. The motor expression of the emotional state increased the power of the felt emotion. The continuous repetition of the essentic expression involved in playing a piece of music increases the intensity of the emotion over time. This principle may explain why loud, aggressive music accompanied by dance movements composed of the essentic forms for those emotions can increase the aggression and violence of some concertgoers.

The sixth biological principle of sentic states involves generated emotion. Clynes' multicultural research showed that a sentic state is experienced and expressed as a pure quality without reference to external situations or symbols

(Benzon, 2001). Emotion is a quality of neurological functioning (LeDoux, 1996). There is a biologically provided coherence between a basic emotion and the motoric form of expression that does not require an external vehicle of meaning. Finally, Clynes sees the communicative power of essentic forms as a function of that form itself. The power of the communication increases as the form of expression reaches its pure essentic form. Music with strong emotional impact likely allows the musicians to more closely reproduce the essentic form for that emotion.

In summary, based on the work of Clynes (1982), emotional expression through music involves the biologically determined motor expression of sentic (emotional) states. These essentic forms are universal and are expressed in a variety of motor systems, including the movements and gestures inherent in musical performance. Music can duplicate the unique patterns of motor responses for each emotional state. Music is fundamental for the venting of repressed emotions because of its ability to create an expression for essentic forms (Rider, 1997; Taylor, 1997).

In contrast to the innate ability of music to express emotions theorized by Clynes, others have looked to the properties of the music to explain music's ability to arouse and express emotion. Theorist Leonard Meyer (1956) postulates that emotion is stimulated by music because of the perceived patterns of the stimulus itself—the formal and structural components of the music, especially those that heighten expectations and postpone resolutions (Storr, 1992). A recent experiment by Damasio (1999) supports this contention. He found that when subjects experienced music, ". . . the skin conductance record was full of peaks and valleys, linked intriguingly to varied passages in the pieces" (1999, p. 50). Meyer based his theory on the ideas of Dewey (1934) and MacCurdy (1925), who believed emotion was aroused when a response pattern was blocked or when a negative or stressful situation, like a dissonant suspension in music, stopped. According to Thaut (1990a),

> Meyer transfers the tenets of these theories into music perception by postulating that listeners develop expectancy schemes when following music patterns. A carefully crafted interruption of the expectation—followed by a period of suspension and resolution in the composition—will evoke an affective experience in the recipient. (p. 4)

Jourdain (1997) further notes that discrepancies in anticipated results creates emotion and states such that ". . . it's easy to see how music generates emotion. Music sets up anticipations and then satisfies them. It can withhold its resolutions, and heighten anticipation by doing so, then to satisfy the anticipation in a great rush of resolution" (p. 312). Clearly, for this to occur, the listener requires some perceptual familiarity with the music, or there would be nothing to anticipate or resolve. Clynes' work and other research support this contention (Radocy & Boyle, 1997).

Berlyne (1971) also postulates that music arouses emotions because of embodied properties of the music. "Berlyne has shown in great detail that art works, including music stimuli, contain stimulus patterns that have specific arousal-influencing potential, and thus can induce affective experiences" (Thaut, 1990a, p. 6). Based on the principles of complexity science, those stimulus patterns can be assumed to be the 1/f spectrum variations found as a universal in nature. Emotion is then aroused when the "chaos" is resolved into a 1/f spectrum pattern. Stress is removed as the anticipated 1/f pattern occurs.

In contrast to these theories, a number of individuals do not believe music arouses specific emotions at all. Langer (1953) sees music more as an "expressive representation" of the state of being emotional. Storr (1992) believes music induces a general sense of emotional arousal. It may move us emotionally, not because it makes us sad or happy, but because we relate to the expression of sadness in the music. As Roger Sessions (1971) notes,

> What music does is to animate the emotion; the music, in other words, develops and moves on a level which is essentially below the level of conscious emotion. Its realm is that of emotional energy rather than that of emotion in the specific sense. (p. 24)

Music may not directly arouse emotion, but it sounds the way emotion feels. Music sadness feels like life sadness even though there may be no life situation to generate it.

Though emotions, as biologic imperatives, are not learned, that which triggers emotions may be. Damasio (1999) states, "While the biological machinery for emotions is largely preset, the inducers are not part of the machinery, they are external to it" (p. 57). These inducers to emotion are learned and conditioned by culture and individual experiences. Music is one of these learned triggers. For example, in Western culture, we are conditioned to hear slow music in a minor key as "sad." Hearing music of this character arouses the emotional state associated with sadness. Whether music directly arouses emotion or enlivens the subconscious emotional state in general, nonspecific ways, it can and does become attached to the conscious memory of emotion.

In summary, a vast body of research now verifies a number of assumptions about music and emotion. Music is an effective means for communicating emotional messages. When musical structures and elements are examined, they are found to correlate with subjective emotional experiences (Thaut, 1990a). Music can influence and reflect the emotional state of an individual. Therefore, music makes an effective tool for increasing emotional awareness, reflecting emotional response, and evoking an emotional state (Gfeller, 1990b). This is explored more fully later in the chapter.

Feelings and Music

Unlike emotion, feelings are conscious, cognitive events. Feelings are individual, highly subjective events that occur when emotions created by the brain are made conscious. "Feelings evolve in tandem with cognition. The achievement of object permanence and the corresponding emergence of mental images as object representations usher in feelings that are no longer just momentary responses to stimuli but are now ongoing affective engagements with enduring objects" (Washburn, 1995, pp. 84–85). Memory of these emotional states is a key factor in feelings. Music influences feelings in many ways.

Music first affects feelings because of the link of music and memory. As explored in the previous chapter, music is closely linked with memory. Music is a highly pleasurable, emotion-laden event that can facilitate memory formation. Music becomes linked with all aspects of a memory, especially the emotional state that is present. The memory of that emotional state becomes a feeling, which, in turn, is associated with the music. Having a feeling response to a particular piece of music comes from a process of conditioned response. The music is linked to certain memories, and we become conditioned to have that certain feeling when we hear the music again. This involves *extramusical associations*. Something other than the musical elements, the memory, is stimulating the feelings. Because of this, feelings are very individual and, therefore, can be used as an effective therapy technique, as explored later in the chapter.

Music further affects feelings because of the mental images (*intrasubjective material*) it evokes. As Damasio (1999) notes, feelings are a matter of creating mental images of the internal states created by emotion. Music may itself be such a mental image of emotion. The flow of emotion becomes a feeling because it is mirrored in the musical event. It conveys the feeling of the emotion symbolically and formally as an external event (Edelman, 1992) and becomes the mental image of an emotional state, and through that process it becomes a feeling. This is the basis of Helen Bonny's Guided Imagery and Music technique (Bonny & Savary, 1990). Supporting Bonny's use of classical music in this technique, Borling and Scartelli (1987) found more vivid imagery and feeling states were produced when classical music was used. Classical music is more rhythmically consistent, which is shown to produce more vivid imagery compared to other music. Music's stimulation of imagery was explored extensively in chapter 4.

Mood and Temperament and Music

The next level of emotional nuance is mood. Moods are more muted and longer lasting results of an emotional state. Mood states alter memories, thoughts, and behavior. Changing mood can have a strong impact on all these aspects of our functioning (Ornstein, 1991). We are culturally conditioned to assign moods to music whether hearing the music actually arouses that particular emotional state in us or not. In Western culture, certain musical elements— tonal patterns, tempo, and rhythm—are associated with different mood states (Radocy & Boyle, 1997). A piece like Tchaikovsky's Sixth Symphony, "The Pathetique," with its slow tempo, minor key, and lush harmonies may create a mood of sadness or contemplation, while a Souza march with its strong rhythmic motifs and major key may create an energized, optimistic mood. Of course, we are also individually conditioned to have a particular mood associated with music just as individual feelings are conditioned.

Music can and does alter our mood (Radocy & Boyle, 1997). In music therapy practice, this was first noted by Altschuler (1954) and identified as the *iso-principle*—music's ability to match and alter mood. Current research shows that when the mood of the music is matched to an individual's mood and then gradually changed, the person's mood can also be altered (Sutherland, Newman, & Rachman, 1982). This is particularly important since mood state affects our cognitive functions. "Good moods, while they last, enhance the ability to think flexibly and with more complexity, thus making it easier to find solutions to problems . . ." (Goleman, 1995, p. 85). Shifting mood states is also an issue in mental health treatment.

Temperament is the final nuance of our emotional life. Temperament is a characteristic of our personality that predisposes us to use a given feeling or mood. It is our emotional disposition. As music affects emotion, feeling, and mood, it can ultimately contribute to this aspect of personality. Personality development and identity are issues of the next level of consciousness development: the personal level.

Personal Level of Development

The next major grouping of developmental levels in Wilber's (1977) spectrum of consciousness is personal development. This involves the development of a sense of self, of identity, and of ego. These attributes are about how to live in and cope with the physical world that surrounds us. It is at this stage that our self-referential consciousness begins to form.

The process of personal development begins with the establishment of a sense of self, an awareness of the "I." Our sense of self is a framework that remains mostly stable in the face of different life situations (Baars, 1997). As Pinker (1997) notes, "The 'I' is not a combination of body parts or brain states or bits of information, but a unity of selfness over time, a single locus that is nowhere in particular" (p. 564). Yet like any self-organizing system, our sense of self is in a constant state of flux. "We are both 'the same' person we were ten years ago and a substantially *new* person" (Briggs & Peat, 1999, p. 4). Our sense of self originally evolves out of the prepersonal developmental stage and, in particular, out of emotion. Ornstein (1991) writes, "The commanding, controlling mental operating system (which might be called the self) is much more closely linked with emotions and the system of autonomic bodyguards than with conscious thought and reason" (p. 153). Damasio (1999) contends that a sense of self is necessary to make the internal changes that constitute emotion known to the organism. Self is that which has access to consciousness. "There seems to be a basic connection between self and conscious experience. They are not the same thing but stand in the relation of context to content" (Baars, 1997, p. 153).

According to Wilber's theory, the sense of self emerges through the three prepersonal stages of development in childhood. The first stage is the physical self where the ability to distinguish self from the physical environment occurs. Simple orientation and response to external sound are basic to this development and form our first consciousness, the auditory consciousness. The second stage in the emergence of self involves the emotional self. In this stage, the ability to differentiate the individual's emotional self from the emotions of others occurs. The link of music and emotion was explained previously. In the final stage, the mental self develops in which the child learns to think, to verbalize, to talk, and to mentally control behavior.

After our basic sense of self is formed, the process of ego development actually begins as the next step in personal development. Ego is our conceptual self, our concept of self as a separate, observing entity. Ego development involves the faculties that make us human. Engler (1986) writes,

> The ego is a collective term designating the regulatory and integrative function. . . . [It involves] the psychological structures that make it possible to think, to plan, to remember, to anticipate, to organize, to self-reflect, to distinguish reality from fantasy, to organize, to exercise voluntary control over impulses and behavior, to love. (pp. 18–19)

The ego has many functions—reality testing, self-control, reflective self-awareness, operational cognition, and personal experience. It is the source of rational thought, volition, and deliberate will (Washburn, 1995). Our ego functions are formed through our experiences with the environment. We try things out, see how we can make things happen, and learn what we can and cannot control. An example of this is when a young child experiments with sound-making instruments.

In addition to this active function of ego, it also allows a receptive mode of operation. Washburn (1995) notes,

> It is the ego or egoic pole of the psyche that has two basic modes, active and receptive. It is the ego that either asserts itself by exercising ego functions (active mode) or "lets go" and opens itself to nonegoic influences (receptive mode). . . . [I]n adopting the former stance [assert itself], the ego takes initiative and exercises its own functions, in adopting the latter stance [surrender] the ego relinquishes hold of itself and allows itself to be influenced by nonegoic or physiodynamic potentials: dynamism, instinctual impulses, affect, the creative process, collective cognitions and complexes. (p. 14)

The ego gives us the capability to make the choice between active and receptive. Ego development can get stuck at a certain stage. Freud called this arrested development, and it is one factor that can develop into mental illness. This is addressed in greater detail later in the chapter.

A large part of ego development is developing self-concept, personality, self-image, and self-esteem. It is these areas in ego development that music therapy often addresses. Collectively, these terms refer to an awareness of being the same over time. It is the experience of continuity and of being unique (Ruud, 1998a). Our self-concept is a coherent story we tell ourselves about ourselves. "It does this by generating explanations of behavior on the basis of our self-image, memories of the past, expectations of the future, the present social situation, and the physical environment in which behavior is produced" (LeDoux, 1996, p. 33). "I'm usually shy in social situations" is a statement of self-concept. It involves both conscious and unconscious processes. Self-concept involves a number of related attributes that frequently factor into therapeutic goals related to this area.

Self-image is the conceptual framework that is used to define the self. It includes our social masks, our inner view of ourselves, our body image (the shape of our body), how we feel about it, the sense of our internal organs, and our awareness of bodily functions. Self-image is how we define ourselves (Davis, 1999). According to theorist A. A. Almaas, self-image ". . . is who we think we are, how we want to be, what we want to have in our lives . . ." (quoted in Davis, 1999, p. 69). Self-esteem, then, is the evaluative aspect of our self-concept. Our self-esteem is the positive or negative value we assign to the aspects of our personality and self-concept (Ruud, 1998a). Self-image is not an innate quality. It develops through our interactions with the world, other people, and our bodies.

The process of making an identity for ourselves is ongoing. It is never finished, nor does it remain fixed (Ruud, 1998a). "It may be that 'identity' is more an issue of boundary than core; that is, one is called upon to represent and define one's personality in certain kinds of social interactions" (Shulman, 1997, p. 25). We are constantly adjusting and re-forming our personal identities in response to the social situations we encounter. As Aldridge (1996) observes, "The dynamic interplay of maintaining our personal identity is an expressive activity akin to improvising music" (p. 23).

Though the basic ego structure is formed and organized in a certain way during childhood, the fulfillment of ego identity or selfhood in the world is ultimately the task of adolescence and young adulthood. "The real work of forging an identity is the task of early adulthood, and it is an indication that adolescence is at an end when a person ceases identity experimentation and embarks upon a long-term identity project" (Washburn, 1995, p. 101). Involvement in music experiences in late childhood and early adolescence can contribute to this development. As explored in chapter 3, music is a cultural phenomenon that conveys societal values, beliefs, and acceptable behavior. Our involvement with music is greatest in adolescence and young adulthood. The music we prefer and become involved with in adolescence reflects our developing values and sense of self (Ruud, 1998a). Adolescents seek recognition and acceptance from peers. "They seek to belong to a circle of supportive friends, a circle in which they can find not only recognition of the newly styled selves they are trying to be but also corresponding confirmation of their value" (Washburn, 1995, p. 103). The music that becomes "their music" is a large part of that peer recognition and personal identity.

> Music, because it is ever present in our daily lives, frames and anchors many of the situations used as raw material in the process of identity-building. In light of the emotional quality of musical experiences, it seems to me that these feeling-filled memories may serve an important role because they highlight and position people's life events significantly. (Ruud, 1998a, p. 37)

Learning to play music may also be important for developing a sense of identity. Guidano (1987) stresses the importance of a sense of mastery in adolescence as a means of social autonomy and development of a strong personal identity. Learning a music skill is an obvious mastery task. Alvin (1975) notes that when we play a musical instrument, the mechanisms slightly resist action. Overcoming this resistance to make the instrument sound provides us with a sense of mastery and control. Ruud (1998a) believes developing musical skill fosters a sense of agency. Agency involves achievement, competency, self-esteem, mastery, and empowerment. In music therapy practice, a number of music skill-building experiences in support of therapy goals are utilized involving these aspects of agency. The idea that skill building in music is a support to positive self-image and self-esteem is a basic principle of music therapy (Gaston, 1968a). Similarly, the flexibility of music as an activity allows the music therapist to structure successful experiences for clients, which also supports positive self-image and self-esteem—vital aspects of personal identity.

Another factor in the development of personal identity and self-concept is a process of external and internal dialogue. Identity is first shaped in relation to others. Ruud (1998a) notes, "The presence of other people seems crucial to making the child conscious of her own perceptions. Other people are necessary for us to be visible to ourselves" (p. 38). Musical improvisation is a form of external dialoging where people express themselves, respond to others, and interact nonverbally.

Internal dialogue is where we communicate, respond, and interact within ourselves. In fact, internal dialogue is the medium of identity construction.

> The internal monitoring adds layers of confirmation or disconfirmation to the elements of the mental ego's identity, [and] from its nuclear components to its more peripheral facets. Internal dialogue during early adulthood is the way in which the mental ego keeps track of how it is doing in the identity project and, therefore, of what its identity is. The identity constructed in this way is always in process; it exists as an ongoing, ever-revisable, never-finished product of the mental ego's self-monitoring efforts. (Washburn, 1995, p. 106)

Music can contribute to this internal dialogue by allowing nonverbal responses to become known. "The creative playing of improvised music offers a holistic form of assessment that is relational, non-invasive, and non-verbal, and that allows the identity of the patient to be revealed and experienced in the world" (Aldridge, 1996, p. 32). Music makes us aware of a private space inside that is not accessible to other people. This "space" involves the basic, nonverbal human functioning of the limbic brain and right hemisphere. Music not only touches that space, it brings that basic response into conscious awareness.

The internal dialogue then becomes a conversation between our verbal, logical processing and the nonverbal, holistic self. This dialogue often takes the form of music-evoked imagery. Interacting with this internally generated imagery becomes a powerful form of internal dialogue. The process of music-evoked imagery and the verbal processing inherent in the Guided Imagery and Music technique are an example of this dialoging with internal imagery (Bush, 1995). I developed a technique I call "Music and Creative Problem Solving" that also promotes this internal dialogue. In this technique, the client is asked to form a question or state a problem. In a relaxed state, the client listens to thirty-five to forty minutes of music selected by the music therapist to evoke emotion, feelings, and imagery. The clients then draw whatever images or write whatever words and thoughts occur while they are listening. This material emerges in direct response to the question posed. When the experience is completed, the client and music therapist explore this internal dialogue as it relates to the question or decision at hand.

Because self-image and identity formation is an ongoing process, we are always developing this aspect of ourselves. Problems occur when we approach situations with a fixed self-image based on past experiences and not from the present reality. Self-image work becomes a process of reality testing. When we approach situations with a fixed self-image based on past experiences, we will be out of touch with the present reality. "Our perceptions, behaviors, and relationships will be less responsive, less appropriate, and less effective. . . . [T]hey will also be more reactive, more forced, and more frustrating" (Davis, 1999, p. 63). We use predetermined patterns of response even when those behaviors become negative or counterproductive. "We become predisposed to certain patterns, and other possibilities continue to elude us" (Davis, 1999, p. 64). In music therapy, problems of self-image can be addressed by exploring feelings, by providing for successful emboldening experiences, and by providing the "space" that will allow self-image to loosen and change. Space in this sense is openness, clarity, and freedom. Music can provide this special form of space. According to Kenny (1989), musical space is an intimate contained space created when the client and therapist begin making sounds together. This is a safe, predictable place where trust is established. In this safe musical space, clients can explore their identity. "Music therapy offers the chance to do something differently. A new identity can be created" (Aldridge, 1996, p. 283).

Transpersonal Level of Development
The third general level of psychological development in Wilber's spectrum of consciousness, the *transpersonal*, involves moving beyond—transcending yet

including—the personal ego. This level of human consciousness development is not traditionally addressed by Western psychology. This level of development is examined more fully in the following section on mental illness and in the next chapter.

Music Therapy and Models of Mental Illness

The possible pathologies associated with psychological functioning are known as *mental illnesses*. Mental illness is as complex as physical illness—and likely more so. There are multiple factors and conditions in which these "diseases" originate (Shulman, 1997). Multiple therapeutic approaches or *models* propose to address the alleviation of these problems and symptoms. All models attempt to change the psychological functioning of the client. "Psychological therapies can be seen as a way of reprogramming the thoughts, emotions and behaviour of a person" (Robertson, 1999, p. 188). Many models are used in this process of reprogramming or repatterning, including organic (neurologic and biochemical), energy, systematic/cybernetic, behavioral, cognitive, psychotherapy, transpersonal, developmental stage theory, and complexity (Gallo, 1999). Each of these approaches is examined with a discussion on how music therapy interventions can potentially contribute to the therapeutic effort in each approach.

Organic Model—Neurologic and Biochemical

Though not identical, for the purposes of this book, neurologic structure and biochemical approaches to mental illness are both placed in the category of organic treatments of mental illness. Organic theories of mental illness and treatment are based on the belief that all mental activity—emotions, behavior, drives, and motivations—are positively or negatively affected by brain functioning, including the manifestations of mental illness. "Behind the symptoms of abnormal behavior there are organic, physiological or biochemical processes which cause the abnormal behavior of patients" (Ruud, 1978, p. 3). In biochemical theories, the cause of mental illness is an imbalance in chemical substances in the brain—neurotransmitters, endorphins, hormones, or neuropeptides. In Pert's (1997) work on neuropeptides, she notes that the receptors for the various brain chemicals are not stagnant and can change in both sensitivity and arrangement. "This means that even when we are 'stuck' emotionally, fixated on a version of reality that does not serve us well, there is always a biochemical potential for change or growth" (Pert, 1997, p. 146).

In this model, the treatment for mental illness would entail changing, balancing, or activating a "normal" chemical balance in the brain. Much of medical psychiatric treatment is based exclusively on this premise. The ever-increasing varieties of psychotropic medications for depression, anxiety, obsessive-compulsive behavior, schizophrenia, and other conditions are evidence of this approach. In terms of music therapy practice relating to this approach, the intervention must influence the production of these brain chemicals in ways that would support normal mental functioning. The impact of sound/music input increasing production of certain brain chemicals, like endorphins, and, as a vibratory input, influencing some level of the neuropeptide receptor/ligand process in emotional behavior was addressed previously. However, application of sound/music as an organic treatment for mental illness is unpredictable at best. It may contribute to the complex web of interactions responsible for the impact of music at this level, but it cannot be seen as a targeted organic intervention like psychotropic medications can be.

The neurological aspects of the organic basis for mental illness and its treatment relate to the knowledge that brain structures are relevant to aspects of cognitive and emotional functioning. The hardware of our neurology is an important aspect of our psychological functioning (Gallo, 1999). As explored previously, brains are shaped and reshaped by our experiences and especially by our emotions. Neural activity, especially when highly charged with emotion, is postulated to alter the synapses of the brain.

LeDoux (1996) found that the sustained, highly emotional states of individuals diagnosed with posttraumatic stress disorder cause irreversible lesions in the amygdala. Depression reduces synaptic activity in the frontal lobe (Robertson, 1999), while individuals who overcome depression learn to increase the activity level in that area (Goleman, 1995). Personality changes require the promotion of more neural activity in the right hemisphere, limbic system, and brain stem (Robertson, 1999).

Since brain activity creates neural circuitry or neural networks, part of the neurological aspects of mental illness and therapy involves exercising and changing these neural connections. "Therapy is just another way of creating synaptic potentiation in brain pathways that control the amygdala" (LeDoux, 1996, p. 265). Exercising the circuitry for emotional awareness and expression is another example. Robertson (1999) notes, "If you are taught never to express emotion, then the emotional circuitry of your brain will wither through disuse. . . . [I]f you never allow yourself to experience a particular emotion, then connections may be lost, making it harder to produce this mood in future" (pp. 207–208). In this view, early life experiences that limit neurological development prevent connections from being formed between the limbic system and the neocortex. Without these connections, the adult is dominated by lower brain processing and early coping mechanisms.

The neural energy patterns engage lower brain centers interpreted through the neocortex most of the time, instead of having the neocortex dominate and suppress inputs from the lower minds. "Without the opportunity to form a 'critical mass' of cortical connections during the first six years of life, certain developmental opportunities are missed, making later adaptation more difficult" (Wade, 1996, p. 79). Mental disorders, like personality disorders, may be created because of such processing.

Fortunately, the brain remains malleable or plastic throughout life. Repeated, intense emotional experiences sculpt and shape our neural circuitry whether through trauma or a therapeutic intervention. In this neurologic model of mental illness, a positive therapeutic change occurs when a highly information-laden stimulation like music is used to ". . . reactivate and reform dormant potentials, a process that is more difficult after the burst of brain growth in early life ceases, and one that becomes increasingly difficult when well-worn neural connections tend to take precedence" (Wade, 1996, p. 78). As discussed, music is a highly complex informational input to our brains. Music therapy techniques that utilize the emotional content of music can function to activate and change neural pathways and levels of brain functioning used in psychological processing. The music experiences become the repeated, emotionally charged sensory input that can reshape the brain and reestablish neural circuitry that has been lost or never developed.

Another aspect of a neurologic approach to mental illness involves the use of the whole brain for fully adaptive and positive mental health. Many theorists (Ornstein, 1986; Ornstein & Sobel, 1987; Restak, 1979; Russell, 1993; Wade, 1996) postulate the importance of "whole brain" activity and functioning in psychological well-being and mental health. These theories state that complex changes in thought processing, necessary in dealing with mental illness, are possible because the hemispheres of the cortex are working in a coordinated fashion. This involves creating similarities or entrainment in the EEG patterns of both the right and left hemispheres.

> Complex changes in mentation are thought possible because the cortical hemispheres are acting in a coordinated manner. . . . This consists of some similarity in EEG patterns in both right and left neocortical hemispheres (entrainment). . . . The two hemispheres of the cortex have similar chemistries but very different physiological lateralization of some gross structures and functions. At any given time, their electromagnetic patterns may or may not be of the same amplitude and frequency. "Whole brain" thinking is a synergistic blend of left- and right-hemispheric styles, integrating intuitive, holistic, spatial, and symbolic processing with linear, rational analysis. . . . [E]ntrainment of both sides of the brain allows an amazing range of creativity and a fuller

range of behavior than was available previously. . . . The coordination of both hemispheres affects the number of solutions available and the experience of temporality. Linear and holistic processing plus the ability to think outside the system increase the possibilities far beyond the infinite, but system-bound alternatives open to [other levels of processing]. (Wade, 1996, pp. 166–167)

Sound input and music, with its patterns of frequency and amplitude, can serve to foster this synchronization or entrainment of the brain hemispheres (Rider, 1985; Russell, 1993). Hemispheric synchronicity is addressed in greater detail in chapter 7.

The thoughts and insights gained from this shift to "whole brain" engagement in consciousness are not readily communicated through language. We are aware that words seldom convey the meaning of the images and symbols from the intuitive right hemisphere. Again, music can serve as a means of this expression, directly through the sound combinations and through the personal imagery that the music evokes. The music therapy techniques of Guided Imagery and Music and Music and Creative Problem Solving discussed previously serve as examples of this processing. In this case, the music serves to support and promote the brain synchronization as well as the integration of the ineffable, nonverbal mental processing of this whole brain consciousness into conscious awareness.

Energy Psychology Model

The theories of the human energy field and how it relates to physical functioning and disease were discussed in a previous chapter. A newly emerging psychological model, energy psychology, postulates that if everything is fundamentally energy, then energy fields—gross and subtle—are responsible for our brains, nervous system, neurochemistry, cognition, and emotions. Energy psychology studies the effects of the energetic system of the body—electromagnetic, quantum, and subtle—on our emotions and behavior (Gallo, 1999). Wilber (1977) sees the levels of consciousness as bands of energy vibrations. Each level has its own vibratory characteristic. Like the theories of disease generation based on energetic fields, energy psychology theorizes that ". . . while psychological disturbance manifests behaviorally, systematically, cognitively, neurologically, and chemically, at the most fundamental level there exists a structured or codified energy component that provides the instructions that catalyze the entire process" (Gallo, 1999, pp. 14–15). For example, depression, which has characteristic neurological and neural chemical correlates, may actually be triggered by slow or disordered energy fields in and around the body.

A therapeutic intervention in this model is designed to influence or alter the energetic template and thus change the emotional, cognitive, or behavioral maladjustment. "Application of the energy paradigm to the field of Clinical Psychology would follow the assumption that psychopathology can be treated by addressing subtle energy systems in the body. . . . [I]n essence psychological problems are a function of energy structures or fields" (Gallo, 1999, p. 14). Therapy at this level is aimed not at the material level but at the underlying energetic level that creates the material. Such therapy techniques would prove to be more thorough and immediate in their effects (Gallo, 1999). Music therapy may be one of these types of energetic interventions. Chapter 4 delineated the numerous ways in which sound, and especially music, impacts the various levels of the energetic system. This influence may very well affect psychological functioning, including emotions, just as it potentially affects various aspects of physical functioning. The sudden changes in affective state and general life outlook that occur in music therapy interventions may be the result of the impact of the complex energy of music on the human energy field.

Systematic-Cybernetic Model

In this model, psychological problems and human behavior in general are theorized to arise out of the context of interpersonal relationships, the family/ community, society, and culture. Psychological problems and mental illness occur as a function of interactions within relationships and systems. In the systematic-cybernetic model, ". . . symptoms are punctuated as responses to relationship problems, as misguided solutions, as ways of exercising control, as structural interactions, and so forth. The treatment, therefore, addresses these variables to promote healthier human interactions, and consequently, mental health" (Gallo, 1999, p. 7). In this model, a psychological disorder like depression would stem from unsatisfactory or disrupted interpersonal relationships. A child may not properly bond with an absent primary caregiver leading to a sense of loss and abandonment. In later life, this may express itself as depression. Or the disorder in relationships may have to do with society or culture at large.

> Sometimes we work with clients whose problems may be deeply interwoven with the material and economic structure of society, or whose problems are shaped more by their own attitudes and reflections, as well as the attitude of others, rather than by their individual or objective biological constitution. (Ruud, 1998a, p. 52)

As explored extensively in chapter 3, music is a social art that plays many roles in society and culture. Music therapy interventions used in this approach

capitalize on the social, relational aspects of music, especially in techniques involving group music making. Music becomes the reason for being together. It
makes it safer and easier to relate to others. As music therapy pioneer E. Thayer
Gaston (1968a) notes, music is a form of nonthreatening familiarity. I experienced this firsthand with a young adolescent boy with whom I worked in an
inpatient psychiatric setting, as presented in the case study at the beginning of
chapter 2. This client had very poor relationship skills toward adult women,
based on the abusive behavior of his mother. He would not interact with any
of the female staff members until I offered him time in the music room. For
weeks, we played side by side (me on piano, him on the drum set) with little
or no interaction. But the music made it safer for him to tolerate my presence
and eventually led to positive interactions around our music making.

In the systemic-cybernetic model, the context of the therapy is vital. Recovery depends on a supportive social network. As Shulman (1997) notes,
being with a client in a loving and supportive way is key to healing mental
illness. Such healing requires human relationship—with another individual
and within groups. Based on extensive research on social context and treatment for schizophrenia, the strongest indicator of good prognosis for this serious mental illness is the extent of the social network the patient had.
"What was most important in a good outcome was social inclusion, meaning
some social network rather than isolation" (Shulman, 1997, p. 53). Shared
music experiences, as structured in music therapy, are inclusive social situations. Everyone can participate and contribute in some way. I have worked
extensively with group percussion experiences as the basis of a therapeutic
group experience. In "drum circle" events, everyone can participate no matter what their level of musical skill. I have facilitated groups with young children, older adults, experienced percussionists, and novice drummers all playing together. The novice players may help keep the steady beat, the
experienced percussionists add complex rhythm patterns, and the young
child and older adults improvise and add to the mix in any way possible. In
such situations, participants immediately feel accepted and valued as members of this social group (Hull, 1998).

Many music therapy techniques positively affect group cohesiveness, peer
acceptance, and interpersonal relationships (James & Freed, 1989). Some of
these approaches include group songwriting (Cordobes, 1997), musical skill
building (Cassette, 1976; Cassity, 1981), group singing (Anshel & Kipper,
1988), and music-based group discussions (Henderson, 1983). This ability of
music to form cohesive social groups and to increase interpersonal relationships has led to music therapy techniques in formal systemic therapy models
like family therapy and group therapy (Borczon, 1997; Plach, 1980).

In general, family therapy involves the exploration and altering of inter-actions and interpersonal dynamics within the family unit. Music therapy techniques like group musical improvisation allow those dynamics to become obvious for all involved. "In this setting, we can observe clients' reactions to others' real behaviors rather than merely hear them describe their reactions. We can explore clients' object relations with a variety of personalities within the group session" (Dvorkin, 1998, pp. 287–288). Improvising together brings out the relationships between family members and provides a means to change those patterns for the better.

Interpersonal relations can also be explored in musical psychodrama, which involves psychodramatic musical improvisation ensembles (Moreno, 1999). In this technique, emotions of members toward others in the group are emphasized. "The role of the ensemble is to create, at any given moment, improvised music to support a wide variety of emotions" (Moreno, 1999, p. 11). Through these improvisational experiences, orchestrated by the psy-chodrama director, intragroup communication, rapport, and responsiveness to group members are emphasized.

Group therapy is another systemic model that is addressed by music ther-apy techniques (Bunt, 1994). According to Plach (1980), music therapy as group therapy ". . . can be defined as the use of music or music activities as a stimulus for promoting new behaviors and exploring predetermined individ-ual or group goals in a group setting" (p. 4). A number of music therapy tech-niques are used in group therapy, including musical improvisation, lyric analysis, and performance groups. Plach (1980) sees a number of advantages of using music therapy techniques as the basis of group therapy. These in-clude music's ability to open up communication, evoke and express feelings, and stimulate verbalization and socialization and its provision of a reliable starting place for the therapeutic work. As Sekeles (1996) points out, music sets up a physical and psychic space for the group process to occur. The mu-sic both creates and contains the group experiences that lead to therapeutic benefit (Whipple & Lindsey, 1999). "An experienced and knowledgeable music therapist can conceivably take any group of clients, at any level of functioning, at any given point in time, and with minimal knowledge of the individual illnesses and group dynamics, design and implement a music ac-tivity that will facilitate exploration and growth on an important issue for the group or its individual members" (Plach, 1980, p. 7).

Plach (1980) identifies three stages of group process fostered through mu-sic activities. Stage one involves developing a sense of group cohesiveness. As explored previously, music helps achieve this through shared common goals (like in drum circles), successful experiences, and the shared pleasure that music affords. Stage two involves the clients' development of personal insight, gaining an understanding of their personal issues, family dynamics, and emotional reactions. Musical improvisation and musical psychodrama are music therapy techniques previously discussed that contribute to this effort. Music therapy techniques like lyric analysis, where lyrics and musical presentation convey meaning to the listener, can provide a form of theme-centered group interaction (Cohn, 1974). The next section explores these therapeutic "uncovering" techniques in greater detail. The third stage of group process, resolving issues and exploring new behaviors, can also be fostered by active music therapy techniques like improvisation. The group music therapy session provides a safe, well-structured situation for using and applying more adaptive behaviors and reactions. The music therapy session becomes a place to practice new insights and new behavioral responses.

Behavioral Model
A behavioral approach to therapy focuses on external behavior and, in particular, the relationship of behavior to environment or context. According to this model, environmental change can produce behavioral change based on principles of stimulus–response developed by Ivan Pavlov and B. F. Skinner. The underlying assumption of behavioral therapy is that all behavior, including maladaptive behavior, is learned. Therapy involves learning new, adaptive patterns (Wheeler, 1981). Behavior change constitutes the therapeutic effort. Using depression once again to illustrate, in this model depression would be caused by changes in environmental factors (loss of a job, divorce, etc.) and would be treated by changing the external behavior associated with the depression (facial expressions of sadness).

The use of music as a behavioral reinforcer and music therapy interventions in a behavior modification approach to therapy is long-standing and extensive. Behavioral music therapy is ". . . primarily concerned with the function of music as an independent variable acting upon dependent variables such as the behavior of the patient" (Ruud, 1978, p. 29). Early music therapy literature advocates for music therapy to be understood as a behavioral therapy with the music itself serving as the environmental cue for behavior change (Carroccio & Carroccio, 1972; Eidson, 1989; Greer, 1976; Madsen, Cottor, & Madsen, 1968; Ponath & Bitcon, 1972; Presti, 1984).

Early research was conducted, demonstrating that music can be used as a reinforcement for interpersonal skills (Eidson, 1989), decrease of inappropriate uncooperative behavior (Hauck & Martin, 1970; Madsen & Madsen, 1968; Steele, 1968), and mathematical behaviors and attentiveness to math problems (Madsen, Cottor, & Madsen, 1968; Madsen et al., 1975; Yarbough,

Charboneau, & Wapnich, 1977). Other research focused on particular forms of music used for reinforcement, such as rock music (Wilson, 1976), and how and where the music is used to reinforce behavior. This "contingent music listening" was studied as an effective reward for a wide range of behaviors and skills from decreasing disruptive behavior to increasing speech production (Garwood, 1988; Hanser, 1974; Harding & Ballard, 1982; Jorgensen, 1974; Madsen & Forsythe, 1973; Reid et al., 1975; Underhill & Harris, 1974; Wilson & Hopkins, 1973). All this research demonstrates that the music is an effective reinforcer for behavioral change and that music therapy can be used within a behavioral approach to therapy.

Cognitive Model

The cognitive approach to therapy for mental illness looks for the internal designs, like language, that allow an individual to feel and behave in a certain context (Gallo, 1999). Cognitive therapy addresses mental "scripts" that are untrue or nonadaptive. Such scripts are the way people habitually perceive and think. In cognitive therapy, the therapist helps the client to discover these maladaptive scripts and replace them with a more realistic interpretation. As Wilber (1996) notes, it is ". . . a more *truthful interpretation* of your interior, so that the false self can give way to the actual self. . . . The idea is, *think* differently, and you will start to *feel* differently" (p. 184). In the example of depression, the problem would stem from a set of false beliefs or self-dialogue that leads to feelings of depression ("nobody likes me"). As Combs (1995) notes,

> We have seen that the state of depression tends to support itself by selecting memories such that we tend to recall oppressive episodes from our past. These memories in turn feed our mood of depression, and so perpetuate a continuous cycle of memory and mood. If we want to break this cycle, we must disrupt the circuit and apply new patterning forces. . . . (p. 68)

Cognitive therapy alleviates psychological stress by correcting faulty conceptions and thought patterns. This approach proposes to reach emotional states through cognitive processing. By correcting erroneous beliefs, excessive or inappropriate emotional reactions can be subdued or changed (Bryant, 1987). Cognitive therapy helps the client move from reaction to action (LeDoux, 1996). The cognitive therapy approach involves exploration of meaning based on verbal processes. Maranto (1996) identifies a number of music therapy techniques used in a cognitive therapy approach, including musical improvisation with verbal processing, lyric analysis, theme-based group improvisation, songwriting, song histories or collage, and overall theme-based sessions. Borczon (1997) outlines a cognitive approach for various mental disorders, including depression and anxiety, utilizing cognitive techniques such as neurolinguistic programming and cognitive restructuring.

Luce (2001) noted that there is little literature on music therapy in the cognitive approach to therapy. Many music therapy techniques seem to involve cognitive strategies, though the vocabulary used in the two disciplines may not match. He postulates that meaning evoked by music may go beyond verbal meaning. However, he sees that the

> . . . essential aspect of meaning-making that is central to the information processing model of cognitive therapy also lies within music therapy. . . . [A]n individual assigns meaning to internal and external stimuli through a cognitive process. Paralleling this meaning-making assignment process, primary music therapy interventions can identify, express, reconstruct, and reintegrate cognitive constellations and modal processes. (2001, p. 102)

Bryant (1987) and Maultsby (1972) also looked at the use of music therapy in the specific cognitive therapies of rational emotive therapy and its offshoot, rational behavior therapy, which teach people practical techniques of emotional self-help. Bryant (1987) notes that the music therapy session is a cognitive microcosm of the patient's beliefs, attitudes, and maladaptive thinking. The client approaches experiences in music therapy in a way that is ". . . identical to his or her approach to any life experience. Values, attitudes, and beliefs, both rational and irrational, are brought to bear in all experiences, and are therefore subsequently projected upon the client's approach to the music therapy setting" (Bryant, 1987, p. 31). The client's musical preferences, approach to activities, and self-evaluation in relation to music making all reflect general attitudes and life scripts. Music therapy in these cognitive models involves a form of reality testing where the maladaptive attitudes are pointed out and confronted. During the music therapy experience, the music therapist can observe and assist the client in recognizing, defining, challenging, and changing self-defeating beliefs and scripts. When I worked as a music therapist in an adolescent psychiatric hospital, I used this form of music therapy intervention extensively. These adolescents would frequently express ideas like, "I'm stupid, I can't do anything." To confront and change those beliefs, I would often record them playing an instrument like guitar so they could hear that they could play, could sound good, and had achieved a real skill.

Arnold (1975) discussed the use of music therapy interventions in another cognitive therapy, transactional analysis (TA). TA uses an interactional approach to psychotherapy where analysis of ego structure and our interpersonal relations brings ". . . a level of awareness which enables the person being treated to make new decisions regarding future behavior and the future course of his life . . ." (Arnold, 1975, p. 106). He notes many parallels between music therapy and TA therapy, including providing emotional catharsis for the child ego, practicing new behaviors with positive reinforcement, providing for play and freeing the natural child, and confronting and examining underlying beliefs and attitudes.

Psychotherapy Model
The psychotherapy model for work with mental illness encompasses a number of approaches and specific techniques. Psychotherapy involves methods of curing mental problems and disorders by *psychological techniques* or processes to help a person make psychological changes necessary or desirable to achieve well-being (Bruscia, 1998b).

Psychotherapyhas numerous goals. These include increased self-awareness, self-expression, changes in emotion and attitude, improved interpersonal skills, resolution of interpersonal problems, development of healthy relationships, healing of emotional traumas, development of deeper personal insight, reality testing, cognitive restructuring, behavioral change, developing a sense of greater life meaning, and fulfillment in life or spiritual development (Bruscia, 1998b). In this model, depression would stem from repressed feelings about past events and traumas. To treat the depression, repressed feelings and memories would be uncovered, intensified in the here and now, and integrated into conscious awareness. The client would relive the past event, reexperience the feelings, and reintegrate that experience so that it no longer generates depressed feelings. The client goes back to move forward (Bunt, 1994).

Music therapy used as a form of psychotherapy impacts on all these aspects of the psychotherapy process. This is known as *music psychotherapy*. According to Bruscia (1998b), in music psychotherapy,

> . . . therapist and client create and listen to music as a primary means of communicating, relating to one another, and working toward goals, supplementing these experiences with verbal discourse as necessary. In short, music psychotherapy is the use of music experiences to facilitate the interpersonal process of therapist and client as well as the therapeutic change process itself. (p. 2)

Music psychotherapy ". . . involves three dynamic elements: the client, the therapist and the music. Within this triad, the therapist and music work together to help the client, serving similar or complementary role functions . . ." (Bruscia, 1998e, p. 76). The music evokes repressed emotions and unconscious memories, represents this psychic material, aids in reexperiencing this in the present moment, and helps to develop a degree of insight (Sekeles, 1996). Music psychotherapy gives the patients an opportunity to explore aspects of themselves from a different perspective by providing a sounding board to amplify and reflect back aurally what is given (Bunt, 1994). These techniques traditionally include sublimation, strengthening of ego structure, uncovering repressed material and emotional catharsis, and insight development and integration of repressed material into current functioning.

Sublimation

In sublimation, music therapy procedures are used to refocus and channel negative impulses and drives into socially acceptable expressions. When clients are beating a drum to express anger, they are engaging in a sublimation process. It is common for adolescents, in particular, to sublimate conflicts and emotional pain into song lyrics and musical improvisation. The current popularity of rap music may, in part, be based on the sublimation of anger and frustration into the often socially negative lyrics of this musical form.

Ego Strengthening

The strengthening of ego structure and mature personality development, or the development of what Goleman (1995) calls "emotional intelligence," involves many skills in self-awareness. These are the skills we need to live successfully and happily in the world. They include identity and self-concept development, self-acceptance, managing feelings and knowing the difference between feelings and actions, impulse control, personal decision making, communication and empathy, delaying gratification, and stress management. As explored earlier, we gain these skills first throughout childhood in exploratory, self-mastery, and successful experiences. This level of psychotherapy addresses individuals who have not done this work or have developed maladaptive or faulty ego structure.

For adults needing this form of psychotherapy work, music therapy offers important experiences for developing ego strength and emotional intelligence. Music therapy techniques allow for exploratory behavior. In techniques like musical improvisation, clients can try out new behavior, experience different ways of being, and experiment with new and more adaptive feelings and reactions. "Music therapy can help adults to take risks, confront changes, reconcile crises and move forward. Adults in music therapy group can use music to explore present issues from a different perspective and to reassess earlier problems . . ." (Bunt, 1994, p. 159). Exploratory behavior like this assists clients in environmental orientation, learning, and developing better coping skills (Gfeller, 1990a). Music skill building also provides for a sense of mastery, self-esteem, and positive peer regard.

The qualities of emotional intelligence parallel the affective attributes of creative behavior. Treffinger (1983) created a model of creativity that delineates both cognitive skills and the affective behavior that constitutes creativity in an individual. The affective behaviors include willingness to take risks, openness to new things, positive reaction to ambiguity, curiosity, self-esteem, and others categorized as "emotional intelligence" by Goleman (1995). Engaging in a creative art like music helps to foster and develop these vital emotional skills. Self-expression and creativity through improvisation, songwriting, and expressive performance allow the client to have structured experiences in skills like risk taking. These creative experiences contribute to developing ego strength and emotional intelligence during this stage of psychotherapy.

Uncovering

The next stage in psychotherapy involves an *uncovering* mode of therapy. Uncovering as a psychotherapy approach involves the identification and re-experiencing of repressed emotions and unconscious memories. "One of the goals of psychotherapy is to make unconscious thoughts and feelings conscious, to make the individual communicate with himself and to the therapist these hidden conflicts" (Ruud, 1978, p. 27). Repressed aspects of the self are then integrated into awareness and present functioning. In this uncovering process, the client regresses to an earlier way of perceiving, conceptualizing, feeling, and behaving during an intense interpersonal encounter with a therapy group or individual therapist (Wilber, Engler, & Brown, 1986). Healing becomes possible when the client lives out, in the here and now, bodily feelings and associated behavior related to past traumatizing events (Schachter, 1993). Music therapy techniques are used extensively for all aspects of this uncovering process.

The initial step in this uncovering process is to evoke and express emotion and feelings, known as catharsis. Catharsis is the remembering, intense reexperiencing, and expression of repressed emotional memories with painful attachments (Winkelman, 2000). Catharsis not only brings psychological release from repressed emotion but alters the brain as well. Reliving psychic pain changes the brain. Studies by Janov (1996) demonstrated changes in brain wave frequency and amplitude after the patient uncovers and resolves a traumatic memory. He further found the brain waves of patients who have participated in uncovering techniques are better synchronized, are slower, have amplitudes more evenly distributed over the whole brain, and have a balance of activity between right and left hemisphere. To be effective, catharsis must involve the same level of consciousness on which the repressed memory occurred and must be a complete experience matching the original emotional event. Further, the catharsis should not overwhelm the individual but, rather, should allow for expression of the emotions in manageable pieces (Janov, 1996).

Music is strongly linked with emotions and feelings in general. When dealing with our emotional life and the psychotherapeutic efforts to change it, emotions are more easily influenced when the person is not aware that the influence is occurring (LeDoux, 1996). Music is such a subconscious influence on emotion and feeling. If emotions and the feeling states that arise from them are mediated and conditioned below the thinking level of the brain, then a therapy like music therapy that uses the same brain pathways is the best way to treat problems arising from early learned emotional reactions. This is because music allows us to experience, identify, and express emotions and feelings in safe, manageable ways. Rider (1997) finds that rhythmical inconsistency, one of the prominent characteristics of classical music, evokes more intense expression of emotions than a regular beat. It also stimulates a variety of emotional experiences. As Rider (1997) points out, no one emotion is desirable all the time. He theorizes we need a continuous shifting of our emotional states to maintain long-term emotional well-being. Music, as movement, provides this shifting of emotional states. That may be, in part, why we like and seek out "sad" music. As Thaut (1990a) points out, "Music, based on its unique stimulus properties and differential processing in the central nervous system (CNS), evokes meaningful affective responses that can be used to modify affect in clinical situations whereby affect modification is considered an essential component of behavioral learning and change" (p. 3).

A true experience of emotion and feeling must be in their own language, which is visceral. Emotion and feeling are body states (Kenyon, 1994). Music provides that visceral experience of emotion. One way emotion is expressed in our bodies is through singing. The act of singing reconnects us with our emotions. Collinge (1998) links breath with expression of feelings: "Fortunately there is a way we can reconnect with our feelings. . . . All we have to do is breathe and keep on breathing *while* we are feeling them" (p. 147). Singing is deep continuous diaphragmatic breathing while experiencing the feelings conveyed by the song.

In emotional expression with music, the structured components of the music first evoke the underlying emotional states. The music, then, becomes a catalyst for feelings as it triggers memories and past associations. Music uncovers the feelings and provides a mechanism for their cathartic expression. My experience during the Guided Imagery and Music session reported in the case study at the beginning of this chapter illustrates this point. While the music evokes the emotion and feelings, it simultaneously expresses those feelings in verbal and, particularly, nonverbal forms.

In the music therapy session, clients can express feelings in a number of ways. They can talk about what they are feeling or express emotional states through art expression like drawing. One of the most important nonverbal forms of emotional expression in music is through the performance itself, especially in improvisational music therapy techniques. An improvisation is a socially acceptable means of expressing even the most inappropriate, extreme, or out-of-control feelings (Bunt, 1994). Improvisation is a way to express oneself through music. It gives nonverbal form to emotional expression (Ruud, 1998a). Musical performance reflects emotion and feeling in a number of ways. These include the timbre of sound used, melodic motifs, dynamics, unique combinations of musical elements, and the emerging whole composition, whether composed or improvised (Sekeles, 1996). The combination of these elements provides an external order for the expression of the seemingly disordered and unorganized inner emotional states (McNiff, 1992).

What is key in music therapy, however, is the shared expression of emotion among the client, the therapist, and others in a therapy group. The emotional expression is witnessed, shared, and validated by the responsive playing of the music therapist and others in the group. The musical mirroring that takes place in an improvisational music experience serves to legitimize and validate the expressed feelings (Sekeles, 1996). This mirroring of the emotions is important in an improvisational technique like Nordoff-Robbins "Creative Music Therapy." When the client expresses emotion or feelings through movement or vocalization, the music therapist improvises music reflecting that emotional state. When this occurs, the client often looks startled and then pleased. The expression of the emotion usually escalates as the clients sense that the therapist is musically empathizing with them. This is a valuable aspect of the uncovering process of psychotherapy—having emotions witnessed and accepted by a caring other (Aigen, 1995a).

In addition to the expression of emotion and feeling, the uncovering process also involves the retrieval of unconscious memories—important psychic experiences that have been repressed and are no longer available to consciousness. It is believed that once an individual is aware of the reasons for a behavior or reaction, one can choose whether to continue it (Wheeler, 1981).

Many repressed memories from early childhood consist of events that occurred in the child's preverbal and precognitive developmental stages. The child's experience of trauma was primarily sensorial. Communicating such a memory through the language of words is extremely difficult. A stimulus (like music) that is itself sensorial and nonverbal (and emotional) serves as a bridge to the early language of sensory impressions. (Skaggs, 1997, p. 36)

The "language" of the unconscious and emotional brain is symbol, image, metaphor, story, and myth.

The logic of the emotional mind is *associative*; it takes elements that symbolize a reality, or trigger a memory of it, to be the same as that reality. That is why similes, metaphors, and images speak directly to the emotional mind, as do the arts. . . . (Goleman, 1995, p. 294)

Jung (1969) believed that dreams and images were the royal road to the unconscious. He postulated a particular kind of imagery, the archetype, which is a basic, inherited image or form common to all humans. "These basic or primordial images represent very common, very typical experiences that humans everywhere are exposed to . . ." (Wilber, 1996, p. 213). These images or archetypal symbols are interfaces between the world and psyche that transcend consciousness and the realm of the unconscious. Jung believed that these images reflected the workings of the psyche. "He felt that the surprising uniformity of images and themes in folktales, myths, and dreams suggests that they are manifestations of dynamics common to the human psyche" (Van Eenwyk, 1996, p. 344). Images can also be very individual and can constitute a form of personal symbol (Kenny, 1982). Whether archetypal or personal images, they serve to reorganize the material presented. The imagery becomes a form of introspection. The client learns something new from the image itself, which leads to understanding beyond previous knowledge and insight (Hunt, 1995).

Art in general and music in particular are acknowledged as human means to access unconscious material (Janov, 1996). "Psychoanalytic theory regards the work of art as the product of a transformation process of drives and desires originating in the unconscious" (Ruud, 1978, p. 16). Many theorists (Bonny & Savary, 1990; Ruud, 1986; Taylor & Paperte, 1958) contend that music reaches unconscious material in the same manner as a dream or meditative state. Music becomes a language that gives symbolic expression to unconscious content (Austin, 1996). Dreams, meditation, and experiences with music, especially when listening occurs in an altered state of consciousness, bypass or suppress the verbal, logical, rational functioning of the upper cortex and allow the holistic, emotional, image-based functioning of the limbic system and right hemisphere to emerge. Music allows us to bypass the ego structure (Ruud, 1986). In so doing, both archetypal and personal imagery can come to the forefront of conscious awareness. Sekeles (1996) has identified "musical archetypes" or simple latent musical patterns that emerge when nonmusicians improvise. She observes that ". . . in the simple creations or improvisations of the non-musician patient, primary symbolism is quite apparent and can thus be perceived as an analogy of sub-conscious psychic experience" (1996, p. 55). I also experienced how music brings out archetypal imagery during my work with the Music and Creative Problem Solving technique. In work with over 100 subjects, I used the technique asking them to answer the question, "What is music?" The images that emerged in answer to that question were highly archetypal in nature—rainbows, bridges, spirals, and undulating lines. The consistency of these images was quite remarkable, as is explored further in chapter 7.

Music first accesses the imagery of the unconscious and then serves as a means to ground the experience so the information can be integrated and used. As music therapy pioneer Helen Bonny states, "The unconscious mind can remember in complete detail everything in an individual's personal history, including events which the conscious mind has totally forgotten. With the help of appropriate music, sets of memories can be resurrected and recombined to produce completely new experiences" (Bonny & Savary, 1990, p. 31). Music can play a vital role in the uncovering of suppressed, unconscious memories and feelings.

Insight Development

Insight development and conscious integration of repressed material can also be addressed in music therapy practice. To review briefly, in psychotherapy techniques, the client revisits old experiences, areas of arrested development, and unconscious material so they can be released from their fixation and dissociation from awareness to allow the continuing development of consciousness. However, these interior or depth dimensions of the psyche require interpretation. The question must be asked, "What does it *mean?*" According to Wilber (1996), all the various psychodynamic or depth psychology approaches are attempts to find a more adequate interpretation for the client's internal experience.

> So these various interpretive therapies, such as psychoanalysis or Gestalt or Jungian, help you to contact and more truthfully interpret your depths. . . . The idea is not to make some sort of more accurate map of the objective world, but

to relax your resistances and sink into your interior depths, and learn to report those depths more truthfully. . . . And this allows your *depth* to begin to match your *behavior*. (Wilber, 1996, p. 110)

These new truths are known as insights. An insight involves learning something new about yourself and understanding unconscious processes that are hindering you (Sekeles, 1996). Insight development is not about trying to "correct" the situations from the past but, rather, to understand them so conscious choices can be made about how to act and respond in the present.

A number of possible approaches are used to help a client develop these new insights based on the principles of whatever school of psychotherapy is utilized. The Freudian approach uses verbal analysis and "talk therapy," while Jung emphasizes imagery, symbols, and the shared human imagery of archetypes as the basis of interpretation of inner experiences. Various music psychotherapy approaches help with interpretation of depth material in both ways. Bruscia (1998f) identifies two general types of music psychotherapy: transformative and insight. In transformative music psychotherapy, the music experience itself leads to the desired change in client insight and behavior. Music provides an experiential change that is therapeutically transformative. Interpretation of the inner psychic materials is intrinsic and nonverbal. Insight music psychotherapy provides verbally mediated awareness. A verbal dialogue between therapist and client extends and consolidates the nonverbal experience of the music (Bruscia, 1998f).

Both types of music psychotherapy are fostered through three basic types of music therapy interventions: improvisation, use of songs, and music imaging. Improvisation can be used as transformative music psychotherapy first in a referential way when the client projects ". . . feelings underlying the words onto the music. The music helps to turn frozen emotions or verbally consolidated experiences into dynamic forms that live in time. The client relives the feelings non-verbally and re-experiences the process by which they unfold" (Bruscia, 1998b, p. 8). The improvisation becomes a means of free association, projecting oneself onto the sounds. The client can also improvise in a nonreferential fashion when a nonverbal projection of the client's inner depths occurs.

A non-referential improvisation then enables the client to non-verbally explore him-/herself and the materials without specific reference to any verbalized feelings or emotions, and to examine the dynamics and processes of his ongoing experience. The in turn helps to clarify the content of his/her feelings. (Bruscia, 1987, p. 562)

Improvisation can also be used in insight music therapy. British music therapist Mary Priestley (1975) developed a form of this that she titled "Analytical Music Therapy." In this method, the client improvises on rhythm instruments and voice while the music therapist ". . . uses the piano from which he can stimulate, control and contain all that is expressed, encouraging the patient to create his own individual music in totally free sound patterns" (Ruud, 1978, p. 22). The musical sounds are used to objectively represent and develop the psychological issue (Wheeler, 1981). The therapist and client then verbally analyze, explore, and interpret the meaning engendered in the improvisation, thus developing the client's insight into his or her behavior and response.

The second music therapy intervention used for insight development is the use of songs. As Bruscia (1998b) notes,

> Songs are the ways that human beings explore emotions. They express who we are and how we feel, they bring us closer to others, they keep us company when we are alone. . . . They are the sounds of our personal development . . . songs provide easy access to a person's emotional world and to the thoughts, attitudes, values, and behaviors that emanate from it. Given the aims of psychotherapy, songs can greatly facilitate the process and provide a very effective vehicle for emotional change. (pp. 9–10)

Transformative experiences with song include song performance and song improvisation where the act of singing brings changes and nonverbal insight. There are numerous uses of songs in insight music psychotherapy. Song recall is when the client is asked to think of a song that relates to a particular therapeutic issue or such a recall occurs spontaneously. Song communication, including lyric analysis, is where the client and therapist verbally discuss the issues expressed in a song, the impact of the lyrics and music, and other issues related to the therapeutic focus. Songwriting and song parody (rewriting existing songs) constitute another possible insight music psychotherapy technique. In writing songs, clients are able to explore issues that are difficult to verbalize (Cordobes, 1997; Ficken, 1976; Lindberg, 1995; Robb, 1996). In my work with adolescents with emotional disturbances, it was quite common for a therapeutic issue, like abuse, to be expressed first in a song lyric before the client explored the issue in the counseling session. In all these techniques, the song provides the basis for therapeutic interaction between the therapist and client. This interaction allows for increased insight as to the issues and concerns of the client.

A third music therapy intervention used in music psychotherapy is music imaging. As previously discussed, images are the language of the unconscious.

Such experiences with music can stimulate and evoke deep images—both archetypal and personal. Music imaging is an ". . . experience that involves listening to music and allowing oneself to respond imaginally—that is, through free associations, projective stories, images, feelings, body sensation, memories, and so forth" (Bruscia, 1998b, p. 11). The most well-established music imaging intervention in music therapy is Guided Imagery and Music (GIM), developed in the early 1970s by Dr. Helen Bonny (Bonny & Savary, 1990). GIM techniques are first used to uncover and evoke unconscious memories and feelings. The technique is then used as a psychotherapy approach allowing for interpretation of the uncovered material. During the GIM session, a transformative process can occur as the client experiences the visual, auditory, and visceral images without verbal interpretation. The direct experience with the images creates a healing system different from the context in which the problem was created. The client can relax into a state of renewed meaning, a place at the center of being where the personality can be restructured and can begin to speak with a new and more authentic inner voice. This new healing context must be created from the material—the images themselves—that autonomously develops from the internal functioning of the individual (Shulman, 1997). The image becomes an "other" that the clients can experientially dialogue with to discover who they are and are not (McNiff, 1992). For example, in a GIM session a client who has been abused by a parent may have imagery of him- or herself beating up the abuser. The imagery and the accompanying emotions are very real and allow that healing act to occur in a context that would not create negative consequences in real life. After the transformative experience of the images, the GIM technique concludes with verbal interaction between the client and therapist to help develop insights as to how the images and experiences relate to client issues and problems. In this dialogue, the meaning of the images and emotions experienced is integrated into conscious functioning.

Role of the Therapist

A vital part of any psychotherapy approach is the role of the therapist. The therapist helps the clients interpret their internal intentions more truthfully. The psychotherapy process is intersubjective dialogue with a therapeutic helper (Wilber, 1996). As noted previously, in music psychotherapy the therapist and the music itself can become such a helper.

Psychotherapy work is best accomplished in an environment of empathy, congruence, and acceptance. The structure and familiarity of music create an atmosphere of acceptance and safety (Gaston, 1968b). It is easier and less threatening to interact when we are engaged in the social and predictable experience music provides. The act of sharing music is a primary act of empathy—the ability to understand or identify with what another person is experiencing.

> Music is a medium par excellence for empathy. In fact, in many ways, it is unmatched by any other medium. When we sing the same song together, we live in the same melody, we share the same tonal center, we articulate the same lyrics, we move ahead according to the same rhythm—moment by moment, sound by sound, through an ongoing awareness of the others, and through continuing efforts to stay together and thereby become one within the experience. (Bruscia, 1998a, p. 60)

Improvisational music is also an empathetic, accepting experience. When the music therapist and client improvise together, adapting to and reflecting the patient's own themes, the music therapist is using a profound expression of empathy (Sekeles, 1996). Empathy is also expressed in the synchronization of movements between people. As Goleman (1995) notes, "The degree of emotional rapport people feel in an encounter is mirrored by how tightly orchestrated their physical movements are as they talk . . ." (p. 116). Within a music therapy experience, the shared music and, especially, the rhythmic elements synchronize our movements so that the sense of closeness and empathy is increased. The motor synchronization to rhythmic pulse verified by Thaut's (1990b) research supports this contention.

In all psychotherapy approaches, it is the dynamic between client and therapist that is the catalyst for therapeutic change. Psychotherapy is an interpersonal process where the relationship developed enables the client to make necessary psychological changes. The dynamics of this interpersonal process are referred to as transference and countertransference.

> Transference *is* the dynamic of the client's conscious and unconscious psyche relating to the therapist, and counter transference *is* the dynamic of the therapist's conscious and unconscious psyche relating to the client. Transference and counter transference, then, are the primary modes of communication and relationship between client and therapist in psychodynamic therapy. (Bruscia, 1998d, p. xxii)

Transference is the reliving of significant relationships from the client's past in the therapy setting, while countertransference is the same dynamic happening in the therapist. In music psychotherapy, then, the relationship developed while the client and the music therapist are interacting within the musical experience is the primary mode of change. As previously explored, a music experience fosters relationship building. Shared music experiences are nonthreatening familiarity (Gaston, 1968b). Being involved in music together provides the vehicle for the interplay of transference and counter-transference to occur.

Transpersonal Psychology Model

The transpersonal model of psychological therapy emerged from humanistic psychology. It is based on two basic assumptions—first, that human development beyond normal ego functioning is possible and second, that a higher, transegoic (beyond ego) stage of life is also possible. "Transpersonal psychology is the study of human nature and development that proceeds on the assumption that human beings possess potentialities that surpass the limits of the maturely developed ego" (Washburn, 1995, p. ix). Transpersonal psychology studies the dimensions of optimal psychological health and well-being and our sense of identity beyond individual ego and personality. Transpersonal psychology is a multidisciplinary inquiry designed as a holistic understanding of human nature. This model is a synthesis of psychology, spiritual studies, and philosophy (Washburn, 1995) and represents the psychic level of development in Wilber's (1977) spectrum of consciousness discussed earlier in the chapter. The chief objective of transpersonal theory is to integrate spiritual experience within a larger understanding of human nature and human development (Washburn, 1995). These transegoic stages of human development have been associated with spiritual development and have been addressed by Eastern spiritual traditions but not traditionally in Western psychology. This aspect of transpersonal psychology will be addressed in the next chapter.

Transpersonal psychotherapy as it relates to mental illness ". . . includes traditional areas and concerns, adding to these an interest in facilitating growth and awareness beyond traditionally recognized levels of health. The importance of modifying consciousness and the validity of transcendental experience and identity is affirmed" (Walsh & Vaughan, 1980, p. 16). This type of psychotherapy involves helping the client to see that problems arise when an individual overidentifies with personal issues and fails to see that he or she is part of an ongoing and greater whole. In transpersonal psychotherapy, the client comes to recognize that the self is "alright" no matter what has happened to him or her individually—that what we do or do not do does not reflect on the essential "alrightness" of the self. For example, one may be a depressed, compulsive drinker, but the core essential self is still whole and valuable. In this model, mental illness or psychological distress comes from an essential and erroneous idea that we are separate from others, the world, and, in particular, the essential unity of all things (May, 1991). In the example of depression, this state occurs when one experiences life as separate and alone because the knowledge of unity and complete belonging is lost. This is often referred to as existential depression.

Psychological work in this model first involves having experiences of unity. As Shulman (1997) notes, "No one needs an image [or experience] of unity more than someone who is fragmented and dissociated" (p. 43). Second, therapy in this model explores issues that arise in nonordinary states of consciousness, such as dreams and paranormal and spiritual events. It provides a means to evoke such experiences in transcending the confines of the ego. These transcendent experiences are essential to transpersonal psychotherapy.

Transcendence involves the ability to extend the self beyond the immediate context of ego and environment to achieve a new perspective. It involves a search for meaning, a sense of what makes life worth living (Aldridge, 1996). One of the earliest theorists in transpersonal psychology, Abraham Maslow (1971), called these transcendent events "peak experiences." Maslow saw peak experiences as innate to human functioning and at the furthest reaches of human nature (Washburn, 1995). He believed true mental health involves transcendent experiences as commonplace. A transcendent experience takes us beyond our ordinarily experienced world of physical environment and material objects and actions. A true transcendent experience is unmistakably beyond the ordinary experience of material reality, so unusual it threatens or destroys previous belief structure and expands or heals some aspect of a person's personality (Brophy, 1999).

A transcendent experience is, by definition, an altered state of consciousness—a state different from the usual state of awareness—and has a number of qualities (Walsh et al., 1980). First, such an experience has an ineffable quality. It is so powerful and so different from ordinary experience that it simply cannot be described with words. At the same time, transcendent experiences offer a heightened sense of clarity and understanding, known as a noetic quality. These experiences energize and motivate the individual. Transcendent experiences usually involve an altered perception of space and time. Hunt (1995) comments, "The human sense of a transcendent reality at the basis of the mystical traditions rests on a direct attunement to time as an experienced flow out of an unknown source" (p. 193). After the experience is over, one may feel that only a short time has elapsed when, in fact, several hours have gone by. Another characteristic of transcendent events is the intense, positive emotion, including a sense of perfection of the universe, that accompanies it. Finally, transcendent events provide experiences of and appreciation for the holistic, unitive nature of the universe and one's unity with it. Transcendent experiences grab your whole attention and envelop you in an indescribable experience.

Literature brings us a wonderful example of transcendent experiences and the effects they have in Charles Dickens's *A Christmas Carol*. Ebenezer Scrooge, the main character, has three transcendent experiences on Christmas Eve in the form of three ghosts who come to him. The three visitations are very real to him, time is altered during the experience, and he has intense and varied emotions. Although initially Scrooge sees his experiences as negative, the subsequent results are overwhelmingly positive—his whole outlook on life changes, he becomes a loving and generous person, and he forges a new relationship with his nephew and family. "In many cases, what began as a negative experience can be seen as a powerful transformative potentiality deep in the center of the human psyche. It can then be sought in a controlled way for its own sake" (Shulman, 1997, p. 187). Music therapy techniques can be one means to seek transcendent experiences in a controlled way. In fact, music may be one of the most common and most acceptable means for individuals to generate transcendent experiences.

One of the most recognized transcendent or peak experiences related to art and, in particular, music is the aesthetic response. An aesthetic reaction is the human response to "the beautiful" in nature and, particularly, in art. Many believe the aesthetic reaction is a fundamental human experience (Gaston, 1968b; Maslow, 1970). An aesthetic experience has all the qualities of a transcendent event. The aesthetic reaction to music is a direct perceptual awareness of flow. In music, sound unfolds over time and carries us into an overpowering, enveloping experience.

> Music arrives in our nervous systems and causes our brains to generate a flood of anticipation by which we make sense of melody and harmony and rhythm and form. By eliciting these anticipations, music entrains the deepest levels of intention, and so it takes us over. . . . For a few moments it makes us larger than we really are, and the world more orderly than it really is. We respond not just to the beauty of the sustained deep relations that are revealed, but also to the fact of our perceiving them. As our brains are thrown into overdrive, we feel our very existence expand and realize that we can be more than we normally are, and that the world is more than it seems. (Jourdain, 1997, pp. 329, 331)

In an aesthetic experience, attention is completely focused on the musical experience at hand. In the aesthetic moment, we are then overpowered with strong positive emotion, a feeling of ecstasy. Ecstasy is a feeling of being overwhelmed but in a wonderful and transporting way. Music is ecstasy in and of itself. "Ecstasy melts the boundaries of our being, reveals our bonds to the external world, engulfs us in feelings that are 'oceanic'" (Jourdain, 1997, p. 327). In other words, it takes us into a transcendent, transpersonal experience. When we are engulfed in oceanic feelings we have a sense of calm and tranquility and an overriding sense of the unity of all. The inherent dynamics of melody, harmony, and rhythm turns raw perceptual experience into a unified whole (Aigen, 1995a). We have aesthetic reactions to things we perceive as an integrated whole.

Transpersonal Music Psychotherapy

The goal of transpersonal psychotherapy is to help the individual move toward what Maslow called self-actualization—the state when the self is unburdened by the deficiencies of personality so that the individual can enjoy the world without attachments and be of service without being self-righteous. Transpersonal psychotherapy works to transcend the conflicts of the ego by expanding identity beyond the ego to a holistic unitive awareness itself. The goal is to ". . . encourage and develop those tendencies which allow an individual to disidentify from the restrictions of the personality and to apprehend their identity with the total self" (Fadiman, 1980, p. 177). This is psychological work at the existential level where the individual confronts basic questions of meaning and purpose in life and disidentifies with roles, possessions, activities, and relationships. This is accomplished by bringing the client into transcendent experiences. The attainment of these experiences is not the aim of therapy per se, but it is a means to bring up fundamental questions concerning the nature of reality and one's true identity (Vaughan, 1980). This is the process of "awakening," which is achieved by enhancing inner awareness and intuition. However, there must be an ongoing "practice" or system to reproduce the insights and new awareness gained (Wilber, 1996). Music therapy techniques used in this therapeutic model can provide some of those practices.

There are several ways in which music therapy techniques can provide a practice to reproduce the insights gained in transcendent experiences. First, the transcendent experience of the aesthetic reaction to music can provide some of the first transcendent experiences. "The aesthetic is essential to our healthful embrace of life" (Aigen, 1995a, p. 242). Listening to music in an altered state of consciousness, such as in GIM, can provide this experience. Though these may not eliminate the symptoms of mental illness at first, they do provide the much-needed sense of wholeness and unity. Second, transcendent experiences with music are safer and more acceptable than other forms. Many transcendent experiences (near-death experiences, spontaneous visions, deep dreams) are frightening and uncontrollable. Music not only evokes the experience but also provides a structure to contain it. The ecstasy of an aesthetic reaction is a socially acceptable and familiar form of transpersonal experience. Another way music therapy techniques provide a practice for transcendent experiences is within active music making, especially spontaneous improvisation. During these experiences, we have a direct, nonverbal experience of transcendence (Rugenstein, 1996). We are focused in the here and now but with a visceral sense of the connection to others and to the greater whole. A fourth way in which music therapy provides a practice for transpersonal insights is in music's ability to facilitate movement between different states of consciousness. This has historically been the use of music in various traditions around the world (McClellan, 1988). From chant traditions, to shamanic repetitive drumming, to use of gongs and metal bowls, music has been used to dissolve psyche boundaries and shift our state of awareness. Music may not be a particular method to lead to transpersonal reality, but it can remove the obstacles to such experiences. This is addressed in greater detail in the next chapter. Finally, as explored in chapter 1, music connects us with "that which is greater than ourselves." It embodies a unity consciousness of Divine Principle. In music, we hear and viscerally experience this principle.

Developmental Model
The developmental model was addressed as it relates to normal psychological growth earlier in this chapter. In this model, arrest at a particular stage in the normal developmental sequence is considered the cause of mental illness. In this developmental diagnostic spectrum, the various clinical syndromes are viewed as originating in specific phases of development. If something goes wrong at any stage in this developmental unfolding, aspects of the self become damaged or "left behind." "This 'getting left behind' is called repression, or dissociation or alienation. . . . [T]his loss results in a pathology that is characteristic of the stage at which the loss occurred" (Wilber, 1996, p. 143). Any number of negative experiences—trauma, loss, abuse, neglect—can cause a person's psychological development to stop at the level at which he or she experiences the trauma. Each stage of development has specific and distinct psychopathologies. For example, a trauma in the earliest stages of Level 1 leads to severe mental illness like schizophrenia; while arrested development at Level 2 could cause a "neurotic" disorder like general anxiety disorder.

In the developmental model, therapy does not treat a disease entity but, rather, ". . . reinstates a derailed, arrested or distorted developmental process" (Wilber, Engler, & Brown, 1986, p. 50). Combs (1995) notes that effective therapy occurs in this model by using a two-stage approach—first disrupting older forms of awareness and second introducing and strengthening new and more mature levels of consciousness. This is accomplished through intense experiences with the therapist guiding and supporting the process. "One of the central tasks of the self is to 'digest' or 'metabolize' the experiences presented to it at each rung of development. 'The basic assumption of developmental theory is that experience must become "metabolized" to form structure'" (Wilber, 1986, p. 79). All the various therapy models and techniques utilize different strategies for addressing a particular problem at a particular level of development. As Wilber (1996) notes, "Different therapies tend to plug into different levels of this spectrum, and use their favorite level as the basic reference point around which they will offer their interpretation" (p. 111). By using the developmental model, seemingly exclusive therapy approaches to mental illness can be reconciled by acknowledging that each treatment modality can be appropriately used at a particular level in the spectrum of consciousness development.

Music Therapy in the Developmental Model

Music therapy interventions, guided by the music therapist, are intense experiences that can effectively be used in this model. Music therapy techniques can both disrupt old patterns of awareness and provide the individual with experiences to help develop and incorporate new levels of consciousness. Sekeles (1996) states, "Music contains the ability to link internal and external processes . . . great importance is attached to this linkage in the process of development and growth" (p. 38). Earlier in this chapter, a number of specific treatment modalities were reviewed, and the use of music therapy in each was explored. Since music influences us on all levels of consciousness, music therapy can work as a psychotherapeutic modality at all levels of development. To complete this examination, mental illness at each level of Wilber's spectrum of consciousness and how music therapy can be part of the treatment at that level are shown.

The three levels of the prepersonal development in stage one involve generation of a basic sense of self, differentiation of self from others, and development of mental and emotional selves. This basic ego development occurs in early childhood. Prepersonal pathologies occur when trauma arrests developmental in this early ego formation, causing structural deficits in the ego through faulty early object relations development.

> Object relations refers to the sequence and quality of one's experience with interpersonal objects, especially with primary caretakers; and the internalization of these interactions in a representation of "self" and a representation of the "object" which are linked by an affect and coded in memory trances as "good" or "bad." (Engler, 1986, p. 26)

In this model, pathologies at this level include psychotic syndromes, like schizophrenia and borderline personality disorder, and neurotic disabilities such as obsessive-compulsive disorder, simple depression, phobias, conversion reactions, and anxiety disorders. In the organic model of mental illness, severe forms of mental illness, like schizophrenia and borderline personality disorder, are believed to be *caused* by chemical imbalance or structural abnormality. In the developmental model, the trauma causing the arrested development is seen to affect the chemical balance in the brain. The problem, including the chemical imbalance, is caused by the arrested development brought on by the trauma. Noted psychiatrist Gerald May (1982) states,

> The fact that certain psychological manifestations are mediated by brain chemicals or may be strongly affected by administrated drugs does not necessarily mean that thoughts, feelings, or moods are *created* by chemicals. Just as thoughts, memories, and behavior can be triggered by certain concentrations and combinations of brain chemicals, so also can thoughts, feelings, and the like trigger changes in chemicals. At the most basic levels . . . the human being is such an intimate joining of mind/brain/body/spirit/energy/consciousness that all arbitrary separations must be fundamentally inaccurate. (p. 156)

Neurotic disorders respond well to uncovering techniques, as discussed previously. However, psychotic and borderline personality disorders require structure-building techniques to build a distinct and individual sense of self. Structure-building techniques help a disordered self to differentiate from others and from early poor caregivers, stabilize as an individual self, and build needed ego structure. Music therapy practice for clients with schizophrenia and borderline personality disorder can provide structure-building experiences in several ways. First, as Sears (1968) postulated, music *is* structured reality. Music is a real event occurring in the environment. Physical sound waves are produced that actually exist. These vibrations stimulate the ear and are perceived by the brain. The music event has a definite beginning and ending. Because of the beat and rhythm, music moves at a set pace over time, making anticipation in a music activity participation in reality. The music provides a moment-to-moment commitment to what is really happening. When I worked in the psychiatric hospital, we often took the patients with schizophrenia out to play softball. This was an excellent activity and had many benefits for their overall well-being and functioning, but reality orientation was not always one of them. Many times, a patient would be standing in the outfield talking to a hallucinated figure, clearly not able to hold a moment-to-moment commitment to the activity. The patients were aware enough, though, to field a ball hit to them, often reporting the event to their nonexistent friend. This does not happen with a music activity. If someone is playing guitar and attention moves away from the reality of the moment, the instrument cannot be played successfully. The chord changes won't happen on time if the performer is not fully aware of what is happening in the present moment. I once learned to predict when a client with schizophrenia was about to have a psychotic episode (a break with reality). I knew because she suddenly would be unable to sing in tune. As she slipped away from awareness of the environment around her, she couldn't match pitch anymore. This demonstrates that music is a real and obvious event in the environment and that successful participation in music requires attention to reality.

A second way music therapy interventions are structure-building activities is when they are used to develop self-concept, as explored earlier in this chapter. In music therapy experiences, the client engages in activities that retrace the basic ego development patterns. This comes through engagement in successful playing experiences with real and obvious standards of achievement. Progress made in music skill building is overt and obvious to the client. No external feedback is needed. We can hear for ourselves when our playing gets better. Music is also a culturally valued activity. We receive acceptance and esteem from others because we have performed a musical skill.

A third way music therapy offers structure-building experiences occurs because music creates a safe, predictable environment with a consistent, empathetic caregiver—the music therapist. Shulman (1997) notes that if a client with schizophrenia ". . .were protected, supported, and understood during this process, a spontaneous rebuilding of personality structure could take place" (pp. 47–48). Music, because of its inherent structure and perceptual predictability, creates the protected, supportive environment while allowing a nonthreatening, interpersonal interaction with the music therapist. In this way, music therapy provides a form of supportive therapy. May (1982) defines supportive therapy as ". . . contacts that help the person handle daily-life tasks and stresses, and that encourage the re-establishment of defenses and understandable thinking" (p. 164). This includes appropriate interactions, basic conversation, responding to external sensory input, following directions, taking turns, and other basic skills and responses. In supportive therapy, the client grows in self-understanding, comprehension of the effects of behavior, and ability to actively change habitual patterns of response. This is accomplished by reexperiencing early caregiver relationships in a new, healthier context. Wilber, Engler, and Brown (1986) contend that the best treatment for clients with schizophrenia and borderline personality disorder is through the medium of a new and different kind of two-way relationship than they had during earlier periods of development. The communication aspects of music provide a means of establishing structure-building interpersonal relationships.

The third level of prepersonal development, the development of the mental self, is the point at which the individual learns to repress the emotional self through mental activity. Trauma at this stage of development leads to what is often referred to as neurosis or psychoneurosis. According to Wilber (1996), this means ". . . that a fairly stable, cohesive, mental self has emerged, and this mental-conceptual self (the ego) can repress or dissociate aspects of its bodily drives or impulses . . ." (p. 170). If the repression is severe and prolonged, these feelings return later in life in disguised and painful forms. These repressed forms are labeled neurotic disorders. They involve symptoms of fear, distress, depression, anxiety, and psychological pain. An excellent example of this process is posttraumatic stress disorder (PTSD). In PTSD, an individual experiences a real traumatic event, such as a plane crash, rape, or war. The psychological effects of that trauma are then expressed months and years later in depression, anxiety, fear, flashbacks to the trauma, and social dysfunction.

Therapy at this stage of development largely involves uncovering strategies to identify repressed memories and emotions. Herman (1992) identifies three steps to recovery from PTSD: regain a sense of safety, remember the details of the trauma and mourn the loss it brought, and reestablish a normal life. Music can contribute to a sense of safety and control because of its predictability and familiarity, but it is the use of music therapy in uncovering strategies as part of psychotherapy that is so essential to work at this level of developmental arrest. It is at this level that music psychotherapy techniques would be beneficial in finding the memories of the trauma, experiencing the emotions associated with it, and mourning the changes that have occurred.

The second stage of consciousness development in Wilber's model is the personal. The three levels of development encompassed at this stage are more concerned with cognitive, identity, and existential concerns. Pathology at this stage includes conduct disorders, social anxiety, and identity disorders; problems of personal autonomy and adult actualization; and existential anxiety over role, meaning of life, and death.

> Existential issues are those crucial and universal concerns all of us face simply because we are human. They include finding meaning and purpose in our lives; managing relationships and aloneness; acknowledging our limits and smallness in a universe vast beyond comprehension; living in inevitable uncertainty and mystery; and dealing with sickness, suffering, and death. (Walsh, 2002, p. 13)

At the first level of the personal stage, the cognitive therapies with their focus on faulty "scripts" and the need to make changes in these cognitive structures would be the most useful. The second and third levels of this stage respond to psychotherapy techniques emphasizing new meaning or personal insights as to the underlying causes of problems and bringing them to conscious awareness. Music therapy in these approaches was extensively examined in the section on music psychotherapy.

The third stage of Wilber's model is the transpersonal stage, which was also explored previously. Pathology at this stage involves spontaneous and unsought transcendent experiences, a sense of aloneness and abandonment, and a sense of the meaninglessness of life. As discussed, music therapy can provide experiences useful at this stage of development. The last two levels of transpersonal development—the subtle and causal—are explored more fully in the next chapter.

Complexity Science Model
A final way in which mental illness and the process of therapy can be envisioned, and of particular interest to the thesis of this book, is from the perspective of complexity science. In previous models, mental illness is assumed to have discrete, objective "causes" often independent of context. Like a virus infection causing a head cold, mental illness is believed to be caused by some factor—chemical imbalance, improper learning, or arrested development. But in complexity science theory, that views our psychological processes as based on complex adaptive systems, such local causes of mental illness are inadequate to explain something as complex as a severe mental illness (Shulman, 1997). Complexity science theory tells us that mental health problems arise from the entire system, not from a discrete factor.

Based on complexity theory, the human psyche, like all other aspects of human functioning, is a complex, dynamical system.

> The lived situation of the embodied psyche is far more complex and ambiguous, with bodily experience, human community, objects, ideas, memories, metaphors, images, symbols, language, and values appearing spontaneously from an unconscious matrix we can know little about because it is more complex and dense than the ego which attempts to know it. (Shulman, 1997, p. 13)

All aspects of mind are emergent properties of this nonlinear dynamical system, as explored in chapter 4. This includes all the stages and levels of consciousness development, our personality structure, ego, and unconscious processing. Complexity is the hallmark of development from biological structures to the subtle evolution of the inner psychic life (Csikszentmihalyi, 1993). As the principles of complexity science tell us, development of the human psyche is not linear. As Shulman (1997) notes, both the body and psyche are ". . . evolving information processing systems that depend on feedback from the environment. They are both complex adaptive systems poised near the edge of chaos, capable of complicated modeling and going through processes of change, though at different time scales" (p. 119). Combs (1995) sees the stages of consciousness development as new bifurcations that emerge as the psyche becomes more complex: "Stage theories in psychology see maturation as proceeding through a series of such bifurcations, each heralding a quantal jump in complexity" (p. 62). As each level increases in complexity through experiences with the environment, it reaches a critical level of complexity and a new type of awareness emerges.

A number of Jungian analysts (Shulman, 1997; Van Eenwyk, 1996) see Jung's theories of ego, consciousness development, and the archetypes as expressions of a complex adaptive system on a psychic level. As Van Eenwyk (1996) writes, Jung ". . . clearly conceived of psychic structure as a function of dynamics, which he defined as energetics. Furthermore, that he conceived of dynamics as generated by (and thus, characterized by) tensions of opposites calls to mind the activity of bifurcations and oscillations" (p. 330). In this view, the ego serves as an attractor. In complexity theory, an attractor is a pattern into which a system settles. It is self-similar across scale. In Jung's own words, the ego ". . . has a great power of attraction, like a magnet; it attracts contents from the unconscious. . . . [I]t also attracts impressions from the outside . . ." (quoted in Humbert, 1988, p. 18). In psychological functioning, such attractor patterns become a person's personality characteristics and level of consciousness. This constantly fluctuating, edge-of-chaos processing is the dynamic of psychic development and mental health. One of Jung's central ideas is that

> . . . consciousness is constantly in the process of being created, that such a process is the result of an intent residing within the psyche—more specifically, in that dimension of the psyche called the 'unconscious'—and that essential to this process are images from everyday life. (Van Eenwyk, 1996, p. 336)

In Jung's theory, these images become archetypes. Archetypal images take the ego from consciousness to unconsciousness and back again in a dynamical system of self-organization and emergence. Because of this constant, dynamic movement between the conscious and unconscious, archetypal images disrupt the linear flow of consciousness, ". . . immersing the ego in the chaotic/non-linear flow of the unconscious and bringing it 'back' again" (Van Eenwyk, 1996, p. 336).

Mental health involves the constant shifting and dynamics of a system balancing at the edge of chaos. Systems at the edge of chaos are immensely flexible, able to adjust to a changing environment while maintaining coherence, and able to create new ways of coping with the unexpected. As a personality structure, the psyche poised at the edge of chaos is not likely to get stuck or arrested at one stage of development. Mental health, then, constitutes a complex dynamical system. Contrarily, mental illness is the lack of dynamic complexity—a lack of movement necessary to generate flexibility, vigor, and the ability to adjust to change and regain equilibrium through the generation of new ways—new bifurcations.

In this model, mental illness occurs when crisis strategies no longer work and the individual becomes "stuck," unable to move from the personality traits that have developed. According to Shainberg (1973), mental illness exists when images of the self become rigid and closed, restricting an open, creative response to the world. Briggs and Peat (1999) see mental illness and negative personality characteristic as limit cycles—systems cut off from the influx of new information from the external environment. To restore mental health, the patient needs to move toward the edge of chaos, a place where potential new order, like a personality trait or coping mechanism, can emerge. In this model, then, as each new bifurcation occurs, a whole new person emerges. "Personal growth becomes less the acquisition of new behaviors (the same person with some added traits) than a total change in the self system (a new person)" (Wade, 1996, p. 168). Therapy for mental illness in the complexity model would involve moving the individual into an edge-of-chaos dynamic through the input of complex information that allows a new way, a new bifurcation constituting mental health, to occur.

The traditional methods of treating mental illness discussed previously are linear and reductionistic. However, in complexity science, they may still positively affect mental health by adding information to the psyche and thus creating a new bifurcation—a state of mental health. Even unconventional and seemingly extreme treatment may be effective from a complexity science perspective. There are some historical examples of this. These methods illustrate the need for intense environmental and sensory information to cause a change from mental illness to mental health. "Unless the environment can overwhelm the individual, he is unlikely to change" (Wade, 1996, p. 265). Perhaps the best historical example of these ancient techniques occurred in ancient Rome in the healing temples of the demigod Aesclepius (Rudolph, 1988). When patients would arrive at the temple, whether for a mental or physical complaint, they would be taken to an underground rock chamber and placed on a couch where they were expected to go to sleep. As they slept, hissing snakes were placed around the couch, monks would chant continuously, and loud horns, flutes, and drums would be played at random. In other words, an extraordinary, unusual, highly sensory stimulating, and emotional event took place. High-order, complex information would be introduced into the patient's psyche. As Wade (1996) notes, one of three things would happen—the patient would ignore the input, essentially being in a state of denial; the patient would dissolve into chaos, psychologically known as regression; or the patient would arrive at some higher level of organization, a new catastrophic bifurcation. This new, higher level of organization would constitute an adaptive state of increased mental health. In the 1940s movie *The Snake Pit*, the central character is "shocked" into sanity when put in a writhing pit of fellow mental patients.

However, we know from complexity science theory that these huge, overwhelming experiences, per se, may not be necessary for these new bifurcations in the human psyche to occur. In fact, small changes in experience can enable complex systems to display new, positive self-organizing behavior. These experiences need to have sensory novelty, should display attention-grabbing characteristics, and must be judged to be highly valuable to the individual.

The experiences in music therapy processes can act as these value-laden, sensory experiences adding to psyche complexity and bringing the individual to a new awareness, a new bifurcation or order of psychic functioning.

> Understanding mental illness through the model of state changes in information processing systems, opens many new possibilities for healing. The world of complex adaptive systems is always open to changes in energy in the environment; it is a world where nothing is "determined" or fixed. To be alive as an organism means to constantly take energy from outside and transform it into morphogenic development. Perhaps, in this model, we can find more creative ways to meet the demoralized spirits of the mentally ill. (Shulman, 1997, p. 202)

We know that music is a highly complex energetic input that brings a high level of excitation both through sensory channels and through the human energetic system. In complexity science theory, higher excitation through information brings a dynamical system to a point of bifurcation. It also evokes the complexity and dynamic movement of internal emotional states. Involvement in and exposure to the information-rich sensory experience of music may bring an individual to such a bifurcation point. Aesthetic reactions may be an example of this. So are the emergence of mental images and emotions in response to music and the creative activity of musical improvisation.

In music psychotherapy, where music is used to reach, express, and integrate deep psychic material, the spontaneous emergence of a deep insight can be seen as an emergent process, a form of catastrophic bifurcation to a new order—the new insight. For these insights to emerge, a threshold, which usually protects the ego, must be crossed. This threshold is the inner phenomenological experience of the edge of chaos, which is a fundamental human possibility touched in altered states of consciousness. In terms of the human psyche, this is a liminal state. A liminal state is an ambiguous state that pulls us out of the conventional into an out-of-time experience where feelings of identification with a whole are intensified (Ruud, 1995). In a liminal, edge-of-chaos state, all possibilities exist, yet none has manifested. It is a state of optimal creativity. In psychological development, it reflects a new maturational window. If successful imprinting occurs during this liminal state, the individual can return to the social world with new energies and a new role. "Such maturational windows can be thought of as 'phase changes' that occur within the organism . . ." (Shulman, 1997, p. 91).

Altered states of consciousness, peak experiences, and aesthetic reactions to music create such liminal states. The music creates a culturally acceptable space separate from language where the images and nonverbal communication of the unconscious are expressed (Ruud, 1995). This occurs in music therapy techniques like GIM, but such liminal experiences are usually seen as frightening, threatening, and difficult by our controlling ego. So to be effective, a liminal experience in psychotherapy must feel somewhat familiar, safe, comfortable, and protected during these periods of transition. Music provides this sense of safety through its familiarity and structure. A music psychotherapy technique like GIM provides an effective edge-of-chaos experience for the psyche because it creates the liminal space, evokes the dynamic energy of emotions and intrasubjective images, and makes the whole experience safe and acceptable. In GIM, it is both music and the regular attention of the guide (therapist) that provide the grounding for these liminal, edge-of-chaos experiences.

> This kind of [musical] harmonic and melodic complexity (or tension) is helpful for a person who opens themselves to the deeper contents of their internal world. The structural complexity is felt as supportive for the person who is discovering and working with deep internal material. (Bonny, 2001, p. 61)

Improvisational music therapy techniques also provide for edge-of-chaos experiences that lead to new personal insights. The improvisation process involves experimentation, self-expression, and creativity. These come from deep places within ourselves and offer an opportunity to experiment with different ways of feeling, being, and expressing. As Ruud (1995) puts it,

> Improvisations in music therapy attempt to create a similar space—a psychic (re)dressing room—where people may try out alternative ways of expression and action in order to find webs of meaning which are in accordance with their own biographical experiences and expectations. (p. 98)

As improvisation proceeds, more complex information is brought to the individual who is then brought to the edge of chaos. Musical improvisation is a liminal experience because it brings in a highly emotionally charged event, physical movement, a sense of community, and numinous symbols. New bifurcations as insights or new awareness then emerge. "This improvisation makes change possible—with or without therapeutic consequences" (Ruud, 1995, p. 107). The guidance and interaction of the music therapist are part of the complexity of information, but a therapeutic change can occur whether the music therapist actively "does" a therapy intervention or not.

During improvisation, spontaneous music making occurs, and a balance is struck between structure and a more unstructured liminal state. The familiar conventions of music—melody, time, rhythm, dynamics—anchor the experience but also constitute the habitual. A partial reversal of the habitual can create a liminal state. In musical improvisation, these conventions of music are stretched, manipulated, and used in uncharacteristic ways. Improvisation becomes an experience of the liminal or the edge of chaos. Shulman (1997) sees specific stages in this general process of movement into the liminal state. These stages are heard in group improvisation experiences. An example of this is the improvisation experience I use as a teaching tool for music therapy students. During a group process class, I engage the seniors in my music therapy program in several weeks of free musical improvisation. I observe these stages clearly during these experiences. The first stage involves the "old order" characterized by stilted, convention-bound improvisation. In this stage of improvisation, there is no creativity and no growth or exploration. The music is very conventional and boring. I refer to this as "rinky-dink" music. This stage, then, gives way to the next—a period of chaotic playing. All musical conventions are lost, and a great deal of banging and noisemaking occurs. No one is playing together or listening to anyone else, but this stage also involves individual exploration where new melodic and harmonic combinations are tried. Toward the end of this stage, the improvisation begins to move away from chaos as a true liminal state is entered. Reordering and reintegration begin. In the final stage of the improvisation, a new, more functional and harmonious ordering emerges as the group crosses back toward the structured. The music becomes more recognizable and more conventional but with a freer, less restricted quality. The students express musical satisfaction and interest during this stage of the improvisation.

Approaching mental health and mental illness from the perspective of complexity science addresses the constantly changing and evolving nature of the human psyche. Information-laden experiences, like music therapy interventions, can provide the movement needed to keep the self-organizing system of the psyche at the edge of chaos and in a flexible, vigorous state to withstand the traumas of our world.

Having added the complex interaction of the human emotional mind to the theory of music and soulmaking, it is time to explore the final area of human functioning—spirit. This exploration of human spirit involves our sense of community and relationships with others, rituals and play, new levels or alterations of consciousness, and, ultimately, the search for a realization of a new way of being. It is this final level of human growth that is addressed in the next chapter.

CHAPTER SEVEN

~

Music Therapy
and Problems of Spirit

A music therapy colleague and I are working with a group of twenty-five sixth, seventh, and eighth grade students in an inner-city school. These kids come from disadvantaged families. Most have problems with attention and impulse control. Each is both a tough, loud teenager and a needy, sweet kid. They are all at risk for involvement in gang activity. Since involvement in gangs provides a means for these disenfranchised kids to belong and feel connected to something, I've developed a music therapy program based on world drumming traditions to provide a positive means of belonging to something. We meet once a week for three hours to learn African, Japanese, and Afro-Caribbean drumming; do arts and crafts; have guest artists teach us international dances; do storytelling; engage in trust-building games; and have some fun. Our activities are meant to foster a positive sense of peer identification and affiliation, personal self-esteem through musical achievement, skills in problem solving and anger management, and tolerance for differences and awareness of diversity.

This is not an easy group to work with. Their attention span is very short, and their ability to practice the various drumming ensembles is limited. They are from different "cliques" and don't like each other. They fight and verbally hurt each other's feelings. And they never, ever let my colleague and me know they're enjoying themselves. But the music therapy interventions we use are designed for them to succeed immediately, and we always include activities like games and arts and crafts they really enjoy. Soon they trust us a bit more and are responding to our structure and discipline. The group names itself "the Village Drummers," and they begin to feel special and important. At holiday time, the Village Drummers perform

*in the school assembly in front of people for the first time. They are terrified of
"messing up," afraid to appear foolish in front of their peers. They act out, goof off,
and have a terrible dress rehearsal. We approach the performance with great trepi-
dation. But they do a wonderful job and are rewarded by the applause and cheers
of the audience. They suddenly develop a sense of pride, a feeling of belonging to
something special. They make connections to us, to their peers, and to the school
community. It is a small step in helping them stay out of the gangs, but it is a step.*

In this chapter, the fourth area of human functioning—*spirit* and issues of
spirituality—is explored. These aspects of human functioning have not traditionally been included in the various therapeutic approaches, including music therapy. More recently, issues of spirit were generally addressed as part of
a therapeutic approach (Dilts & McDonald, 1997; Faiver et al., 2001; Frame,
2003; Washburn, 1995; Wilber, 1998) and specifically in music therapy practice (Aldridge, 1996; Bonny, 2001; Lipe, 2002). There is increasing evidence
that the impetus for this interest in spirituality is biologically based (Cook &
Persinger, 1997; Hooper & Teresi, 1986; Newberg, d'Aquil, & Rause, 2001;
Saver & Rabin, 1997; Siegel, 1977). "Spirituality is far more than a psychological and emotional need: it is an inherent biological need" (Myss, 1996,
p. 64). Anthropologist Michael Winkelman (2000) sees human involvement
in experiences of spirituality as a neurophenomenological occurrence, linking neurological structures, physiology, and neurological processes with cultural practices and personal experiences of spirit. Such an approach acknowledges the complex interaction of neurophysiology, psychology, and
culture in this aspect of human functioning.

The term *spirit* has a number of meanings and definitions derived from
many cultures and belief systems around the world. For the purpose of this
book, a Western definition of spirit is used with the word having two meanings both derived from the Latin root word *spiritus*. *Spiritus* means "breath,
life force, vigor, and animating principle." However, it also implies "otherness" (Frame, 2003). With these two meanings *spirit* implies first the "otherness" of a greater whole, known as the Divine Principle, Great Creator, Divine Spirit, or God. In this sense, spirit involves living life in a perpetual
reaching out for *Divine Spirit* (Freeman, 2001a). The second meaning of spirit
implies the *human spirit*, your individual portion of the greater whole that is
manifested and expressed in an individual's life as vitality and life force
(Davis, 1999). This distinguishes self from other people, another form of
"otherness."

Experiences with Divine Spirit and human spirit are vital to the process
of soulmaking (Dilts & McDonald, 1997) because they help us explore issues

of purpose and meaning. "It is these spiritual elements of experience that help us to rise above the matters at hand such that in the face of suffering we can find purpose, meaning and hope" (Aldridge, 1996, p. 225). The links of spirituality to health and well-being and why this aspect of human functioning is important in a holistic approach to therapy, like the theory of music and soulmaking, are examined later. Music was linked with issues of spirit since the earliest human cultures. As the composer Igor Stravinsky (1947) noted, "The profound meaning of music and its essential aim . . . is to promote a communion, a union of man with his fellow man and with the Supreme Being" (p. 21).

This aspect of music and soulmaking is within the realm of deeply subjective experiences. This chapter introduces theories related to these subjective experiences from transpersonal psychology, spirituality, and the tools to stimulate and evaluate subjective experiences culled from the wisdom traditions of the world. Music in some form has always been a part of those traditions. The importance and relevance of these techniques and experiences related to music therapy practice and to the theory of music and soulmaking are explored.

Issues of spirit are deeply personal relating to reconnection to our essential wholeness as a state of being. This involves another form of healing not related to "fixing" problems but to experiencing that wholeness as pure love (May, 1991). "If we do not make room in our diagnosis and medical models for spirit, exactly that which can never be fully known because it is more creative than 'knowing,' the most important healing function of the human personality is not recognized" (Shulman, 1997, p. 206). Perhaps music therapy and spirit are about allowing music to take you to a state of pure being. Though complete separation from cultural and personal influences may never be possible for human beings, a closer experience of Divine "at-oneness" may be the next stage of human potential.

The Nature of Spirit

To begin, let's explore the use of the term *spirit* in its two definitions—as the metaphysical source of "all-that-is" or Divine Spirit, and as the manifestation of that metaphysical source in every person known as human spirit (Davis, 1999).

Divine Spirit
Divine Spirit is an extrapsychic, metaphysical cosmic force variously referred to throughout history as the Divine Principle, the Great Creator, Spirit, the Universal Mind, and God (Washburn, 1995). This is traditionally the area of

the numinous, the nonrational, mysterious aspects of the Divine (Lipe, 2002; Otto, [1923] 1958). Divine Spirit is the potential out of which all-there-is in the universe emerges. It is the impetus for all-there-is to emerge from the void of potential (Brophy, 1999). That impetus for emergence from the void comes from an intention. The basic tenant of Divine Spirit is that the universe did not form by accident. There is an intention behind it. One could say the universe is not random (Brophy, 1999).

Though Divine Spirit has traditionally been mysterious, unknowable, and beyond scientific investigation, the new sciences of quantum physics and complexity science give new perspectives on its nature and origin. As Wade (1996) notes, "The extreme reaches of science ultimately lead to spiritualism; the two are not necessarily different paths . . ." (p. 275). There are several theories from these sciences as to the nature of Divine Spirit.

Many quantum theorists (Brophy, 1999; Capra, 1975; Wolf, 1999) see Divine Spirit or Potential as quantum potential that allows one outcome to occur over another. On the subatomic level, phenomena cannot be predicted with certainty because subatomic particles are not "things," only tendencies to exist. Only the probability of an event can be predicted. The outcome of a quantum event is based on what property—position or movement of subatomic particles—we choose to measure or observe. All possibilities exist as a potential for occurrence waiting for some factor (the observation) to create something out of the potential. In a real sense on the subatomic level, all possible "realities" exist as potential waiting for some event to create or actualize any given reality. Divine Spirit is equated with this potential out of which reality emerges and with the reason one reality emerges over another (Zukav, 1979). Brophy (1999) defines Divine Spirit as ". . . that aspect of reality that is not contained in, or described by, or arising out of the mathematical equations of physics" (p. 131). It is that factor, other than chance or randomness, that causes one potential to occur over another. These "mysteries" are those aspects yet to be explained.

Physicist Fred Alan Wolf (1999) believes Divine Spirit lies in *zero-point energy* or the "vibrations of nothing," which have the potential for everything. These are the subtle vibrations that exist in the great cosmic void. To illustrate zero-point energy, he uses the example of a pendulum swinging back and forth past a point of rest. When the pendulum seemingly stops, it still jiggles with quantum potential around the point of rest. It is this type of vibration in the vacuum of the universe that he defines as Divine Spirit.

> The vacuum is alive with these vibrations. They contain the potential for anything. The process for realizing anything, becoming aware of anything, results

from reflection of these vibrations in the form of waves. To accomplish this re-flection some form of resistance that bounces these waves back in the direction from which they came must arise. (Wolf, 1999, p. 268)

This theory implies that this resistance is Divine Spirit.

From the perspective of complexity science, Divine Spirit is defined as a field of meaning, animation, or flow (Peat, 1992b). Davis (1999) sees spirit as a nonphysical subtle energy, while Goswami (2001) believes this subtle energy is a form of consciousness. In a broader sense, Divine Spirit is the pri-mordial force of complexity, the waxing and waning of chaos and order poised at the edge of chaos (Shulman, 1997). Ainslie (1995) points out that the word for chaos used in the Bible is derived from the Greek word mean-ing "gap or yawning chasm," often translated as "void," and the Hebrew word for "formlessness." This implies that the biblical meaning of chaos is a state of readiness to create order or the potential for all-that-is. Ainslie (1995) also states that, in chaos theory, Divine Spirit ". . . can be thought of as an 'at-tractor'" (p. 311). In fact, Briggs and Peat (1989) state that Divine Spirit may be all types of attractors—point, limit cycle, torus, and strange—depending on the types of creation needed. Ainslie (1995) also postulates an unknown attractor, a *numinous attractor*, as another way to conceive of Divine Spirit. To consider Divine Spirit as an attractor, a creative and flexible definition is required, defining it as a verb rather than a noun (Ainslie, 1995).

Music Therapy and Experiences of Divine Spirit

Traditionally, a direct encounter with Divine Spirit is known as a mysti-cal or *numinous* experience. The term *numinous* was first used by Rudolf Otto ([1923] 1958) to describe the nonrational aspects of Divine Spirit. Though the form of the numinous experience is influenced by cultural expectations and conditioning, it is the cross-culturally common *feeling* core of religious experience (Hunt, 1995). Numinous feelings are perceived as a direct expe-rience of the realm of the sacred (Shulman, 1997). True mystical, numinous experiences are more than and different from a mere altered state of con-sciousness (ASC) associated with human spirit. ASC are addressed later in this chapter. An ASC is another form of restricted response with its own type of narrowed awareness. The true mystical experience is an open awareness where information experienced is immediately integrated into awareness without psychological processing. The experience has a sense of realness and authority beyond psychological problem solving. It involves information not available to ordinary senses (Hunt, 1996). "With nothing specific that it is about, it is sensed as about everything" (Hunt, 1995, p. 29).

The numinous mystical experience is the direct sensing of our vitally streaming aliveness (Reich, 1949). It is our direct, living connectedness with Divine Spirit (May, 1991). As such, it is the experience of Divine Spirit in its fullness—in ecstasy and despair, in beauty and ugliness, in light and dark. According to Washburn (1995), the numinous is a

> ... dynamic presence that is ineffable, overawing, and compellingly magnetic.
> ... [T]he numinous is dramatically bivalent in that it has both light and dark
> manifestations and engenders in the mental ego both ecstasies and agonies,
> both exaltations and abasements. . . . [T]he numinous is experienced by the
> mental ego as an incomprehensible, ego-eclipsing, entrancing, and disconcert-
> ingly bivalent force. It presents itself as a reality that is daunting as well as
> transporting, a source of engulfing gravity as well as uplifting grace (pp.
> 125–126).

We both seek and deeply fear the mystical encounter.

In chapter 6, the connection between music and music therapy tech-niques and transpersonal experiences was explored at length. The numinous mystical experience is the ultimate transpersonal event. Music is one of the tools of spirit that can open the door to a mystical experience. It engenders and reflects mystical experiences. Music is a link to Divine Spirit, a glimpse of the spiritual world. As Rudolf Steiner notes, "In music, too, he [the per-son] experiences the image of a higher world" (quoted in Godwin, 1987, p. 259). Music provides us with a tangible means of remembering Divine Spirit. It gives us a glimpse of the infinite source of love and wholeness through felt moments of connection to the unknowable (May, 1991). As recognized since the earliest days of human culture, there is a metaphysical correspondence between music and Divine Spirit (Daniélou, 1995). Music opens the lines of communication between humans and Divine Spirit (Lipe, 2002). Many the-orists contend there is no straight line from the mind of humans to the Di-vine (Smith, 1989). Perhaps music, in all its complexity, is a form of com-munication that, in fact, provides such a connection.

Human Spirit

Divine Spirit is the creative force of the universe, the greater whole. This force is expressed in each individual. Wolf (1999) believes that the reflection of spirit in *time* is soul and the reflection of spirit in *space* is matter. Our individual por-tion of Divine Spirit, expressed in both soul and matter, is human spirit.

Human spirit is Divine Spirit expressed in each person. As Huston Smith (1989) notes, human spirit is the "thing" that is similar to or even identical with the Divine. Bateson and Bateson (1988) see Divine Spirit as the larger mind of which each individual is a subsystem. Human spirit is the Divine life force manifested and expressed in each person. The meaning of the word *spiritus* as "breath and wind" implies that human spirit is an animating principle. Breath and wind are the internal and external manifestations of movement (Abram, 1996). Human spirit implies movement as the life energy (Diamond, 1985). It is a vital, dynamic force of being and implies energy and power (May, 1982). Human spirit is vitality, a sense of the person coming alive.

Human spirit has a tangible quality. It is an actual palpable presence that serves to amplify experience. Human spirit magnifies and energizes all dimensions of human psychic life—mental images, insights, emotions, bodily sensations, intuition, and personality. It is something that is actually, substantially present. Human spirit is manifested in experience but is not itself that experience or our reaction to it (Davis, 1999). As psychologist Michael Washburn (1995) notes, referring to spirit as the Dynamic Ground, "When the power of the Ground flows, experience quickens, becoming alive and acute, if not tumultuous and overwhelmingly intense; when the power of the Ground ebbs, experience slows, becoming pale, distant, and dull" (p. 121). This aspect of human spirit is summarized by the words of the philosopher A. A. Almaas:

> Essence (spirit) is not alive, it is aliveness. It is not aware, it is awareness. It is not the quality of existence, it is existence. It is not loving, it is love. It is not joyful, it is joy. It is not true, it is truth. (quoted in Davis, 1999, p. 87)

Human spirit is a multidimensional aliveness that has many aspects. In fact, it is a whole world of qualities (Peay, 1999). Human spirit has the quality of love and compassion. According to psychiatrist Gerald May (1991), love is ". . . the fundamental energy of the human spirit, the fuel on which we run, the wellspring of our vitality" (p. 3). According to Ken Wilber (1998), human spirit is about the Good, the True, and the Beautiful as the faces of Divine Spirit expressed in the world: "Spirit seen subjectively is Beauty, the I of Spirit. Spirit seen intersubjectively is the Good, the We of Spirit. And Spirit seen objectively is the True, the It of Spirit" (p. 201). Human spirit is also full of joy, laughter, and exuberance. It is expressed in the human ability to play, sing, dance, create ceremony and ritual, tell stories, and laugh at jokes, but it is also all other human experiences—emptiness, longing, withdrawal, and despair. Human spirit embodies a deep awareness of the total human condition.

Human spirit involves a relatedness to all existing things (Fox, 1995). This relatedness springs from human spirit's ability to move out from the individual into the world. Human spirit searches for communion and connection. We see this search for connection in our social structures, group affiliation, and forms of community. It is about needing others in our lives and actively reaching out to them. Human spirit is inclusive in the deepest sense of belonging and participating (Remen, 1998).

Human spirit is a luminous intelligence. As intelligence, human spirit involves our search for the meaning and purpose for our life (Dilts & McDonald, 1997). The search for spirit is the search for our true identity—who I really am and what I exist for (May, 1991). Spirit brings us through the final stages of psychological development and healing as wholeness. Jung saw spirit as the secret source of healing and balance (Shulman, 1997). The urge toward true healing is seen in human creativity, symbolic and ritual healing, and transcendent experiences. As Remen (1998) notes, "Spirit is an essential need of human nature" (p. 64).

Music and Spirit

As explored in chapter 1, music has been linked with breath, spirit, spirituality, and religious expression since earliest human history. According to Rudolf Steiner (1983), music is not a symbol of spirit—it *is* spirit. He believed that the music of the "great composers" gives us a reminder of the spiritual realm:

> The composer conjures a still higher world; he conjures the Devachanic world [spirit realm of tone and absolutely true meaning]. . . . If we are at all capable of experiencing a foretaste of the spiritual world, this would be found in the melodies and harmonies of music and the effects it has on the human soul. (quoted in Godwin, 1987, p. 257)

Music becomes a direct earthly expression of Divine Spirit, reflecting its nature in a way understandable to humans. Numerous similarities exist between experiences of spirit and music.

Human spirit is equated with breath, vitality, movement, power, and force. These qualities also relate to music. In music, the use of the voice for singing, chanting, and toning makes the overt use of breath more obvious and pronounced, while the rise and fall of the harmonic structure and phrasing give an experience of gentle cycles of inhalation and exhalation. As extensively noted throughout this book, music is movement on all levels of organization and experience. Music also embodies the flow and power of spirit.

As we experience the movement in music, we are immersed in a direct experience of the vital life force (Diamond, 1981).

As movement and force, spirit reaches out from the individual to connect to others. Faiver et al. (2001) note, "Although this life force is deeply part of us, it also transcends us. It is what connects us to other people, nature, and the source of life. The experience of spirituality is greater than ourselves and helps us transcend and embrace life situations" (p. 2). Music could be described in exactly the same fashion. Music reaches out to others and helps us interact and relate to each other.

Another way music and spirit are related is in their rhythmic nature. O'-Donohue (1997) equates being spiritual with being in rhythm with the primal rhythmic nature of the universe—a state of dynamic equilibrium and readiness much like the edge-of-chaos dynamics of complexity science. This nonlinear sense of rhythm and time is another characteristic shared by spiritual experiences and music. They both are ". . . very rarely encoded in terms of linear time. In fact, spiritual experiences are typically characterized by a very altered perception of time, such as having a sense of 'timelessness'" (Dilts & McDonald, 1997, p. 49). Spirit rides on the nonlinear movement of music, which gives an experience of openness, receptivity, and clarity (May, 1982).

Experience of spirit is also an experience of the overflowing fullness and joy of unconditional love. "Spiritual love has no desire to get but only to give, no goal except to awaken itself within others, no need except to share itself. Being unconditional, it never falls or falters; being boundless, it embraces everyone" (Walsh, 1999, p. 75). We experience this boundless love when we are enveloped by music. The aesthetic response to music is clearly a time when we experience this openness, increased clarity, and sensation of boundless love through music. The aesthetic reaction is one of engrossed joy, a peak experience when we have an awareness of and closeness to Divine Spirit (May, 1991). "The musical self is the aesthetic entity in each and every individual. It is the 'life spirit' of the person" (Amir, 1995, p. 53). The need and desire for spirit are manifested through the human need and desire for the aesthetic response. Many writers believe that the need for the aesthetic is a basic human need (Gaston, 1968b; Maslow, 1970). The need for the spiritual is also a fundamental need. Experiences with both Divine Spirit and human spirit are part of ultimate healing and consciousness development into wholeness (Wilber, Engler, & Brown, 1986). Having explored the nature of spirit and how it relates to music, it is time to examine human spirit from a music therapy perspective.

Music Therapy and Expressions of Human Spirit

The vitality and élan of human spirit make up our personal life force and are expressed in human functioning in a number of ways—through experiences of belonging and affiliation, play, creativity, general quality of life, and spirituality and religious expression.

Belonging and the Need for Affiliation

Spiritual awareness is generated in relation to "others." Work in this area involves strengthening our relationship to the larger systems of which we are a part (Dilts & McDonald, 1997). These systems include the family, community, social groups, and the broader community of humans. Being part of a group, feeling affiliated, and developing social bonds are important for mental and physical health and healing. Therapy groups function to ". . . enhance health and well-being through heightening group identity, strengthening community cohesion and commitment to the ill person, reintegrating them into the social group, and resolving difficulties among members of the community" (Winkelman, 2000, p. 98). We are social beings. We need each other. A lack of social affiliation negatively affects us physically and psychologically. "Good social support supports us biologically. Its absence is dangerous to our health and contributes to our early death" (Gordon, 1996, p. 206). Involvement in a closely affiliated group is a natural expression of human spirit and is therapeutic.

Music, especially shared music making, is an important tool for developing a sense of affiliation, belonging, and group identity (Feld, 1994; Lomax, 1968; Merriam, 1964). Music helps create group affiliation through synchronizing breath and movement, through shared cultural values, and through shared experiences and emotions. Music therapy practice in this area of human spirit uses this principle to create an instant therapeutic community. For example, group singing allows for synchronization of breathing and movement while sharing emotional expression and affirming shared beliefs based on lyrics (Anshel & Kipper, 1988). "This limbic-based communication system [vocal chanting] provides information about visceral states linking members of a group" (Winkelman, 2000, p. 149). Group musical improvisation also engenders a sense of group belonging, shared emotions, and community (Ruud, 1998a).

Group percussion experiences can also be used to create group cohesiveness (Hull, 1998). The shared rhythm experience can help to entrain group members' movements. Geissmann (2000) notes that the introduction of a steady beat may make it ". . . easier to assess a group's cohesiveness and therefore its strength based on group display" (p. 119). The case study at the beginning of this chapter illustrates the use of this music therapy technique for junior high school students at risk for gang involvement. I developed this program specifically to address the needs of these students for a positive sense of affiliation and belonging to counter one of the motivations for involvement in gangs. Needing to belong, to be a part of a group, is recognized as a factor in joining gangs (Byerly, 1967). Norris (2000), in her work with criminals in prisons, found that a large number of them ". . . do not feel connected to anything. They have little connection, with their families; have no connections with school, the community, the government . . . and actually have no felt sense of belonging anywhere" (p. 5). The drumming group I created for the at-risk students at the beginning of the chapter helped the students gain an instant peer group and a heightened sense of affiliation.

Need for Play

A second expression of human spirit is experiences of pleasure and play. Playing for children is recognized as an important activity but is not always acknowledged as equally important for adults. Adults need to play and to be playful (May, 1982). Play is a stress reducer. It increases our vitality and decreases preoccupation with the day-to-day stresses of life. When we play together, we counter isolation and alienation through shared pleasure (Pert, 1997). Active play helps individuals develop receptivity and balances seriousness with sincerity (Faiver et al., 2001). Play has the outgoing, exuberant, joyful, and free qualities of a child that are equated with human spirit. "In order to become fully human, one has to get rid of the intellectual perspective, one has to become a child. The perspective of the playful shall counteract all fragmentation and intellectualization" (Ruud, 1995, p. 101). Playing directly reconnects us with spirit because it is a natural ecstasy (Fox, 1981). "In forgetting themselves in play . . . individuals give themselves over to something greater than themselves" (Faiver et al., 2001, p. 37). When we are playful, we are expressing the élan and vitality of spirit.

Adults often forget how to play. Making music, as a shared pleasurable activity, is a way in which adults can easily and naturally play. Music therapy techniques are designed to make it possible for people to play music with little or no musical training or background. Improvisation techniques using percussion instruments, electronic instruments, and adaptations like special guitar tunings make playing music possible for everyone. I have experienced some of my most playful experiences while participating in drum circles. In these experiences, all play to the level of their ability. Trained drummers play complicated rhythmic parts, while novices play the steady beat or improvise whatever they like. Everyone plays with enthusiasm, joy, and abandon. The group leader ensures that the playing "hangs together," so the experience is positive for all involved (Hull, 1998). The experience of shared, joyful play is exhilarating. The flow of human spirit is obvious during these events.

Need for Creativity

The need for creative expression is the third aspect of human spirit. Creativity as a cognitive skill was explored in chapter 4. Expressing creativity and living creatively are expressions of human spirit. Creativity may be seen as a bridge between mind and spirit. "Creativity cannot be separated from the processes of life" (Kenny, 1982, p. 11). Wilber (1996) sees creativity as another name for spirit because it engenders so many of its qualities. Jung (1922) saw creativity as an active, dynamic process linked to play. It is related psychologically to spontaneity and freedom (Combs, 1995). Creativity is a form of intuitive knowing, which moves us beyond what we know to the ultimate truth of things.

> Our creative moments . . . are moments where we are in touch with our own authentic truth, when we experience our unique presence in the world. But, paradoxically, the experience of a unique presence is also often coupled with a sensation of ourselves as indivisible from the whole. (Briggs & Peat, 1999, p. 28)

Creativity, then, is life-giving spirit as a means to true health or wholeness. Becoming healthy is a creative act. "When we introduce form and order into the creative act then we promote a higher form of human articulation. This is the process of healing; the escape from emotive fragmentation to the creative act of becoming whole" (Aldridge, 1996, p. 18). It is spirit expressing itself in the world.

Music is a creative art. We think of musical creativity when we consider composers and songwriters, but creativity infuses the entire musical process. Playing music, re-creating the music from a written score, is a creative process. This is musicality as creativity. Certainly, musical improvisation is creative whether in a formal jazz composition or a simple rhythmic ensemble without written music. Musical creativity, in whatever form, is about projecting one's created sounds into the world, about moving the expression of human spirit from the internal to the external realm. It is a spirit-filled, mystical act.

Because of this connection of creativity and human spirit, creativity plays a major role in music therapy practice. Music therapy techniques provide structure and encouragement for experiencing the creative process (Kenny, 1982). From formulas for composing blues songs to musical improvisation of feelings, music therapy techniques make creative expression possible and keep the creative spirit alive (Amir, 1995). A good example of the therapeutic benefit of creative expression is the use of songwriting in music therapy practice for clients with a psychiatric diagnosis, adolescents who have been abused, and individuals with traumatic brain injury. Songwriting is used to promote self-expression, self-awareness, and self-empowerment (Clendon-Wallen, 1991; Ficken, 1976; S. Goldstein, 1990; Lindberg, 1995; Robb, 1996). Engagement in the creative process of songwriting stimulates self-awareness and self-expression because creativity is about expressing what we uniquely feel and believe. Creativity as spirit is about expressing what is unique about ourselves and making that uniqueness manifest in the world. Songwriting is an organized, structured way to do this.

Need for Quality of Life
The fourth expression of human spirit is *quality of life*. Quality of life is a complex phenomenon and involves a number of subjective evaluations of well-being and happiness. These include self-concept and self-esteem; general life satisfaction; opportunities for socialization, interpersonal relationships, and belonging; activity involving vitality, energy, and freedom; a sense of personal well-being and safety; joy and happiness; and a sense of life meaning and fulfillment (Ruud, 1998a). All these qualities clearly relate to issues of human spirit.

Ruud (1998a) sees an important role for music in fostering quality of life because ". . . it strengthens our emotional awareness, installs a sense of agency, fosters belongingness, and provides meaning and coherence in life" (p. 49). Music helps us to be aware of feelings and fosters a sense of belonging. Music engenders a sense of agency through awareness of our own possibilities of action, feeling of mastery, and increased social communication. Music fosters a sense of meaning in our lives through a flexible, coherent identity. Music therapy practice in this area of human spirit has focused on quality of life issues for older adults (VanderArk, Newman, & Bell, 1983). Active participation in music groups has been shown to positively influence the quality of life for older adults in community band programs (Coffman & Adamek, 1999), in group percussion activities (Reuer & Crowe, 1995), in intergenerational choirs (Bowers, 1998; Wise, Hartmann, & Fisher, 1992), and in organ instruction (Clair, 1996). Participating in a goal-oriented, pleasurable, social interaction like playing music together positively affects the quality of life as an expression of human spirit.

Need for Spirituality and Religion

The final areas for expression of human spirit are *spirituality* and *religion*. There is much debate and little agreement as to the definitions of spirituality and religion (Albanese, 1992). For the purpose of this book, the term *spirituality* refers to one's direct experience of the sacred, of Divine Spirit. It focuses on the direct and immediate feelings, thoughts, and behavior related to a person's search for the Divine (Lipe, 2002). Tillich (1959) defines spirituality as the meaning-giving dimension of culture, while Cervantes and Ramirez (1992) believe it is the search for harmony and wholeness. Hinterkopf (1994) contends that the spiritual experience is felt in the body, involves an awareness of the transcendent dimension of life, and brings new meanings leading to personal growth. Spirituality is a quest for an authentic inner life and personhood (Roof, 1999). It is about experiencing joy and vitality, connectedness, ultimate belonging, and the Divine source *for ourselves* (Walsh, 1999). The key to spirituality is the *experience* of Divine Spirit and not just *knowing* about it (Dilts & McDonald, 1997). Spirituality is a real, true, personal experience with Divine Spirit. As Davis (1999) points out, "Spiritual doesn't mean 'airy fairy.' Spiritual means what's real, what is" (p. 55). Walsh (1999) sees spirituality not as a discovery of something "new" in our lives but as a recognition that the spiritual is already present in ourselves and the world around us.

The direct experience of spirit requires a spiritual system or practice. Such a system ". . . invites us to live in a way that both reflects and develops wisdom, love, joy, vitality, power, peace, authenticity, passion, curiosity, appreciation, stillness, pleasure, trust, gratitude, and an unrelenting engagement with what is" (Davis, 1999, p. 3). Religion is one form of spiritual system (Frame, 2003). Shafranske and Maloney (1990) define religion as a set of beliefs and practices of an organized religious institution. It is a social institution (Roof, 1999). Religion and spirituality are not necessarily the same thing. Spirit and spirituality can be addressed as part of the therapeutic effort without involving an individual's religion or religious beliefs. In fact, experience with spirit may or may not involve the concept of a Supreme Being (Frame, 2003).

Experiences with spirit are important aspects of human functioning. Music is linked with experiences of spirit, first as direct links to Divine Spirit and, then, through experiences with human spirit. Because these expressions of spirit are vital to a perspective of wholeness in human functioning, they are an important part of the therapeutic effort for an individual.

Problems of Spirit as Part of Therapy

Issues of spirit should be included in the therapeutic effort for clients for a number of reasons. Issues of spirituality are a psychological fact of human interest. Human involvement in spirit and spirituality is an early development historically (Eliade, 1964). Whether based on psychological, social, or cultural needs, humans have extensively addressed issues of spirituality from the earliest human cultures. In a therapeutic intervention, clients cannot divorce themselves from their spiritual belief system. It is, in fact, unhealthy to do so. To see a person as a whole and to address therapy holistically, spirituality must be included (Faiver et al., 2001).

Because spirituality is an important part of human functioning, positive effects of spiritual experiences are noted in mental health (Bergin, 1983; Gartner, Larson, & Allen, 1991; Shumacher, 1992) and in physical health (Borysenko, 1998). As Lipe (2002) points out, "Within a holistic health paradigm, spirituality and health/healing appear to share a number of common terms and concepts" (p. 230). The effects of spirituality on mental and physical health occur largely because of the impact of spiritual experiences on the limbic system related to the mind/body connection. These forms of healing are based on manipulation of processes and functions in the midbrain area, relating to personal and social identity, emotions, and values and meanings (Winkelman, 2000). Spiritual experiences also lead to continued psychological development, personal growth, and fulfillment (May, 1982). Such work addresses the existential issues of aging, disease, physical decline, death, pain, injustice, evil, and the need for meaning (Faiver et al., 2001). In this sense, spirituality leads to "ultimate" healing. This ultimate healing or healing work with spirit involves the search for meaning and purpose, discovery of our inner unity with all life and with the Divine Principle, and consciousness development in the upper levels of the consciousness model (Aldridge, 1996; Bonny, 2001; Grossman, 2002; Wilber, Engler, & Brown, 1986). Ultimate healing is about the search for our true selves, our intrinsic nature and possibilities (Davis, 1999). "'Health' is an idealization of a kind of self, and 'healing' is part of the process by which growth toward that ideal is achieved" (Roof, 1999, p. 107). Resolution of the contradiction between our personal life and our spiritual life is the discovery of our core or true self—the integration of both points of view without distortion by our personal histories (Almaas, 1988b). This is the work of all people striving for wholeness and authentic adult consciousness. Wilber, Engler, and Brown's (1986) consciousness development at Levels 8 and 9 serve as examples of this form of healing.

Consciousness development at Level 8 of Wilber's (1977) "spectrum of consciousness" is the subtle level of transpersonal growth. This is the level of transcendent insight and absorption. The processes at this level are more subtle than gross, waking consciousness. "Personal development at this stage becomes a spiritual quest to escape the objectification of the ego and the appearance of reality . . ." (Wade, 1996, p. 177). In this stage of consciousness development, deity mysticism is experienced. The forms of this mysticism ". . . include luminosities and sounds, archetypal forms and patterns, extremely subtle bliss currents and cognitions . . . expansive affective states of love and compassion . . ." (Wilber, 1996, p. 211). Personal experience and relationships with Divine figures, like spirit helpers of shamanic practitioners, are common (Harner, 1982).

Wilber's Level 9 is the causal level of consciousness development. This is a state of awareness characterized by formless mysticism, the unmanifested source. This is a consciousness of nonduality where distinction of self separate from the world is meaningless. You, the observer, and the object you are observing are one and the same experience—two sides of the same reality.

> Across the board, the sense of being any sort of Seer or Witness or Self vanishes altogether. You don't look at the sky, you are the sky. . . . precisely because awareness is no longer split into a seeing subject in here and a seen object out there. There is just pure seeing. Consciousness and its display are not two. (Wilber, 1996, pp. 227–228)

Work on these levels of consciousness brings a person to a place of equanimity—the capacity to experience the inevitable ups and downs of life without being thrown into wild emotional swings. The multiple layers of the psyche are explored, and the powerful transpersonal forces are experienced, integrated, and expressed (Walsh, 1999). The dynamic process of love working in one's life is acknowledged (May, 1982). Equanimity also allows the development of the human qualities that bring happiness to self and others. These qualities include love, compassion, patience, tolerance, forgiveness, contentment, a sense of harmony, and personal responsibility (Gyatso, 1999).

This form of healing work is often termed "spiritual growth" and involves creative, dynamic, expansive ways of living in and experiencing the world (Wade, 1996). Psychological growth becomes inseparable from spiritual growth (Davis, 1999). This form of healing involves true transformation—a radical shift in identity, a process of death and rebirth (Wilber, 1999). "Contemporary spiritual quests give expression to the search for unity of mind, body, and self" (Roof, 1999, p. 46). As Bonny (2001) points out,

> Spirituality is the personal act or process of transformation that takes one from an ego-centered, exclusionary attitude toward life to one filled with inclusionary attitude of love, acceptance, adoration, appreciation for all life forms, a sense of unity and purpose that extends into the past and into the future. (p. 60)

This ultimately is a lived experience of chaos. "One must enter chaos to attain a new being" (Ainslie, 1995, p. 314).

To have this transformation, the individual must enter a chaotic state—one where the familiar order of identity, ego, beliefs, and "knowns" is destroyed. This is the state of the "dark night of the soul." It is this chaotic state out of which the new spiritual order arises (Ainslie, 1995). Such chaotic states are terrifying, but spiritual growth requires a commitment to the process no matter how difficult or uncomfortable. Spiritual growth requires ". . . a willingness to stay with the process and be personally engaged in the resultant chaos" (Ainslie, 1995, p. 314).

Ultimately, spiritual work must be included in therapeutic effort because it helps us understand how and why we have abandoned our true nature (Davis, 1999). In a holistic approach to health and healing, the discovery of our true nature is an essential component. This is again the area of transpersonal psychology, first introduced in chapter 6. The transpersonal is about human development beyond "normal" to the full, true potential of each individual. However, these experiences are used differently in this type of healing than for problems of emotion and feeling. In spiritual healing, the experiences and insights are observed but not analyzed. In this sense, transpersonal work is about repairing our disconnection or alienation from spirit as a part of development (Peay, 1999). Like a true complex process, this healing is creative and unpredictable—in both its process and its outcome (Quinn, 1998).

Music and Spirituality and Healing

Music has always been linked with experiences of spirituality and religion (Blacking, 1973; Bonny, 2001; Merriam, 1964). Music is ". . . a way to access clients' spiritual resources for the purposes of optimizing wellness and moving toward wholeness" (Lipe, 2002, p. 233). Because there is a strong link among music, medicine, and spirituality, music is a likely avenue for spiritual experiences and the associated health effects.

Music fosters experiences in spirituality related to health in a number of unique ways. First, it opens individuals to the spiritual while at the same time grounding and confining the experience. Music is a socially acceptable way to evoke spiritual experiences yet, at the same time, bring them into other aspects of functioning for practical use. Music helps us subjectively experience Divine Spirit, while the rhythm and structure of music keep those experiences grounded. The active engagement in music helps individuals *experience* very abstract concepts. "As individuals engage with music, abstract concepts such as hope, meaning, and purpose are made concrete in the person's lived experience, opening up paths to growth and healing" (Lipe, 2002, p. 233). Music therapy techniques like "Guided Imagery and Music" (GIM) utilize this feature of music. When I developed the "Music and Creative Problem Solving" technique, it was to utilize this dual aspect of music to help clients solve problems using the transpersonal and spiritual experiences fostered by listening to music in an altered state of consciousness. The music chosen first evoked spiritual experiences but was rhythmic enough to ground that experience in conscious awareness. Participants were able to record and examine their responses and experiences. In this way music became a spiritual practice or, as Wilber (1998) describes, ". . . a tried and tested practice for *reliably reproducing* the transpersonal and super-conscious insights . . ." (p. 112), especially those relating to health and healing.

Second, music fosters spirituality as it relates to health through altered states of consciousness. Explored at length later in this chapter, music is one way to create the altered state of consciousness known as relaxed wakefulness, which creates an openness to spirit (May, 1991). Listening to a composition like Ralph Vaughn Williams' *Fantasia on a Theme by Thomas Tallis* can create this mind state. The piece is an intricate weaving of tonality among a full string orchestra, chamber strings, and a string quartet. The sonic interplay pulls the listener into a state of deep relaxation, yet the return of the theme and the underlying rhythmic structure keep you grounded and cognitively alert and aware.

The third way music stimulates spirituality as it relates to health is because it embodies the universal concept of love as belonging and connectedness. Because of this, music provides an effective means to address issues of ultimate meaning.

> When we facilitate the creation of music in the clinical setting we are simultaneously fostering the client's capacity to create and discover how to find meaning in life. As clients in music therapy integrate the materials of their medium into a unified whole, they gain the ability to experience themselves as a part of a greater whole and experience their relationship and connection to the social and physical environment. Thus, as they learn to express themselves through an artistic medium they gain a sense of their place in the world. (Aigen, 1995a, p. 250)

Music provides a lived experience of this connectedness and ultimate meaning. Music therapist Anne Lipe (2002) completed a survey of the literature on music in relation to spirituality for health and healing. She found that 52 percent of the authors writing on music, spirituality, and health were credentialed music therapists. "This illustrates that music therapists are addressing issues of spirituality within the framework of clinical practice" (Lipe, 2002, p. 216).

Music Therapy and the Tools of Spiritual Healing

Many specific tools to access spirituality have been identified throughout history. These tools include altered states of consciousness, myth and ritual, dreams and images, meditation, and the arts, including dance, visual arts, storytelling, drama, and music (Dilts & McDonald, 1997). May (1982) categorizes spiritual experiences as either unitive in nature, in which our identity is suspended, or those experiences where our personal identity is maintained. The traditional tools of spirituality potentially provide experiences in both. All spiritual experiences involve a process of letting go and the evocation of images and symbols (Bonny, 2001).

Music, Symbols, and Symbolic Healing

Tools of the spirit require the language of symbols and dreams (Dilts & McDonald, 1997). A *symbol* is a tool for comparing experiences. It is a sign with which to infer meaning (Skaggs, 1997). Symbols are a form of emotionally charged thinking that predates language. They facilitate conceptual and emotional change by integrating different forms of meaning. This is accomplished because symbols link activities from different levels of the brain. Symbols are culturally determined and are linked through experience with the vast variety of neural networks.

> A symbol may evoke any neural network or neurocognitive model with which it has been entrained, including autonomic and endocrine systems, brain structures, emotions, and abstract ideas. This is symbolic penetration, the effects of the neural system mediating a symbolic precept or associated physical systems. Evoking and entraining associated physiological systems allow meaning and symbols to influence physiological processes and allow physiological process to evoke meaningful associations. (Winkelman, 2000, p. 244)

Symbols, then, penetrate the various neurocognitive systems and reorder them to produce a physical and physiological effect. Symbols can simultaneously operate on many levels of consciousness.

> Symbols, therefore, pull together. . . . the many fragmented aspects of self into related patterns—patterns that become an integrated whole. Symbols also infer and suggest meanings that stimulate reflection and contemplation. . . . Any or all of the meanings derived from the different levels can be accurate. They open the door to perspectives from many viewpoints. (Skaggs, 1997, p. 29)

Perception itself is a symbolic process because it is a representation of current sensory input compared to memories based on previous experience

(Winkelman, 2000). As a basic component to perception, symbols can have a profound effect on human experience and functioning. This is symbolic healing, which is ". . . based on the human capacity for interpersonal communication derived from a prior capacity of humans to communicate with themselves through emotion" (Winkelman, 2000, p. 239).

Music is an important means of symbolic healing. First, it stimulates emotions and is an intrinsic emotion/meaning system. As a symbol system, music serves to mediate between sensory input and behavior as output (Winkelman, 2000). Music also is a culturally determined symbol of wholeness, of the relationship of many parts, and of various levels of human functioning.

> Music as a symbol consists of a relationship of one process to another. Every tone is a whole. Each of the overtones created by the sounding of a fundamental tone is a different aspect, yet a part of the fundamental. We could say that each overtone is within the context of the whole. No fundamental tone and no overtone is independent of the other, and each is affected within the relationship. (Skaggs, 1997, p. 34)

The various musical elements provide profound symbols. They are socialized to symbolize everything from emotional states (happy, sad), values (patriotism, justice), and human character (for example, the hero's theme from *Star Wars*), linking music with memories and associations. We also develop a set of personal symbols to specific music. For example, a particular song may remind you of your first love or become associated with a painful time in your life.

As the tools for transformation utilizing symbolic healing are explored, it is clear that a variety of music therapy techniques is effectively used for this level of healing. The uses of music in the various methods of symbolic healing allow and facilitate change rather than force it. "True growth is a process which one allows to happen rather than causes to happen" (May, 1977, pp. 70–71). All the traditional tools of spiritual healing involve symbolic healing in one form or another. These traditional tools include altered states of consciousness, myth and ritual, dreams and imagery, and meditation. Music is used in each.

Altered States of Consciousness

An *altered state of consciousness* is one tool frequently recognized in fostering spiritual growth. The search for the spiritual and the transcendent to foster consciousness growth involves the destabilization of ordinary consciousness and the establishment of another mode of awareness (Wade, 1996). A mode of consciousness is biologically based and represents a system of operation among brain structures to meet the organism's needs. Different brain areas work in different combinations for each of the modes. There is no single brain area responsible for a given mode of consciousness.

Winkelman (2000) identifies four modes of human consciousness— working consciousness, deep sleep, dreaming (REM activity), and integrative. Working consciousness is the active, alert state we identify with "consciousness." In working consciousness we learn, adapt, and survive in our environment. Deep sleep is the consciousness of physical recuperation, growth, and regeneration. All animals experience deep sleep, indicating this state is essential to survival (Shulman, 1997). Dreaming or REM sleep, as discussed in chapter 4, is an important state for memory integration, consolidation of learning, and psychosocial adaptation. The fourth mode of consciousness, *integrative*, provides for psychodynamic growth and social and psychological integration (Winkelman, 2000). The first three modes of consciousness were discussed in previous chapters. Before exploring integrative consciousness and its role in consciousness development and spiritual growth, let's look at brain wave production as it relates to modes of consciousness.

Modes of Consciousness and Brain Waves

The four modes of consciousness are associated with particular combinations of brain wave activity. A brain wave is the speed of the electrical activity in the brain. The frequency of the wave is related to the mode of consciousness, usually designated delta (0–4 Hz), theta (4–8 Hz), alpha (8–13 Hz), and beta (13–30 Hz [Wise, 2002]). Some writers (Kenyon, 1994; Russell, 1993) also postulate higher frequencies of brain waves, up to 150 Hz above beta. Every state of consciousness equates with a particular combination of brain waves. "The combination of frequencies your brain is producing determines or underlies the state of consciousness that you are experiencing" (Wise, 2002, p. 8). Each brain wave has unique characteristics.

Delta waves correspond to the frequencies of brain stem activity and core consciousness. They are associated with deep sleep and the unconscious mind. When delta is present with other brain wave states, it acts as an unconscious scanning device that underlies intuition, empathy, insight, and instinctual action. Delta helps us get information not available on the conscious level. "The nature of delta is such that it can act like an antenna of perception, allowing us to sense the emotions, moods, nuances, and mental states of those around us" (Wise, 2002, p. 106). Delta waves are present in greater numbers in healers and people in helping professions. They seem to help these individuals reach out to others on an intuitive level. The presence of delta waves promotes empathy by allowing the helper to enter into another's mental, psychological, and emotional functioning (Wise, 2002).

Theta brain waves are produced by the limbic system and are associated with subconscious processing, dreams, and REM sleep. Theta is the experience of deep meditation, strong imagery, spiritual connection, and peak experience. It is also associated with heightened creativity and the psychoneuroimmunology phenomena (Kenyon, 1994). "Accessed through theta brain waves, these ordinarily subconscious parts of the mind hold the key to creativity, insight, spiritual awareness, and a variety of experiences of mastery" (Wise, 2002, p. 74). When alpha and some beta are added to theta, unconscious material is made available to consciousness processing. The combination of brain waves allow one to

. . . get in touch with the most profound depths as well as have the vividness and clarity of imagery provided by the alpha to transmit this experience in a tangible way so that the conscious thought process of beta can interpret it, understand it, and act upon it. (Wise, 2002, p. 74)

Alpha brain waves stem from the neocortex. This state is associated with relaxed, detached awareness. "The presence of alpha as the predominant rhythm is characterized by feelings of well-being, a capacity to be absorbed by and get pleasure from simple activities. . . . Alpha is sometimes referred to as 'a natural high'" (Norris, 2000, p. 4). Alpha brain waves are the link between the conscious and unconscious and are important in combination with other brain wave states as stated above (Wise, 2002).

Beta brain waves stem from upper cortex activity producing thought processes. Beta is needed to be active and alert in the world. Higher frequencies of brain waves above beta are just now being researched and are associated with ecstatic and out-of-body experiences and accelerated learning (Hunt, 1996; Kenyon, 1994).

It is interesting to note that there are only a few discrete states of consciousness produced out of a huge potential for such states. The principles of complexity science may offer an explanation. Each state of consciousness is accompanied by an attractor in the complex brain processes and a corresponding attractor in the structure of consciousness by which the various aspects of the mind–body system are drawn into patterns of activity, like a mode of consciousness (Combs, 1995).

The alpha rhythm appears as oscillation within the range of 8–13 Hz. This rhythm corresponds to an attractor state associated with maintained, alert relaxation. The alpha rhythm displays deterministic chaos; it is globally stable, but there is an exponentially fast loss of predictability in the detail of the alpha rhythm's trajectory. The human brain returns to the alpha rhythm after transitory perturbations caused by external stimulation or purposive mental activity. The alpha rhythm is hypothesized . . . to be a global state of great sensitivity to incoming sensory stimulation, enabling the system to easily flip into a new regime. (Alexander & Globus, 1996, p. 44)

Tools to alter consciousness, like meditative practices and music, alter the large but finite array of potential states of consciousness by stimulating some brain regions and making them more accessible while diminishing others. Such activity, then, creates the attractor, the ". . . pattern to which a system is drawn according to its own nature" (Combs, 1995, p. 59). The impact of sound/music on brain wave states is discussed later in the chapter.

Integrative Consciousness

Having explored brain waves and states of consciousness, it is time to return to the fourth mode of consciousness, integrative. The integrative mode of consciousness is typically identified as an altered state of consciousness, although any mode other than working consciousness could be considered "altered," including REM sleep. The mental state involved with integrative consciousness represents the maximum synthesis and integration of cognitive functions available to humans (Hunt, 1995). In this state, an integration of information processing across the functional areas of the brain occurs. This produces a limbic-cortical integration and synchronization of the activity of the two cerebral hemispheres (Winkelman, 2000). Information processing from the lower brain is integrated into cognitive functioning and conscious awareness. While in a state of integrated consciousness, information processing between the reticular formation and the limbic system, between the limbic system and the frontal cortex, and between the hemispheres of the cortex is integrated and available to conscious awareness.

Integrative consciousness constitutes a true integration of cognitive, emotional, and behavioral abilities. "These experiences reflect the simultaneous elicitation and integration of normal modes of information processing and consciousness that do not ordinarily occur together" (Winkelman, 2000, p. xii). Integrative consciousness is a highly adaptable mode of awareness and problem solving because it promotes the ability to simultaneously access a greater range of mental processes.

Numerous physiological mechanisms are involved in integrative consciousness. These include the hippocampus, the hypothalamus, the limbic structures regulating emotion, and the entire parasympathetic nervous system. In this mode of consciousness, the frontal cortex is entrained to high-voltage, slow-wave activity originating in the brain stem, hippocampus, and related areas of the limbic system (Winkelman, 2000).

In terms of brain wave states, the integrated state of consciousness is a combination of the four brain wave patterns in the particular relation and proportion typical of it.

> Someone in the awakened [integrated] mind brain-wave pattern has access to the unconscious empathy, intuition, and radar of the delta waves; the subconscious creative storehouse, inspiration, and spiritual connection of the theta waves; the bridging capacity, lucidity and vividness of imagery; and the relaxed detached awareness of the alpha waves; and the ability to consciously process thoughts in beta—*all at the same time!* (Wise, 2002, pp. 15–16)

The presence of all four types of brain waves shows the integrated processing of this state.

Integrative consciousness is characterized by mental functioning that is clearer, sharper, quicker, and more flexible. It constitutes a state of greater psychological organization and increased introspection and creativity. High levels of attention and awareness are experienced. This state alters our sense of perceived time and promotes deep relaxation. Emotional bliss and euphoria are common (Walsh, 1999). Peak or transcendent experiences and increased awareness of being part of a greater whole is common during integrative consciousness (Russell, 1993). Vivid perceptual imagery occurs, and conscious control of biological and mental systems is possible. "Emotions are more available, understandable, and easier to transform. Information flows more easily between your conscious, subconscious, and unconscious, increasing intuition, insight, and self-healing abilities" (Wise, 2002, p. 5).

All human cultures studied by anthropologists have techniques for achieving this state of consciousness (Winkelman, 2000). The cross-cultural commonalties in experiences of altered states of consciousness ". . . seem to indicate that such nonverbal states have a common underlying brain structure. These states can plausibly be interpreted as exemplifications of the 'deep structure' of a kind of intelligence that directly reuses and reorganizes the structures of perception" (Hunt, 1995, p. 28). The integrative state of consciousness is a natural part of human consciousness and is based on neurological functioning. It constitutes a normal integrative form of functioning.

Tools for Achieving Integrative Consciousness

A change in state of consciousness requires two agents—a disrupting force and a patterning force for the new state (Tart, 1975). For an altered state of consciousness to occur, the working mode of consciousness has to be destabilized and suppressed. This allows the symbolic and emotional aspects of integrative functioning, usually suppressed by working consciousness, to emerge (Winkelman, 2000). Once working consciousness is destabilized, the new pattern, likely of brain waves, must be established. Both destabilization and patterning occur through changes to sensory input—sensory overload or deprivation, novel or unusual input, or extended exposure. These sensory experiences depress left hemisphere activity and disinhibit the right (Wade, 1996). Such sensory experiences also activate the parasympathetic nervous system and promote temporal lobe discharges, which lead to decreased stimulation (Winkelman, 2000).

The agents of destabilization and patterning are psychophysiological manipulations of the human brain (Winkelman, 2000). Traditionally, these manipulations include drugs and other psychoactive agents, sensory stimulation or deprivation, physical exertion, and the combination of sensory experiences, symbols, physical activity (dancing, singing, and playing instruments), storytelling and drama, and ritual. The influence of music/sound in fostering the integrative or altered state of consciousness is the focus here.

Sound/music has been used by humans to alter consciousness since the beginning of recorded history (Eliade, 1964). In complexity science, if normal or working consciousness is thought of as an attractor state, then any simple uninterrupted repetition of sound could be seen as a disruptive factor to ordinary consciousness by adding complexity and destabilizing the current attractor (Combs, 1995). The complex input of music could then serve to repattern consciousness by creating the attractor for one of the other modes of consciousness. As sound pioneer Robert Monroe stated, "Certain patterns of sound will induce distinct states of consciousness not ordinarily available to the human mind" (quoted in Russell, 1993, p. 14).

Five music/sound elements are traditionally used to alter consciousness (Crowe, 1991a). The first involves the rhythmic element of music. These practices involve repetitive, monotonous sound or complex rhythmic patterns. The use of the repetitive element such as drumming and rattling is prominent in traditional shamanic practices (Harner, 1982). Complex rhythms are seen in traditional music to engender trance states. Examples of this include African dancing, Balinese trance dancing, and voodoo ceremonies. Normal consciousness is disrupted because the sound is too boring or too complicated to process through normal thought. The linear left hemisphere functioning shuts down in favor of right hemisphere and limbic system response.

Melodic subtlety is the second musical element used to alter consciousness. Melodic subtlety is the slight variation of pitch prominent in the raga tradition of India and in vocal chant traditions of many cultures, including the island of Bali. In these traditions, the small changes of pitch fall between the notes of our Western scale. Such small changes are processed in the brain stem, bypassing cognitive processing.

The third musical element for altering consciousness is sound timbre. Timbre reflects the unique complexity of sound produced by a particular instrument. Musical traditions using struck and rubbed metal instruments, like Tibetan singing bowls and gongs, utilize this musical element for transformation of consciousness. Timbre is also a brain stem perception.

The fourth musical element may be referred to as "ear tricks." These often involve the generation of combination tones—tones that are heard by the ear but are not present in the sound input. This is a phenomenon of the basilar membrane in the inner ear. When two loud sounds of different frequency enter the ear, they set the basilar membrane into such a large vibration that another area on the membrane is also activated (like a wave effect in a waterbed). Because the cilia above that area of the membrane are being activated, the brain "hears" a sound (Radocy & Boyle, 1997). This element for altering consciousness is present in the low-frequency chanting of Tibetan monks and in the high-frequency sounds of Peruvian healing whistles.

The final musical element for altering consciousness is full-spectrum harmony. This element is most fully developed in Western music. With this element, the highly developed vertical structure of the harmony bombards the listener with complex sound characterized by rapid shifts in the harmonic structure. An excellent example of this use of harmony is the presence of large pipe organs during worship services. The highly resonant sound produced by the organ in a large, stone cathedral creates a prayerful and worshipful mental state in the participants. Compared to normal, working consciousness, such a state is altered by definition (Levenson, 1994).

Acknowledging that music/sound has been used to alter consciousness since earliest human history, the question is how these effects occur. As noted in chapter 3, the auditory nerve innervates a large portion of the brain. The auditory nerve first affects various areas of the reticular activating system (RAS). This structure regulates the electrical rhythms of the cortex. Abundant connections exist between the RAS and the auditory pathways and among the RAS, the cortex, and a significant number of lower brain structures. Any impact on the RAS has a profound impact on all aspects of brain functioning, including modes of consciousness (Tomaino, 1998). Also noted previously, the auditory nerve has direct connection to both the sympathetic and parasympathetic nervous systems. An altered state of consciousness is a parasympathetic-dominated brain state. To inhibit the sympathetic nervous system and promote the parasympathetic, sensory input must ". . . manipulate the sympathetic nervous system to the point of exhaustion and collapse into a parasympathetic dominant state . . ." (Winkelman, 2000, p. 125). This is accomplished through monotonous auditory stimuli like loud repetitive drumming, harmonic shifts, and subcortical pitch processing (Harner, 1982; Maxfield, 1994; Neher, 1962; Winkelman, 2000).

Another reason why sound/music can alter consciousness is that sonic input can alter brain waves in the characteristic patterns of a particular state of consciousness. In these states, the slow-wave discharges of the limbic system synchronize and dominate the frontal cortex (Winkelman, 2000). ASC are characterized by brain wave shifts to low-frequency such as alpha yet high-amplitude activity in the temporal lobes. Theta waves are also present.

Music and Brain Waves

Music has been associated with the production of various brain wave states, especially production of alpha waves (McElwain, 1979; McKee, Humphreys, & McAdam, 1973; Wagner, 1975). A classic early study by Neher (1961) showed that regularly occurring drumbeats produced alpha brain wave shifts in exposed subjects. Traditional shamanic techniques that alter consciousness use this technique (Harner, 1982). Research has shown that listening to music tends to increase alpha production in musicians versus nonmusicians, which may indicate the impact of training, experience, or learning on music's ability to produce alpha waves (McElwain, 1979; Wagner & Menzel, 1977). Additionally, musical training affects musicians differently than nonmusicians, with musicians showing increase in alpha in the right hemisphere, while nonmusicians show alpha increase in the left hemisphere (McElwain, 1979). Similarly, Bruga and Severtsen (1984) found that EEG slowing and alpha production depended on the subjects' judgment of the music as "relaxing," whether the music was judged to have "sedative" characteristics or not. Borling (1981) found the same degree of alpha production for both sedative and simulative music during a focused attention task. The production of the "relaxing" alpha rhythm to music may not be due to any characteristic of the music per se but, rather, to learned relaxation response to a particular music for each individual (Rider, 1997). A Japanese study (Kabuto, Kageyama, & Netta, 1993) found that EEG shifts were significant when the subjects liked the music regardless of the musical genre (New Age or classical) used. One study (Dostalek et al., 1979) measured brain wave production in subjects chanting "OM." "Singing the syllable OM led to the appearance of theta and delta rhythms as well as increases in the amplitude of alpha and beta activity" (Rider, 1997, p. 106). This combination of brain waves is typical of a meditative state of consciousness (Wise, 2002). The chanting of OM is a standard meditative practice. The typical brain wave production for this chant may be due to the direct impact of the sound on brain waves or, more likely, may reflect the learned response to this particular stimulus.

Musical activities like chanting and repetitive drumming induce brain waves in the theta and low alpha range (Rogers & Walters, 1981; Wright, 1995). The brain wave state characteristic of meditation—alpha, theta, and beta—can be produced in music therapy techniques like GIM where the music input induces the alpha/theta activity while the verbal reporting brings beta into the system.

Another way in which sound/music can generate an ASC is the process of entrainment. Entrainment was introduced in chapter 4 when discussing rhythmic entrainment of physical activity. Entrainment of brain waves is addressed here. "Entrainment is a term in psychoacoustics that refers to the effects of a repetitive sound pattern on brain wave patterning" (Kenyon, 1994, p. 192). In music both the frequency and rhythm can provide for entrainment. Brain wave entrainment to sound has been researched extensively by the Monroe Institute. It developed a system called Hemi-Sync that entrains the brain waves of the two hemispheres using binaural beats. "Binaural beats are produced within your physiology when different audio frequencies are introduced into each ear. The brain discerns this difference and seeks to bridge the gap. In so doing, it produces a third frequency—the difference between the two" (Russell, 1993, p. 16). It is this third frequency that entrains the hemispheres and brings the brain into coherence. This state of hemispheric entrainment creates the integrative state of consciousness. Sadigh and Kozicky (1993) verified the production of hemispheric synchronization using the Hemi-Sync frequency following technology but were unable to find the synchronization using other auditory input.

Finally, music may alter consciousness because of its ability to alter the time sense. "Music shapes time because it marks it with the experience of change and transformation. . . . Music commands time; it determines whether time seems to rush forward or hang suspended . . ." (Rothstein, 1995, p. 125). All experiences, including modes of consciousness, involve some form of sensed temporality (Hunt, 1995). ASC involves a sense of virtual and, therefore, changeable time. Music has the ability to create that sense of virtual time typical of ASC. Blacking (1973) reports on the people of Bali who speak of "the other mind," a state when people become keenly aware of the true nature of their being, of the "other self" within themselves and other human beings, and of their relationship with the world around them. This state of mind is created by the virtual time of music engendered during their intensive dance and music forms (Blacking, 1973).

During a research trip to Bali, I personally experienced this altering of time during many different musical events. One musical form in particular, the *Kecak* dance, was particularly effective in producing an altered sense of time. The Kecak is performed at night by the men of a village. Up to 150 men sit in concentric circles around a large fire chanting a highly complicated, multipart rhythmic composition that accompanies dancers depicting one of the great Hindu myths. The chant shifts and changes numerous times though there is no "conductor" to keep this large vocal ensemble together. The complex rhythms and the bodily movements that accompany the chant create an ASC in the performers that allows them to entrain and synchronize with each other. They become especially sensitive to others in the group. As an audience member, I also experienced this ASC, and my sense of time shifted completely. As the performance ended, I was amazed to realize that close to two hours had gone by. Real time had been changed to virtual time.

Myth and Ritual

The next traditional tool for transformation through symbolic healing is *myth* and *ritual*. Myths and rituals have been associated with symbolic healing since earliest human history (Campbell, 1968; Eliade, 1964; Harner, 1982; Winkelman, 2000). A myth is a widely held cultural story that conveys a message about how to live, to interact with others, and to heal. Though the current Western cultural definition of myth is as "an untrue story," myth serves as a powerful symbol that speaks to the entire culture or community.

> Myth can be considered a synthetic mode of experience which travels through our holistic awareness. It connects us and relates us to our surrounding world through perception, which is not always empirically testable. It comes to us through patterns and archetypes which affect life indirectly through symbolic activity. . . . (Kenny, 1982, p. 35)

Myths allow us to share our internal symbolic reality with others from our group and make it a shared phenomenon. We share these myths through ritual.

Rituals are symbolic statements of basic cultural values. They create a sense of commonality, express the basic structure of society, set rules for social behavior, and outline the best relationship of the individual to other humans, nature, and the greater whole. Ritual links experience, feeling, intuition, and reason to provide interpretation of and shaping for experience (Winkelman, 2000). A ritual involves a series of actions—a ceremony—that symbolizes or expresses the intention for the event (Dilts & McDonald, 1997). The intention is brought into action through the ritual. "Ritual brings together action and idea into an enactment" (Hillman, 1975, p. 137). Rituals may be cultural, religious, or social. Some rituals, such as weddings and funerals, birthday parties, and retirement parties, overlap in their function.

Rituals as forms of symbolic healing are important in both psychological and physical healing. A ritual affects all levels of human functioning. "Although the classic analyses of the function of rituals have emphasized their psychological, social, or symbolic functions, the physiological effects of ritual must also be considered as a basic level of action on the body" (Winkelman, 2000, p. 231). The use of ritual to affect physiological functioning is one way in which the psychological influences the physical. Ritual creates this effect on physical functioning for a number of reasons.

Rituals first affect physical functioning because they are designed to evoke strong emotional states. Ritual symbolization affects the brain's reticular formation and limbic system (Winkelman, 2000). Early in development, the symbolic language of emotion is entrained to ritual behavior and external symbols so that the experience of the ritual changes or restructures the feeling states. In previous chapters, the importance of emotion in behavior, memory, cognitive functioning, and consciousness was explored.

The most profound impact on people's emotional state is the sense of community support and value of the individual the ritual brings to the patient. In a healing ritual, the patient is the focus of everyone's intention and effort. It conveys a sense of the importance of the event and brings hope to the patient. The ritual declares that something important is happening and that the person involved is valued. Like the healing ritual at the Greek temples of Aescelepius, the ritual is an event out of the ordinary, designed to bring the patient to the edge of chaos where new order and direction can emerge.

Ritual also contributes to the mental state affecting the physical because of its direct impact on physiological functioning. This is accomplished through experience. "An essential function of ritual is to both produce and control human experience" (Winkelman, 2000, p. 97). Experience is what shapes our brain, programs our behavior, and sets our individual psychology. Ritual brings us new experiences that can help reprogram our responses. "Participation in ritual drama evokes and programs experiences, activating developmental sequences for the individual" (Winkelman, 2000, p. 97). It helps us control the operating structures of consciousness, break barriers to unconscious material, and retrain our cognitive organization. "Rituals may reelevate, transform, and integrate latent or suppressed neural networks through symbolic penetration techniques that bypass normal inhibitory functions" (Winkelman, 2000, p. 245). Ritual used in this way becomes a tool of depth psychotherapy.

Ritual, as an expression of human spirit, is also important to human growth, whether a physical or psychological "problem" exists. For all of us, it marks periods of transition and transformation. We have weddings and funerals, birthday parties, and bar mitzvahs and first communions for this very reason. Life's transitions—physically, emotionally, intellectually, socially, and spiritually—are marked by ritual (Dilts & McDonald, 1997). As expressions of human spirit they reintegrate the individual into the social group and establish group cohesion by reducing social tension and resolving conflict (Winkelman, 2000). The rituals in our everyday life maintain our connection with Divine Spirit and serve to connect the everyday with the sacred (Faiver et al., 2001). Overall, rituals allow us to rethink, reorder, reconnect, and re-create ourselves and our lives (Shulman, 1997).

Music Therapy and Myth and Ritual

Music has long been associated with myth and ritual (Rothstein, 1995). Music therapist Carolyn Kenny (1989) has written extensively about this link. She notes that both music and myth are nonverbal forms of expression, involve a holistic awareness, connect individuals to the world through perception, create externalizations of feeling that become shared phenomena, and promote a shift from the individual to the group. As the *experience* of myth, music also serves as ritual. In fact, music may be one of the few currently acceptable forms of ritual in Western culture (Kenny, 1982). Examples include the importance of music during opening ceremonies for the Olympics and in the continuing drum circle movement (Hull, 1998).

Music functions as ritual for a number of reasons. As Shulman (1997) notes, traditional healing rituals are based on feelings of kinship and culturally held beliefs. Participation in music making is a modern ritual of kinship. It is a shared community experience expressing the beliefs of the group (Dissanayke, 2000; Farnsworth, 1981; Gaston, 1968b). Ritual experiences are highly emotional and involve bodily experiences. As Shulman (1997) observes, "The rituals are effective exactly because a powerful bodily experience is connected through symbol and ritual with social values and religious feelings" (p. 60). This also describes the participatory music experience.

Rituals create a special environment, a time and place outside the ordinary. It is this liminal or edge-of-chaos place and time that leads to transformation (Faiver et al., 2001). Rituals transform space and time by promoting altered states of consciousness. As previously explored, musical experiences create those ASC and open this liminal space, a space that has emptiness and spaciousness connected to the dissolution of boundaries (Davis, 1999). One of the best examples of this in music therapy practice is the use of improvised music sessions (Ruud, 1998a). In this form of music participation, experimental and creative possibilities are allowed and encouraged, as is characteristic of healing rituals (Shulman, 1997). The loosening of boundaries and the creation of a liminal space allow for the emergence of new ways of being, new self-organization.

Dilts and McDonald (1997) believe healing benefits come from the interaction of three elements—an intention, a relationship, and a ritual: "When these three elements are aligned, the deep structure behind healing may be activated and healing occurs in a natural, self-organizing manner" (p. 83). The music therapy session as a healing ritual brings together these three elements. The music therapist and the group members hold the healing intention. The music brings the group together and fosters relationship. The music experience, structured by the music therapist, then engenders the sense of relationship and becomes the ritual.

> The intention to heal and the relationship which supports that intention are manifested through a ritual of some kind. . . . The most important factor in the success of the ritual seems to be its degree of congruence with the level of intention and the relationship it is supporting. (Dilts & McDonald, 1997, p. 83)

The music therapist structuring and guiding a music therapy experience, like group improvisation, can provide that flexibility to meet the level of intention and relationship needed. It must also have creativity. A predetermined or rigid ritual may not provide the flexible, creative experience necessary to meet the specific needs of the client. The music therapist must structure the session as a ritual for the unique needs of each client.

Dreams and Imagery

Another traditional tool for experiences of spirit is dreams and *imagery* (Cowan, 1996; Doore, 1988). The importance of dreams and imagery in psychological functioning was addressed previously. In chapter 4, the brain state of REM sleep was detailed for solidifying memory and learning. In chapter 6, the use of imagery when dealing with the psychological problems of emotion and feeling was explored. Now let's turn to how dreams and imagery are associated with issues of human spirit. Dreams and imagery emerge from ASC and are our first experience with spirit and the nonlinguistic symbolic processing of human functioning. The REM sleep that spawns dreams is right hemisphere activity, so that it has a different symbolic form of presentation. "Dreams [and imagery] appear bizarre and illogical from the point of view of waking consciousness because dreams involve a different system of information representation, processing, and consolidation" (Winkelman, 2000, p. 138). The images and symbols that emerge during ASC frequently involve archetypes of spirit and spiritual issues. I learned this when developing the music therapy technique of "music and creative problem solving."

To develop this technique, I asked a number of music therapists and music therapy students to participate in creative problem solving sessions to answer the question, "What is music/music therapy?" Participants listened to forty-five minutes of music I selected with the intent of evoking images and responses. After a relaxation induction, participants listened to the music and then drew the images they experienced in response to the stated question or wrote the words that emerged. What emerged were images and expressions that were profoundly spiritual in nature. According to their drawings, music was symbolized as a rainbow, a column of light, radiating colors, and a shimmering bridge. These images emerged over and over again. The written responses were very poetic, much to the surprise of the responders. They wrote that music is an unfinished wholeness, the ultimate source, and the universe in every soul. Here are some specific examples.

Music is:
  bonding with nature
  allowing creativity to express itself
  refreshment of spirit
  a development of the spiritual within us
  getting in touch with eternal flow
  resurgence of self
  reconvening of life
  spiritual bonding
  involvement—an "at-oneness" with the rhythm of living

Music therapy seeks to connect human rift to uncover the universe in every soul. Music therapy is being a complete being and celebrating joy and sorrow together, in expressing from the true wordless source of what we are. (Crowe, 1991a, p. 118)

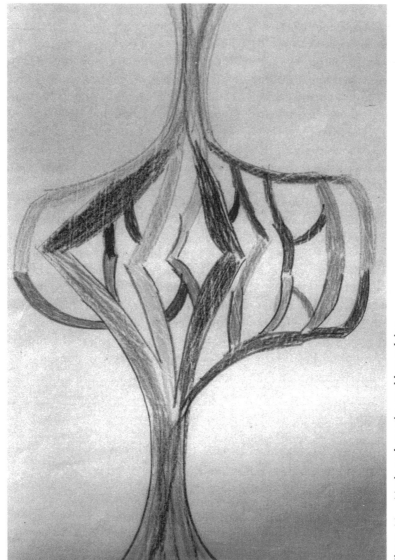

Figure 11. Music and creative problem solving.

As explored in chapter 6, the most well-developed music therapy technique utilizing imagery is Helen Bonny's Guided Imagery and Music (Bonny & Savary, 1990). Though developed to deal with problems of emotion and feeling, the technique has also been associated with spiritual practice, spiritual growth, and the direct experience of Divine Spirit (Bonny, 2001; Clark, 1998–1999; Warja, 1994; Wesley, 1998–1999). In this usage, the music serves to break down ego boundaries, foster a sense of receptivity, and open the individual to a broader experience of spirit. "Music seems to induce a heightened empathy with others, a sense of unity among people and things, a sensitivity for the divine" (Bonny & Savary, 1990, p. 17). These are again the transformative, peak experiences of transpersonal psychology stimulated by the GIM process (Lewis, 1998–1999).

Meditation

Meditation practices are another traditional tool of spirituality (Wilber, Engler, & Brown, 1986). Meditation allows the practitioner to focus attention on internal processes. "The mind is brought home instead of being engaged in constant search and analysis in the external world" (Srinivasan, 2001, p. 6). Meditation involves deliberate suspension of cognitive activity, especially the verbally organized thought of the left hemisphere. This suppression of left hemisphere activity allows another synthesizing capacity of self-awareness to emerge (Hunt, 1995). Meditation practices promote an increase in voluntary attention and concentration (Walsh, 1999).

> Meditation practices bring about a greater awareness by disrupting habitual conditioning and identification with thought and behavior. The development of greater attention and awareness and a dishabituation from one's habitual identifications and reactions reveal that the appearance of a continuous sense of self is a selective and arbitrary construction from fluctuating mental contents, and only one of many possible ideal selves that the individual presents to the social world. (Winkelman, 2000, pp. 172–173)

Two types of meditation with different focuses of attention are identified—concentration and insight meditation (Wilber, Engler, & Brown, 1986).

During *concentration meditation*, attention is restricted to a single object or phrase, like a spoken mantra or visual focus point. This leads to a withdrawal from sensory input and an increasing sense of tranquility and bliss. During *insight meditation*, attention expands to all physical and mental events as they occur in time. This leads to a ". . . process of *observation of sensory input in progressive states of 'knowledge'* . . . of the impermanent, unsatisfactory and non-substantial nature of all phenomena" (Engler, 1986, p. 20). Both practices bring spirit into conscious awareness. In concentration meditation awareness is fostered through an experience of bliss and unity. During insight meditation changes in intrapsychic structure move an individual beyond identification with personal ego to the greater reality of spirit.

The psychological and physical benefits of meditation have been substantiated by research. Meditation can help in managing stress, anxiety, depression, and the physical diseases, like high blood pressure, aggravated by stress (Benson, 1996; Cuthbert et al., 1981; Shapiro, 1990; Taylor, Barry, & Walls, 1997; Walsh, 1979, 1983, 1988). It also generally improves psychological functioning, the sense of well-being (Walsh, 1999; West, 1987), and a better understanding of psychological needs and attributes (Carrington, 1987)

Music Therapy and Meditation

Music therapy techniques are not considered meditation practices per se. Yet there are similarities between some music therapy techniques, like GIM, and meditation that would support the conclusion that involvement in these techniques could have the same benefits as meditation. As explored previously, music can foster the ASC characteristic of the meditative state. As Wise (2002) summarizes, music that is noninvasive and unfamiliar melodically with a quiet dynamic and with an underlying but not prominent rhythmic structure fosters the alpha brain waves of the meditative state. These characteristics identify sedative music (Radocy & Boyle, 1997). Wise also notes, however, that the meditative state needs beta brain wave activity. "The best way to add beta to your meditation pattern is through words—thinking, talking, writing—anything that adds conceptual articulation" (Wise, 2002, p. 128). The verbal reporting done by the client during a GIM session likely adds the beta brain waves to the music-induced alpha of the meditative brain state to produce a meditative effect.

Like psychodynamic processing, insight meditation involves uncovering techniques. Wilber, Engler, and Brown (1986) identify four uncovering techniques used in insight meditation that parallel the processes observed in GIM. The first technique utilizes technical neutrality, which involves only a basic awareness of mental and physical events as they are observed. In GIM, the client is placed in a comfortable position to decrease awareness of the body and the environment. Sensations, bodily reactions, and mental imagery are then observed and reported without analysis or processing during the experience. The second uncovering technique of meditation is the removal of censorship. "Any and all thoughts, feelings and sensations are allowed into awareness, without discrimination or selection" (Engler, 1986, p. 35). This is also a basic tenet of GIM. Clients are encouraged to report all experiences without censorship or editing. The third technique involves abstinence from gratification of wishes, impulses, and desires. When GIM is used in this way, it emphasizes the pure experience and not the catharsis of emotional expression or the acting out of problems or conflicts when GIM is used as a psychotherapeutic technique. Finally, meditation techniques allow for a therapeutic split from the ego. The participant becomes a witness to his or her own experience. Some GIM experiences also allow for this sense of detached observation. Part of the self can objectively observe the imagery and reactions as they occur. In my own GIM experiences, I frequently report, "*She* is seeing a person," indicating the reporting "me" is observing an experience that another aspect of "me" is having. A music therapy technique like GIM may provide an experience equal to a meditative practice in terms of providing the opportunity to expand awareness and develop consciousness to the higher levels.

A holistic approach with any client requires attention to issues of spirit as part of the therapeutic effort. Music therapy techniques are used as part of the traditional tools of spiritual healing, including altered states of consciousness, myth and ritual, dreams and imagery, and meditation. Music makes significant contributions to our experiences of spirit and issues of spiritual healing.

Specific Applications of Music Therapy and Spirit

Throughout this chapter, how music therapy meets the needs for spirit in clients with physical and mental difficulties as well as for the general growth and evolution of consciousness for all humans was noted. This aspect of human functioning can have relevance for most clients served by music therapy. There are two areas of music therapy practice—dealing with addiction and grief work—where issues of spirit are particularly important. These serve as illustrations of music therapy practice in the area of spirit.

Music Therapy and Addictions

Addiction is a state of compulsive, habitual behavior characterized by attachment of desire to specific objects, substances, or behavior. Addiction limits an individual's freedom, will, and true desire. "Addiction exists whenever persons are internally compelled to give energy to things that are not their true desires" (May, 1988, p. 14). Tombs (1994) believes addiction has multiple causes based on biological, psychological, behavioral, and social factors. Spiritual needs are often not mentioned in traditional therapy approaches to treatment for addiction. However, many experts are now addressing addiction, in part, as a longing for the Divine source, as a misguided search for the whole (Grof & Grof, 1993; May, 1988; Skaggs, 1997).

Addiction may truly be a problem of complexity—the complex interaction of numerous factors giving rise to the compulsive behaviors of addiction. For example, substances, like drugs and alcohol, directly affect the brain in the forebrain area and influence emotion and the pleasure response through release of dopamine (Johnston, 1999; Robbins, 1998). But biology is not enough to create an addiction. Attachment, a psychological process of learning, is also needed. As May (1988) notes,

> The process of attachment takes place psychologically as a form of learning. This learning happens through reinforcement and conditioning, and it is accompanied by physical and chemical changes in the brain and elsewhere in the body. Since multiple functional systems are involved, the learning becomes entrenched. (pp. 89–90)

There is a sense that people with addictions are striving to cover unconscious pain or trauma and to "fill a hole" in themselves. The perceived emptiness may involve problems of psychological development and arrest and inadequate social systems, including the family and community at large. The spiritual aspect of addiction, however, also involves the quest for ultimate meaning and Divine love characterized as the search for the spiritual.

There is likely no one cause and, therefore, no one form of treatment that could address this complex problem. Treatment for addiction must address all possible causes (Skaggs, 1997). Music therapy techniques can address a number of these areas, especially the spiritual needs.

In terms of the physical aspects of addiction, these is no evidence that the brain chemicals produced in response to music listening (see chapter 5) can block the effects of drugs or alcohol on the brain. However, music may influence the physiological component of addiction in several ways. As addressed earlier in this chapter, music listening can induce the production of alpha brain waves. Norris (2000) found that alcoholics and people with other substance abuse problems have a low level of alpha and theta brain wave production, possibly based on genetic predisposition. Slower brain rhythms help the brain produce the natural substances, like endogenous opiates, endorphins, and dopamine, that give people a sense of happiness and well-being. Since people dealing with substance abuse may not produce the slower waves naturally, they often feel that the only way to experience happiness and well-being is to use a substance. They need other ways to produce the alpha and theta brain waves

(Norris, 2000). Music listening and participating in music can induce both alpha and theta brain waves and may serve as an alternative to the ingestion of the substance. Research (Prince, 1982; Scarantino, 1987) demonstrated that endorphin levels are increased in response to music listening.

Music may also relate to the biological components of substance abuse by stimulating the pleasure pathway and inducing the release of dopamine. Dopamine now is known to underlie almost every form of pleasure that animals experience (Johnston, 1999). Again, music may serve as an effective substitute for the pleasure response. "The intensity in the musical interaction seems to replace the need for drugs" (Ruud, 1995, p. 104).

The psychological needs of the client with an addiction can also be addressed by music therapy techniques. As explored extensively in chapter 6, music therapy techniques provide means for uncovering repressed emotions and feelings, catharsis of these affective states, and psychotherapeutic processing of the emotional material. Soshensky (2001) believes music therapy techniques can address the psychological and emotional concerns of people with addictions, giving them experiences where they can ". . . step outside of habitual non-productive and painful emotional patterns" (p. 45).

Music therapy interventions can also provide therapeutic transpersonal experiences. As explored in the previous chapter, transpersonal experiences move the client beyond the issues and restrictions of personal self and ego and bring an awareness of a broader and deeper reality. Addiction is a rigid, narrow behavior focused on limited sense of self and restrictive ego boundaries. The suffering of addiction comes from a belief that we are what we think we are (Wolf, 1999).

> Transpersonal therapy can teach people to regulate their desires so that they are not controlled by them. . . . [A]ny therapeutic intervention which decreases the centrality of the personality will in turn decrease the compulsive effects of desire and the debilitating effects of unfulfilled craving. (Fadiman, 1980, p. 179)

Music therapy techniques have the ability to loosen rigid, entrenched behavioral patterns, expand client's perception, and provide an experience with deeper realities (Skaggs, 1997). The "high" of substance abuse is a pseudo-transcendent experience (Metzner, 1994). Music provides a true transcendent experience.

As noted, the spiritual causes of addiction are not usually addressed by traditional therapeutic approaches (Skaggs, 1997). Jung (1987) saw addiction as a spiritual thirst for wholeness, for the Divine, for one's spiritual nature. We all have a longing for wholeness, completion, fulfillment, and love that comes from our experience with Divine Spirit. *"For many people, behind the craving for drugs, alcohol, or other addictions is the craving for the Higher Self or God"* (Grof & Grof, 1993, p. 145). Woodman (1993) sees addiction as a response to the despair and alienation of the emptiness of the soul. The "emptiness" comes from a sense of disconnection.

> Present experience is an embodied experience, related to our body, mind, and emotions. When we come upon a dimension of our experience that has to do with disconnection from our true nature, we experience that disconnection as a kind of emptiness, a hole. (Peay, 1999, p. 23)

People with addictions use external things and substances to try to fill the hole. Addiction is more than repression of past pain and conditioned learning; it is also attaching the ultimate desire for Divine Spirit to human behavior or things (May, 1988). In a fundamental way, recovery from addiction involves the individual self finding who it really is—spirit—and reestablishing contact with the Divine source (Wolf, 1999). This is accomplished through experiences of grace.

Grace is the direct experience of Divine Spirit. According to May (1988), grace ". . . is the dynamic outpouring of God's loving nature that flows into and through creation in an endless self-offering of healing, love, illumination, and reconciliation" (p. 17). Twelve-step programs, like Alcoholics Anonymous, are based on a spiritual principle and a belief in a higher power that will assist in overcoming the compulsive urges (Skaggs, 1997). Through grace, spiritual growth becomes a process of transformation not education. "It is, if anything, an unlearning process in which our old ways are cleansed, liberated, and redeemed" (May, 1988, p. 105). Transformation through grace can only be expressed and appreciated in an ". . . actual, immediate experience of real life situations. Finally, it can only be 'lived into'" (May, 1988, p. 125).

Music therapy is extensively advocated as a spiritual therapy for clients dealing with addiction (Bonny, 2001; Skaggs, 1997; Walker, 1995). Music therapy relates to the spiritual needs in treatment of addiction in several ways. The first spiritual need is to belong to and feel part of a community. People who are addicted feel isolated and alone. They frequently are alienated from family, community, and support systems. "It is often a sense of separation from one's larger self, and from others, from our oneness, that brings people into drugs and alcohol, crime, and prison" (Norris, 2000, p. 5). Community is vital in treating addiction because the struggle with an addictive substance can never be a private thing (May, 1988). This is a fundamental belief of twelve-step groups (Alcoholics Anonymous, 1976). Earlier in this chapter, how music can create a sense of belonging and affiliation, how participation in participatory music experiences can promote involvement in groups, and how music experiences allow for participation at the client's level of functioning and comfort were explored. Music therapy techniques address this aspect of spirit effectively. For example, music therapists are successfully using group drumming experiences with clients dealing with drugs and alcohol in Veterans Administration Medical Centers (Barry Bernstein, personal communication, February 24, 2003) and in other substance abuse treatment settings (Winkelman, 2003).

Another aspect of human spirit, creativity, can also be addressed for clients with addictions. Small (1982) and Leonard (1990) see blocked creativity as a primary cause of addiction. All the avenues for creativity in various music therapy techniques provide both the means and the opportunity for exploring and expressing creativity. From songwriting, to improvisation, to performance, participation in music brings creative opportunities to everyone. The music therapist structures the musical intervention to insure that everyone can participate and have a satisfying, successful, creative experience.

Symbolic healing and ritual are other aspects of human spirit that are important in treatment for people with addiction. As explored, music can evoke the personal and spiritual symbols through imagery needed in the process of spiritual transformation. Symbols and images give people new ways of thinking and being (Skaggs, 1997). Individuals dealing with addictions have lost the ability to image. "By reconnecting individuals with their image-producing capacity we start the long process of returning them to their true nature—to a sense of wholeness within self and the world" (Skaggs, 1997, p. 28). Music therapy techniques not only evoke the images and symbols of spiritual healing but then become the rituals needed to further the healing on this level. Healing an addiction is a process of transformation because addiction itself is a process (Wolf, 1999). Ritual provides direction for this process while allowing the openness and spaciousness needed for the transformation to unfold. "Through the spaciousness will come some homeward call, some invitation to transformation" (May, 1988, p. 149). Music is just such a transformative ritual—structured and familiar, yet providing space and openness to explore, risk, and discover.

Finally, music offers individuals dealing with addiction a direct experience of Divine Spirit through grace.

> When surrendering to music . . . the addicts are often set free in a sense of peace and joy, experiencing anew, or for the first time, something greater than

their lives have been. In this respect, the surrendering connects the addict with the redemptive force within, the force that supports the ascent from death to re-creation. (Skaggs, 1997, p. 2)

Music becomes the direct experience of Divine Spirit—the life-enhancing, vital, pleasurable joy of connection, love, and celebration.

Music Therapy and Patients with Terminal Illnesses

Music therapy techniques are used in supporting clients through the grief process (Hilliard, 2001). This is certainly true for individuals facing the end of their lives. Music therapy practices for patients with catastrophic or terminal illnesses or those facing death due to advanced age also need to include experiences in spirit. A number of music therapists have advocated the use of music to handle the spiritual issues of terminal illness (Aldridge, 1995; Gilbert, 1977; Krout, 2000; Martin, 1991; Munro & Mount, 1978). Doka (1993) identifies three spiritual tasks for people who are facing death. First, the people need to find meaning in life and come to terms with the life they have lived in a unified, integrated manner (Erickson, Erickson, & Kivnick, 1986). This involves embracing a wider view of life, whether through religious faith, personal philosophy, or significant relationships. This process may involve reconciliation (Callanan & Kelley, 1992), a process of "making peace" with one's life and completing unfinished business. The second spiritual need is to make sense of death so that the individual can die with integrity. Finally, the person dealing with death needs to overcome suffering and find a hope that extends beyond death (Frame, 2003).

Music therapy techniques related to spirit can address all these needs. Finding meaning in life first involves a process of life review. Music triggers memories that can be shared and processed. Karras (1985) has developed a systematic approach to life review using music, particularly songs, to begin the process of reconciliation. Songs can also be used to illustrate the stages of an individual's life (Bruscia, 1998b). I recently had a student who was working with a client in the hospice unit of a long-term care facility. They worked together on a life timeline where songs represented each stage of the client's life. By experiencing the songs from each era of his life and determining why a particular song was the best to illustrate his life at a certain point, he engaged in a deep life review. Techniques used in music psychotherapy, discussed in the previous chapter, can contribute to the clients' process of "making peace" with their life. Finally, the link of music and religious/spiritual values can be part of reaffirming a wider view of life (Blacking, 1973). As discussed in chapter 3, music/songs are used to affirm and communicate beliefs (Merriam, 1964). Transpersonal experience with music can also be a part of this process.

The second spiritual need of patients who are dying, making sense of death, can also be addressed through music therapy experiences. Music and imagery techniques can make significant contributions to this process. Music therapist Kenneth Bruscia (1992) reports on his work with patients with AIDS in making sense of death. In his work with numerous patients with AIDS, he found that the final step in the healing process was for patients to ". . . embrace life while dying, and to embrace death while living" (Bruscia, 1992, p. 202). This was accomplished during GIM sessions with imagery of "visits from the other side" and deeply felt experiences of compassionate, encompassing love.

The third spiritual need of persons with terminal illness, finding and supporting hope, is addressed in music therapy. Hope is the belief that things make sense no matter how they turn out (Hibbard, 2002). Aldridge (1998) believes that active engagement in music moves hope from an abstract concept to a lived experience. The music therapy group becomes a community of support where joy and celebration are a large part. Though not a music therapy technique per se, music can be used to accompany the death process to comfort and support individuals as they transition into death (Schroeder-Sheker, 1993).

Spirituality as experiences of both Divine Spirit and human spirit is the fourth component of human functioning addressed in a holistic approach to therapy. Experiences with spirit help us explore issues of meaning and purpose and bring us to a greater sense of wholeness and consciousness development. This is a vital part of the soulmaking process. Through the sense of breath, movement, and rhythm, music has been associated with spirit throughout human history. Music therapy techniques address this basic human need and provide therapeutic effort in this area when required. Having explored the four areas of human functioning and how music therapy has effects in each, the music therapy theory of music and soulmaking can now be fully developed.

CHAPTER EIGHT

~

Toward a New Theory
of Music and Healing

There is no truer truth obtainable by Man than comes of music.

—Robert Browning

Music is a higher revelation than all wisdom and philosophy.

—Beethoven

Let's briefly summarize the developments of previous chapters, so we may continue to journey into the complexity of our world with music as our map. The amazing complexity of music derived from the multiple layers of sound production and perception was explored. The organization of sound over time led to the intricate human behavior known as music. This fundamental human behavior affects human functioning in mind, emotions, body, and spirit. From this investigation, reasons why music is a good tool for therapy and health were delineated and the underlying processes involved when music affects human functioning were summarized. Extensive research demonstrates the effectiveness of music therapy treatment interventions. Throughout the book, the fact that human involvement with music is an immensely complex, interactive system was emphasized. Based on this information, a music therapy theory of wholeness from the perspective of complexity science—music and soulmaking—can be fully developed. This chapter explores how this new theory influences music therapy practice and research. It concludes with an exploration of music as a map to human knowledge and wisdom.

Theory of Music and Soulmaking

The profession of music therapy has struggled with what theoretical model, paradigm, and research approaches are most appropriate to substantiate and explain the effects of music therapy interventions for clients. In the late 1960s, an effort was made to standardize the theoretical approach to music therapy based on behaviorism (Carrocio & Carrocio, 1972; Madsen, Cottor, & Madsen, 1968). Others have supported a psychodynamic model as the most useful (Bonny & Savary, 1990; Bruscia, 1998g: Priestley, 1994). Kenny (1989) proposed a phenomenological theoretical basis for music therapy, while Ruud (1978) explored music therapy processing from the perspective of several different theoretical models. Thaut (2000) proposes a theoretical model based on vigorous, empirical research to "prove" the impact of music therapy. Taylor (1997) advocates a theory of music therapy based primarily on neurophysiology. A number of people have recently proposed a "holistic" approach to theory and research for music therapy (Ruud, 1998b). Such an approach urges consideration of the clients in their wholeness and encourages the use of many theoretical models and research methods based on the unique characteristics and circumstances of the clients. Bruscia (1998a) believes one theoretical base or one research approach for substantiating music therapy practice would not be appropriate. Kenny (1998) identifies eight "cultures of inquiry" appropriate to music therapy practice—phenomenological, hermeneutic, theoretical, empirical/analytical, evaluation, action, historical/comparative, and ethnographic. She writes, "To assume one approach is 'it,' is dishonoring the wholeness, the complexity, the richness of being" (1998, p. 215).

Does this mean that there can be no agreement, no unification of music therapy theory?

> If the reconciliation of the various approaches within the field of music therapy is to be regarded as impossible, would this necessitate one day, that one of these theories is proclaimed to be the model of understanding upon which all further research is based? Or, can the variety of approaches within the field of music therapy be maintained without causing any loss of the "scientific standard" to the field of research? (Ruud, 1978, p. 70)

A new scientific theory of music therapy is needed that is inclusive of all the approaches and processes observed in the highly complex interactions of music and human functioning found in music therapy. It is proposed that this new scientific theory of music therapy is music and soulmaking, based on the principles of complexity science.

This new theory of music therapy must include the analytical components of empirical research, both qualitative and quantitative, but also requires a larger context that accepts and encompasses the necessary wholeness and interrelatedness of all complex systems. An expanded scientific paradigm of music therapy is needed—one in which the old elements, theories, and research methods are included as components of a broader, more balanced perspective (Wilber, 1996). Complexity science is such a paradigm because it can encompass all music therapy approaches and theoretical orientations. Borysenko (1998) notes, "The new paradigm is really about the mind, the body, and the spirit coming into harmony. About relationship, about connectedness, about having that intention" (p. 6). Music therapy's influence is in its complexity and wholeness. This is the theory of music and soulmaking developed here.

What Is Soul?

To begin a definition of music and soulmaking, the term *soul* must be defined. Throughout human history philosophers, theologians, and great thinkers of all kinds have asked the question, "What is soul?" It is not an easy question to answer. The quotes from the great thinkers of history listed below show the diversity of these answers:

> The soul is a breath of living spirit, that with excellent sensitivity, permeates the entire body to give it life.
>
> —Hildegard of Bingen

> You could not discover the frontiers of soul, even if you traveled every road to do so; such is the depth of its meaning.
>
> —Heraclitus of Ephesus

> The soul, which is the first principle of life, is not a body, but the act of a body.
>
> —Thomas Aquinas

> The soul is in a sense all things, because it has been created in such a way as to have the whole order of the universe inscribed within it.
>
> —Aristotle

> For the soul is the beginning of all things. It is the soul that lends all things movement.
>
> —Plotinus

> For soul cannot, indeed will not, be caught in our net of words. Butterfly-like she eludes our every attempt to grasp her conceptually.
>
> —John Sanford

> Soul is a perspective rather than a substance, a viewpoint toward things rather than a thing itself. Soul is a world of imagination, passion, fantasy, reflection, that is neither physical and material on the one hand, nor spiritual and abstract on the other, yet bound to them both.
>
> —James Hillman

Soul is not a "thing." It is not an object. It is not any kind of entity, not even a nonmaterial entity (Sardello, 1995). From a psychological perspective, it is a point of view, a capacity, or a quality of human functioning. Soul is what is most unique and genuine about us. It is the focus of our personal individuality. Soul ". . . reflects the essence of one's existence . . . the whole, living being of an individual person. Thus it is manifested through, rather than divorced from, body, mind, or any other facet of one's being" (May, 1982, p. 7). The word *soul* derives from one of the Hebrew words meaning the essence of a person. Soul is the fundamental nature of who we are, our true selves, our deeper aspects (Walsh, 1999). Soul describes the entirety of the individual (Davis, 1999). Though related, soul and self are not the same thing. Wolf (1999) contends that the self is the soul's reflection in matter. Soul is broader and more encompassing than self.

Soul is a never-ending quest for information. It is a passionate, hungry fire, a thirst for knowledge, truth, and enlightenment. Soul involves a compelling search for meaning, depth, and genuineness. It becomes a way of being, a way of living. Soul is about creativity and subjectivity and yet has a noetic quality, which involves a heightened sense of clarity. Soul is about imagination, the ". . . imaginative possibilities in our nature" (Sardello, 1995, p. xiv). It is not about mind, logic, and reason. It expresses itself in images, dreams, and metaphors. It is ineffable—beyond the ability of words to describe.

Soul is malleable, sensitive, receptive, impressionable, and alive with possibility. The soul can and does learn, change, and grow. It does this through experiences with the world. Soul is a dimension of experiencing life and ourselves. Subjective experiences are the basis of the soul process. "My soul is not the result of objective facts that require explanation; rather it reflects subjective experiences that require understanding" (Hillman, 1975, pp. 15–16). Interactions with the world are imprinted on the soul. These experiences change, mold, and transform the soul. All aspects of human experience involving the body, mind, emotion, and spirit form and deepen soul. It is the complex energy of individualization that vitalizes the person and is then projected into the world. Soul enlivens the body but is not confined by it. Our interactions with the world come back to us to make and shape soul through deepened experiences creating the sum total of our uniqueness, our individuality.

Subjective experiences relate soul to the essential humanness of emotion. It is expressed in joy and enthusiasm yet deepened and shaped by pain, crisis, and tragedy. The emotion of love in all its forms—love of self, love for other humans, love of nature, love of God—is a large part of soul. But the essential humanness of emotion also requires the very human emotions of deep pain, anguish, grief, and rage. Soul is also about the ugly and the pathological.

> We need to revalue what we consider to be negative. The poet, Rilke, used to say that difficulty is one of the greatest friends of the soul. Our lives would be immeasurably enriched if we could but bring the same hospitality in meeting the negative as we bring to the joyful and pleasurable. (O'Donohue, 1997, p. 115)

All emotions relate to humanness in its most profound depth. Emotions provide soul with its energy, its potential to do work. "In the strength of its emotions, the soul is a gun, full of potential power and effect" (Moore, 1992, p. 135).

Soul has the characteristic of connection. It is about relationships—of the soul to the numinous force of creation, of the inner self to the outer self or ego, and of the self to other people. Soul has a relationship with the Divine through the action of spirit. Soul plays a ". . . dual role in linking us to our most enlightened possibilities here on Earth, as well as to the higher levels of conscious awareness that . . . are the source of everything we are and can become" (Bordier, 2001, p. 23). Spirit relates to soul but is not soul. Soul is temporarily trapped spirit (Wolf, 1999).

> Some people use the words *soul* and *spirit* interchangeably. But in fairy tales [deep metaphors of human experience] . . . the spirit is a being born of soul. The spirit inherits or incarnates into matter in order to gather news of the ways of the world and carries these back to the soul. When not interfered with, the relationship between soul and spirit is one of perfect symmetry, each enriches the other in turn. (Estes, 1992, p. 292)

Soul and spirit nurture each other. Spirit becomes the Divine spark moving soul and enlivening the body. Soul relates our inner being to our outer, conscious self.

> From the point of view of psychology, the soul is that within us that connects our consciousness to our inner depths. The soul's primary function is relationship, and the relationship between the ego and the inner world is the most important relationship of all, for if this is broken, relationships with other people and God are impossible. (Sanford, 1987, pp. 122–123)

Soul provides the link between the external self and the deep essential nature of individual being. Soul engages. It reaches out to make contact and seeks experiences in all human realms through the action of movement. Soul is a circular movement of continuous becoming on one hand and deep inner stillness on the other. "Soul has a flowing quality like water that can be shaped into an infinite variety of forms" (Davis, 1999, p. 47). Soul is not "in" the body per se but is that which moves out from us (Moore, 1992). As Wolf (1999) notes, it is ". . . somehow outside the body and inside the body at the same time" (p. 244). The healthy life of soul depends on continual movement—a flowing out and gathering in (Holdrege, 2002). Soul receives from the wisdom energy of spirit and moves from a place of matter and the body back out to spirit. A healthy soul moves from inside to outside and between self and others (Pressman, 2002). On all levels, connectedness, relationship, and kinship characterize soul.

In keeping with the explorations of complexity science, soul can be considered a higher frequency of information that is nonlinear in character. It is a nonmechanistic vital force—a process with no mass and no energy (deQuincey, 2002). Like a quantum wave potential, it has effect without being a "thing" (Wolf, 1999). Soul works in wholeness as a complex, nonlinear process. Having an energetic property, soul is a dynamical system in motion—not the outward kinetic energy of spirit but the constant iterative feedback of newly energizing information. From a nonlinear perspective, soul is a field of energy as information. It is continuous movement, movement as information. "[Your soul] is a positive, purposeful force at the core of your being. It is that part of you that understands the impersonal nature of the energy dynamics in which you are involved, that loves without restriction and accepts without judgment" (Zukav, 1989, p. 31). Like all complex systems, soul is immeasurable. As John Polkinghorne (1993), the great chaos theorist, writes,

> The soul is not an extra spiritual ingredient injected at some stage into the body, and in principle separable from it, but rather it is that holistic, almost infinite information-bearing pattern, carried by the body and maintained as the locus of our personal identity—through all the unending changes of the atoms actually comprising our bodies at any particular instant of time. (pp. 113–114)

Soul, like deterministic chaos, is associated with structure and creation where matter is manifested out of the movement of soul (Wolf, 1999).

Music and Soul
Extensive connections exist between music and the characteristics of soul. Soul is defined as a capacity or ongoing process of living. In chapter 3, mu-

sic was defined as an ever-unfolding process as well, one that has to be realized on a moment-to-moment basis. The philosopher Rudolf Steiner wrote,

> Musical creations, however, must be generated anew again and again. They flow onward in the surge and swell of their harmonies and melodies, a reflec-tion of the soul, which in its incarnations must always experience itself in the onward-flowing stream of time. Just as the human soul is an evolving entity, so its reflection here on earth is a flowing one. The deep effect of music is due to this kinship. . . . Out of music the most primordial kinship speaks to the soul; in the most inwardly deep sense, sounds of home rebound from it. (quoted in Godwin, 1987, p. 259)

Soul and music have a kinship because they are, in essence, one and the same process implying movement. Soul movement is a living movement of expanding information. This is also a good definition of music. There is no sound, no music, and no music production without movement. Vibration gives us tone, kinesthetic movement of the human body produces the tones, and organization of tones over time gives us music. Soul and music are both special kinds of rhythmic vibration, a process of movement.

Soul is about our essential humanness, the fundamental properties that make us human beings. Music is a basic human behavior. Music has been a part of all human cultures on this planet. As far as we know, it is exclusively a human behavior. Soul and music are both fundamental to our essential humanness.

Another characteristic of soul is the quality of connection and relationship. As defined in chapter 3, music is the *relationship of tones over time*. Isolated tones are never music. From this basic definition of music, we also learned about music's power to form groups, interact in positive ways, and relate. Music allows for the connection of communication and expression. It is a social activity. Music is also our connection to the Divine. As discussed in chapter 7, music embodies and expresses spirit. Sufi philosopher Hazrat Inayat Khan writes,

> The best use of it [music] is made in spiritual evolution; by the power of sound or word one can evolve spiritually and experience all the different stages of spiritual perfection. Music is the best medium for awakening the soul; nothing is better. Music is the shortest, the most direct way to God. . . . (quoted in Godwin, 1987, p. 263)

The ancients linked music with the Divine order and used it in worship.

Soul grows and deepens through human experience in all its forms. Music is a fundamental yet all-encompassing human experience. Music is organized sound meeting human consciousness. It is the perception of a multiple sensory input (music) being processed by elaborate brain functioning. Experiences with music involve hearing, of course, but they are also experiences of sight, of muscle movement and position, and especially of touch. Music flows from your fingers and dances on your skin in waves of tactile sensation. Music is a total experience with the body. "Your senses are the guides to take you deep into the inner world of your heart. . . . The senses are our bridges to the world. Human skin is porous; the world flows through you" (O'Donohue, 1997, p. 58). Music gives us other experiences of the body by stimulating movement. It inspires us to dance, to coordinate action, and to tap our toes. Through music, we have all human experiences—meaningful connections with others, the emotions of pain and pleasure, and the aesthetic experience of the numinous.

Soul involves the deeply subjective experience of imagination. Indeed, soul is a process of our imagination, it ". . . is the activity of imaging rather than the momentary results of this ongoing activity" (Sardello, 1995, p. xiv). Playing music itself requires this ongoing process of imagination. To play, we create an image of the sounds produced from the musical notation (notes, etc.). We are in a constant process of imaging every time we re-create a piece of music. We also know that music deeply touches our personal images and fantasies. Techniques like "Guided Imagery and Music" show how profoundly music evokes the imaginal realm. "The soul thinks in symbols. It is not literal-minded. Developing a process language nourishes the soul" (Artress, 1995, p. 133). Music is such a process language, mirroring soul's character and quality.

Finally, soul is a nonlinear process as a complex, dynamical system in motion. This also characterizes music. Soul and music are information-laden. As such, both are the source of creativity, expansion, and new forms. "Chaos is the source of all form and creativity, the mother of invention, the soul" (Abraham, 1994, p. 149). Chaos is the potential out of which everything emerges. Soul and music also have this quality.

Music as Soulmaking

Thus far, the many reasons why music is therapeutic were explored. In some instances, like rhythmic music in rehabilitation of patients dealing with strokes, the effectiveness can be "proven." The use of music as an effective treatment for various clients with wide-ranging problems and disabilities was reviewed. This gives us a clear picture of the complexity involved with music as therapy and healing. It is time to explore the concept of soulmaking as a therapeutic process.

The term *soulmaking* has been around a long time. The poet John Keats was the first to coin the word soulmaking, referring to the human need for mystical and imaginative experiences. For Keats, soulmaking involved defining ourselves by struggling with the difficulties of experience. The psychiatrist C. G. Jung (1933) wrote about soulmaking as individuation, the process of becoming a unique individual as a creative experience. According to philosopher Albert Camus, soul is not given to us fully formed but is created through all the experiences of living (Grosso, 1992). The idea of soulmaking was formalized by psychologist Dr. James Hillman (1975), who saw "soul" as a perspective, a way of seeing the world, and the true province of psychology. Soulmaking for Hillman is a lived quality of human experience but not a divinely given life force as others define soul. In fact, soulmaking is seen as a way to psychological health. It is an important process in the fully developed human psyche. Soulmaking implies human development, maturation, and evolution of humanness in its complete and fullest sense (Davis, 1999).

The theory of music and soulmaking postulates soulmaking as an ongoing process of *health* in mind, emotion, body, and spirit. In this definition, health, from the perspective of complexity and wholeness, implies a harmonious relationship among all elements of human functioning. Health, then, involves being in a dynamic process of "right relationship" at or among any one or more levels of the human experience (Quinn, 1989). In a state of health, this right relationship is a coherent state where natural and logical connections exist as a result of being a part of the whole. Coherence is not a static state, however. This right relationship of coherence is an ever-changing process Health is a dynamical system in motion. In biology, when an equilibrium is reached, you're dead (Gleick, 1987). According to complexity science, health is a nonlinear state of chaos. Physiologists now

> . . . identify chaos with health because nonlinearity in feedback processes serves to regulate and control. In other words, a linear process, given a slight nudge, tends to remain slightly off-track. A nonlinear process, given the same nudge, tends to return to its starting point. (Shepherd, 1993, p. 94)

Health is constant movement, keeping all aspects of human functioning in right relationship. It is the ability of living systems to continue to self-organize (Shulman, 1997).

As explored, optimum "fitness" and vitality in living systems rest at the edge of chaos. The edge of chaos is a place of phase transition, a boundary that, when crossed, creates a sudden change of state. The shifts from health to illness or disease to health are such transitions. In complex systems, the edge of chaos is the point of maximum information, maximum creative potential.

"A system poised at the edge-of-chaos is neither too ordered and thus un-changing, nor too chaotic and so incoherent" (Alexander & Globus, 1996, p. 39). Perhaps health itself is a state of the right relationship of body, mind, emotion, and spirit dancing at the edge of chaos, the point of optimum fitness. Health, then, is not the absence of disease but, rather, the process by which individuals maintain their ability to function optimally in the face of change, trauma, and challenge (Schlitz, Taylor, & Lewis, 1998). This requires contin-uous input of new information. "Systems that self-organize out of chaos sur-vive only by staying open to a constant flow-through of energy and material" (Briggs & Peat, 1999. p. 16). As the complexity of the system increases, as more information is added, new properties emerge. A particular state of health is such a property. As a self-organizing system, growth of the human body/mind is inevitable, including movement toward health. Health becomes the optimal complexity: optimal vigor of the highly complex, recursively or-ganized system that is the human body/mind. Health becomes an emergent property of the human system pushed to the edge of chaos by increased com-plexity but stabilized by the right relationship of the four components of func-tioning. Health is then seen as a process in a dynamical system in motion poised at the edge of chaos.

As a new theory of music therapy, music and soulmaking emphasizes the ancient idea of wholeness and the complex relationships of all functioning as requirements for health. Soulmaking is a holistic process.

> We are a totality of body, soul, and spirit. . . . If any one part of our being suf-fers, the total human organism suffers. If the total person is to live, to be free, to come into expression, all sides must be consciously recognized and joyfully received. . . . (Sanford, 1987, p. 131)

Wholeness implies unity, connection, and congruence. It is an aesthetically pleasing relationship among all the elements of the whole. "Wholeness is a dynamic process of the human experience. Wholeness is not an endpoint or a state, but rather a process that is alive in us. It's dynamic; it's always chang-ing. It's never beginning and it's never ending" (Quinn, 1998, p. 5). The root word of wholeness is *hal*, "to be or become whole" (Crowe, 1991a). Human beings' earliest intuition about health recognized the need for wholeness.

Music therapy is a process of soulmaking for a number of reasons. Music is a fundamental, all-encompassing human event involving the complete range of experiences that deepen and challenge the soul. Music is a sensory expe-rience, a physical experience, and a perceptual experience. It is an event of deep emotions—of joy and pleasure, of grief and pain, and of numinous transcendence. Music is the human experience of the spirit—the sense of belonging and community. Music is also an imaginal experience. Forming music requires imagination itself. It evokes deep, vivid images in us. Soulmaking is an experiential process. Music is also an ever-unfolding process. Music is a safe, nonthreatening, and easily accessible means of experiential self-understanding on all levels.

Soulmaking is also about movement, energy, rhythm, and the right relationship of harmony. These four qualities virtually define music and certainly constitute it. Music is the organization of those sounds in patterns of harmony—right musical relationships—and movement over time. Musical harmony creates a state of coherence among the moving musical elements. This becomes the perfect model for the harmony among human functions required to maximize the energy needed to interact with our world—the state of optimum fitness. Soulmaking involves becoming fully ourselves in order to move in the world powerfully. In soul work, we shed the hindrances to our full participatory capacity, whether it be unhealthy bodies, psychological trauma, an impaired memory capacity, or social isolation. C. G. Jung stated that only something overwhelming, no matter what form of expression it uses, can challenge the whole man and force him to react as a whole (Grosso, 1992). Through the engagement of multiple sensory channels and its highly emotional impact, music becomes that overwhelming experience—an event of wholeness pushing us to the evolution of the soul. "Experiences that nudge us out of the rut of everyday consciousness are roads to recapturing the soul" (Grosso, 1992, p. 83). Music is that extraordinary event that gives us that nudge. Music influences human functioning in numerous ways and helps us explore who we really are.

Soul is an attitude, a certain capacity for being in the world. The fully enlivened soul is creative and has an openness to wonder. Soulmaking requires this creativity. Music is a creative art. Even when we're playing composed music, the very act of playing is a new creation every time. Music opens us to wonder. We are awed and overwhelmed during the aesthetic reaction to music. We experience ". . . the bliss of sacred time—time transformed by music into ecstasy" (Grosso, 1992, p. 197). Music takes us out of linear time and opens a sense of expanded reality, of expanded possibilities.

> Music uses time in such a way that it can fill us with feelings of eternity. Most of us have known moments when music swelled the boundaries of ourselves, transporting us to other worlds. Music seems a natural ally of soulmaking, and there are great lessons to learn from it. . . . (Grosso, 1992, p. 197)

We learn an expanded capacity for living. If soulmaking is an ongoing creative process that is used in the structure of our lives, music becomes the perfect teacher. As we've learned, music is highly structured yet allows unlimited, unfettered process. It is creativity rooted in forms understandable to all. The processes of music and of soulmaking are the same.

The purpose of soulmaking is to evolve as human beings, including developing our mystical, spiritual nature. "I believe the soul's goal is to evolve to the highest level, spiritually, emotionally, intellectually, and physically—this requires the full development of one's mystical nature" (Hunt, 1996, p. 181). Of course, our mystical nature is our direct experience of the Divine. The experience of music becomes soulmaking as it moves us beyond human concerns and touches the Divine source. Because music can and does affect all these areas, as explored extensively, it becomes a primary tool for soulmaking.

Exposure to and, particularly, involvement in the complex, holistic experience of music, then, are human soulmaking. Soulmaking is the simultaneous engagement of the essence of a person—mind, emotion, body, and spirit—in the right relationships that constitute health. Soul is our connection to the world around us and to the infinite source of life energy. Music is a gift, a remarkable tool, for humans to remember, touch, and actualize that force in the world. "The soul needs a guiding structure upon which to grow, one that is large and complex and beautifully constructed" (Whelan, 1999, p. 24). Though not intended to be, Whelan's quote is a lovely definition of music because of the complexity of music and its impact.

Role of the Therapist

There is one more relationship, one more aspect of complexity, to consider in the new theory of music therapy—the presence, interactions, and intention of the music therapist. As previously noted, music therapy interventions have the greatest effect when a trained music therapist uses live music in interactions with clients (Standley, 1986). In a holistic theory of music therapy, this makes sense. The experiences needed for music and soulmaking to be effective must be guided and facilitated over time. For music experiences to be therapy, the music therapist must understand the complexities of sound and music and be able to use those in a systematic yet holistic fashion over time. As Thomas Moore (1992) writes, general soulmaking can be done on our own. But soulmaking as a treatment or therapy needs the external intervention of a trained professional. Is music alone a powerful tool for therapy, or do the particular context and intention for its use matter? Based on complexity science, even the smallest elements matter in the overall outcome. The active participation of the music therapist with specialized training in music, scientific inquiry, and therapy methods and interventions is an essential element in the effectiveness of music therapy.

True therapy requires two dimensions—continuity of effort and interaction where process unfolds as ever-changing interrelationships. The trained music therapist provides both. The continuity comes from the goals and objectives set. The interaction derives first from the music itself and then from the music therapist and the client making music together. This process of ongoing relationship around and through music making allows music therapy to be an art.

> Therapy has often been described as an "art" which requires creativity on the part of both client and therapist, and active engagement of both parties in a creative process. This is particularly true when an art form such as music is used as the modality of therapy. (Bruscia, 1995, p. 196)

The music therapist creates the musical environment that meets the abilities and needs of the client and facilitates the interaction with the client. As the session progresses, creative response, engagement, and interaction with the client are ongoing (Aigen, 1995a).

The general *intention* of the music therapist for the client is an energy form that also impacts on the complex system and is a vital part of music and soul-making. Intention is a clear understanding of our purpose, a wish one means to carry. Intention is a planned choice that holds attention on a desired outcome (Laskow, 1999). For intention to have an effect as an energy form, the music therapist must first create a general mental state where his or her mind is quieted and a connection or coherence is established with the client (Hibbard, 1999). Kenny (1989) notes that the state of consciousness for the music therapist ". . . is a field of focused relaxation and intense concentration, yet playfulness" (p. 106). Once in this mental state, the music therapist needs to hold the intention that the music and the interaction around the music can make changes in the client, that it can provide the complex information necessary for the shift into health. The most effective intention is first to focus lovingly on the client and then add a directional intention, a specific outcome for the therapeutic intervention (Laskow, 1999). That directional intention can be based on the therapeutic goal established and can take the form of an image. When thought is added to imagery or imagery to thought, the impact of healing intention is doubled (Laskow, 1999).

Therapists should hold the best intention for the clients. The most effective and, perhaps, the ultimate intention is compassionate love. The ability to do healing is an expression of a deep inner desire by the therapist to help the other person. It is an intention of pure compassion, an expression of love at the highest level (Gerber, 1988). Love is deep interpersonal resonance. It is a universal pattern of resonant energy that can influence other energies to move toward wholeness and healing (Laskow, 1992). Love as a therapeutic intention is a skill that can be cultivated and developed by reducing barriers to love such as fear and anxiety, by cultivating an attitude of trust and empathy, by cultivating love directly through a practice like meditation, and by exploring all aspects of the human experience (Walsh, 2002). Music is a culturally acceptable embodiment and expression of universal love and compassion. It is itself love and compassion. Because of this, it may be easier for the music therapist to hold this intention of healing love. As a physical waveform, music can serve as a carrier wave for the therapist's intention to help and for the directional image of what is expected to happen.

Music Therapy and Health as an Emergent Property
The ultimate goal of soulmaking is a state of health—that state of right relationship of all aspects of human functioning, that energetic "dance of opposites." Soulmaking, then, is the process of bringing information, complexity, into the human system to create the emergent property of health. What single human experience brings more complexity into the human system than music? Music may add so much complex information to an ailing system (unhealthy body or unsettled mind) that it is pushed to the edge of chaos, the place of maximum creative potential and activity. Music is likely a strange attractor, creating health as a new organization emerging out of chaotic movement. Strange attractors emerge from the presence of multiple oscillating systems. Music certainly has such oscillating systems—in complex sound, in multiple frequencies, and in numerous sound sources. Music potentially affects human functioning on all levels of recursive organization. As one level is influenced, the effects can move up or down the levels of organization. Effects on the DNA level can impact the much higher level of consciousness, while changes of consciousness can impact the cellular level. Because human functioning is nonlinear, a small input to the system from music can have large consequences. Music as soulmaking is an intricate, ongoing nonlinear process where healthy patterns emerge out of webs of relationships. Schneck (1997) envisions this process from the engineering perspective of physiologic adaptation. In his model, he sees music as continuous disturbance that can move an individual to a new, more adaptive response—health.

Music therapy, like music itself, is more than the sum of its parts. We can gain some understanding, some reasons why and how music heals, but reducing this process to small, measurable effects does not explain what is actually happening. Just as our bodies and how they function are recursively organized layer within layer, so to are the reasons why music therapy works. It has impact from the simplest, basic levels to the overall complexity of effects built layer upon layer, recursively adding to the effect it has on human functioning. Music has effects on each layer. Each layer of effect, then, adds to the overall impact and is changed as the layers stack up. Because influence can come at any point in the recursive organization and because even a small influence can be compounded by iterative feedback, the impact of music therapy can be profound. We may be able to demonstrate that influence through analytical methods in complexity science, but we cannot "prove" it happens or how it happens. We can verify some of the layers through empirical research but not the complex overall effect of the music therapy interventions because of the nonlinear dynamic involved. The therapeutic effects of music therapy are a process of creative emergence, which cannot be reduced to component parts to re-create the emergent whole—health and healing benefits. We must look at the whole process in all its frustrating, beautiful complexity. "Perhaps the most significant factors of music therapy experience are embedded in the interconnecting webs of factors which we cannot directly observe much less quantify" (Kenny, 1998, p. 209).

We may never totally know how and why music therapy works because chaos theory implies there will always be missing information that, through feedback, may profoundly affect the outcome.

> Chaos theorists have been quick to point out that, both in principle and practice, there will always be missing information, a limitation to our knowledge, a hole in the data. Our data-gathering abilities can never be sufficiently extensive to know all there is to know about a complex system. . . . (Briggs & Peat, 1999, p. 170)

Based on the principles of complexity science, it is impossible to find any therapeutic intervention, including music therapy, that will affect every client in the same way consistently. This does not mean that the intervention is not effective, beneficial, or useful, only that our standard of "proof" is impossible and unrealistic based on the real, complex nature of the world.

A New View of Music Therapy Practice and Research

The theory of music and soulmaking will dramatically affect music therapy practice and research. Where does complexity science take us as it relates to music therapy? In this book, various forms of music therapy practice were introduced. How these are effective in treating many kinds of problems and disabilities was delineated. Current music therapy practice certainly considers total client functioning in formulating treatment objects. However, music therapists typically work within the principles and procedures of behavioral science. In this approach, the music therapist assesses specific, often isolated client needs and functioning. Based on this information, goals and objectives are set. A music therapy treatment intervention is then created to target those need areas (Hanser, 1987). For example, if I were working with a patient with dementia of the Alzheimer's type, I would assess his or her attention span, memory, verbal skills, and many other abilities affected by this disease. If I note poor attention to task, I would set the following treatment objective: "During singing activity, the client will sing one song verse to show increased attention." I would then plan my session, picking songs that would motivate this client to sing at least one verse. For an older person, such songs would be rhythmic, easy to sing, and already known to the client.

Though this reductionistic approach has its uses, the theory of music and soulmaking will require an approach based on a "science of wholeness." *Wholeness science* sees the world not as a machine but as a living, open-ended system where every part of our universe is connected to every other. Wholeness science does not assume objectivity. It acknowledges human consciousness, feelings, and attitudes as important factors. It accepts subjective reports and human intuition as valid forms of information gathering. In wholeness science, the interconnectedness of everything is assumed and the futility of identifying which causal factors create a certain effect is recognized. With this new belief, it will no longer be said that a certain chemotherapy regime will always cure stomach cancer or that New Age music is always relaxing for everyone. Cause can only be determined in a specific context for a specific, limited purpose.

> Let us imagine for a moment what science would look like if we start from the holistic assumption that everything—not only physical things but all things experienced, including sensations, emotions, feelings, motivations, thoughts—is really part of a single unity. If things are so interconnected that a change in any one could affect all, then it follows that any accounting for a cause is within a specific context, for a specific purpose. In the broadest sense, there is no cause and effect, only a whole system evolving. (Harman, 1994b, p. 377)

Wholeness science tells us we can no longer predict outcomes from reductive analysis because of the interconnectedness of everything. The complexity science paradigm gives us a scientific approach to wholeness.

Wholeness science is inclusive. It does not replace reductionistic science. It expands it. Empirical science is not a wrong answer. It is just incomplete (Pert, 1997). "But an even more complete approach is to also consider information from beyond the boundaries of present science, while accepting everything science tells us" (Brophy, 1999, p. 157). Willis Harman (1994a) postulates that wholeness science will not throw out or ignore the current scientific approach but, rather, becomes a model where the present scientific approach and newer scientific models like quantum theory and complexity science are particular aspects of knowledge acquisition. Wholeness science would also involve depth psychology, which includes representations of reality through metaphors, symbols, and images. It would embrace information from the intuitive, the aesthetic, and the imaginative (Tarnas, 1998). This mind-set concerning scientific inquiry ". . . proposes a restructuring of science in which nothing is lost, but many present [scientific] puzzles appear to be resolvable . . ." (Harman, 1994c, p. xxviii).

The insights gained from complexity science require this kind of shift. This model is the unification of empirical and descriptive science. "Descriptive science is as old as the human race" (Smith, 1989, p. 169). Future development of science will require a shift toward the "old way" of knowledge based on direct experience. This approach toward knowledge acquisition involves careful observation of data. The emphasis is on *what* is happening, not *how* or *why* it is happening. Descriptive science is not involved with establishing causes. It uses observed information gathered on what is working and what gives the results desired. Specific qualitative research methods provide this descriptive approach. Wholeness science unifies our modern science and all it has brought us with the descriptive approach of our ancestors. In this way, the approach of the scientist and the shaman meet to guide us through to a new paradigm.

Music Therapy Practice Based on Complexity Science
In a music therapy approach based on the principles of complexity science, the therapist will act as an agent or catalyst for change by adding aspects of complexity to the intervention. This will be accomplished by adding new and unexpected musical elements to break up rigid patterns of client behavior and routines by providing multiple options, flexibility of response, and immediate adaptability. As should always be the case in music therapy, the therapeutic process will be playful, exploratory, and spontaneous (Fink & Bettle, 1996). Music therapy interventions will intensify the moment and call attention to absurd or maladaptive client responses. Therapy will be based on mutual transactional patterns of responding with a back-and-forth quality. Certainly a number of music therapy activity interventions currently utilize such an approach, including improvisational music therapy methods. Increasingly, music therapists will recognize that the three-way interaction of

music, music therapist, and client has its own unique, emergent property. In this approach, the music therapist focuses on the immediate present and allows the structure to emerge rather than having the therapeutic approach structured in advance. "Instead of imposing a specific plan or system, chaotic therapists would try to react to what is happening with the client at the moment . . ." (Fink & Bettle, 1996, p. 126). Because a complex system is in constant movement, the shifts and unexpected changes occurring in the therapeutic dynamic will be better understood and accepted. Clients' reactions will be observed closely, with the music therapist responding musically. This will become a form of iterative feedback amplifying and enhancing the therapeutic effect.

A music therapist working from the perspective of complexity science will use a number of basic techniques and approaches. Such a music therapist will first use mindfulness—an openness to alternatives and a willingness to accept uncertainty (Langer, 1989). He or she will notice everything and see meaning in the seemingly meaningless as an acknowledgment of the vast connection of things. A music therapist using a complexity approach will do the "outrageous" and unexpected, emphasizing playfulness and creativity to add stimulus and complexity to the therapeutic process. For example, during improvisation sessions, I will often throw an instrument like a tambourine or play an instrument in an unusual way to prompt a reaction from the clients. Further, the music therapist will "go with the flow," using the naturally occurring events in the session as part of the process. He or she will vary responses musically and verbally to add information into the interaction. Further, the music therapist will act on the holistic tool of intuition without regard for the outcome.

Intuition is the immediate knowing or learning gained without evident input from the senses or rational thought (Borczon, 1997). Pressman (2002) defines intuition as ". . . the high mind which gives credit to and looks into the subtle, invisible realms" (p. 13). Intuition is an organ of perception that reaches beyond the five basic senses (Collinge, 1998). It is the key to making significant changes in complex systems (Briggs & Peat, 1999). A therapist's intuitive ability is the natural consequence of self-esteem and trust in his or her own abilities and belief in music therapy as a vehicle for change (Myss, 1996). Through intuition, music therapists will perceive all aspects of therapy as possibilities. By opening ourselves to all the physical and non-physical senses, a global impression of the client is received (Morris, 1993). Intuition will give a holistic awareness of the unfolding process of therapy. The therapy session will be guided by this deep inner sense of what is happening and how to proceed as the session unfolds (Fink & Bettle, 1996). As it should be, music therapy will then become a true creative process, a dance of interaction among therapist, client, and the music.

Music therapy practice in wholeness science will be less concerned with predicting the results of therapy and more involved with the process as it occurs.

> In music therapy, we can see this unity of means and ends when we adopt a dynamic conception of the purpose of clinical process. Client outcome is not a static state of being achieved at the end of therapy, but is instead something that unfolds within the clinical process itself. A deep level of involvement in music therapy process . . . is simultaneously the vehicle and goal of the process. (Aigen, 1995a, p. 239)

Music therapy will become less prescriptive in terms of results and more involved with the unfolding process of self-organization leading to change and improved health.

With an understanding of the complexity of this therapy, the music therapist will address client's functioning as wholeness. Client's overall functioning will be considered, not just the area of disability. The reductionistic goals will be part of the process but won't constitute the entire therapeutic effort. In this practice, the music therapist will consider all four aspects of client functioning when forming goals and interventions. The overriding goal will be soulmaking for all our clients. "If we are to even come close to true care for souls, we must try to at least *attend* the whole person even though our primary work will be with specific dimensions of that person's being" (May, 1982, p. 203). A number of music therapy theorists have already proposed this holistic approach to music therapy practice (Aigen, 1995c; Hesser, 1995; Kenny, 1985, 1989; Ruud, 1998b).

With increased understanding of music therapy's sensitivity to initial conditions and small changes, the importance of all the musical factors present in the music therapy session will be acknowledged. In nonlinear systems, small things can have big consequences. There are many "small things" in music. The music therapist's knowledge of the music used in sessions will be critically important. Effective therapy could depend on a repeated rhythm pattern, the melodic contour, or any other musical property. Intensive musical training and background will continue to be a critical factor in educating music therapists. A truly effective music therapist will need to be completely familiar with all aspects of the music.

More attention will be paid to the elements and qualities of the music used. The importance of certain intervals, melodic contours, and rhythm patterns will be considered as important elements of music therapy interventions. These are not always considered in current music therapy practice.

Other musical elements will also need to be considered, including timbre, dynamics, and duration of exposure to the music. Both quantitative and qualitative research needs to be done to provide information on these effects.

Within the new model, music therapists will emphasize live music making with the best-quality instruments for themselves and their clients. As noted earlier, an analysis of medical music therapy research concluded that a live performance by a trained music therapist created the greatest effect on whatever medical factor was tested (Standley, 1986). Clearly a live performance has different initial conditions than a recording. These could include a fuller spectrum of vibration, greater impact on body resonance, and changes in pitch and tone quality. With a live performance, specific intention for a healing effect can be set. As explored previously, this could be an immensely important component in therapy. Live music making also allows the music therapist to immediately respond to the energetic needs of the client. Daniélou (1995) gives an example of how live music playing creates a flexible space that can meet the energetic needs of the client. He notes that ". . . the twelve regions of the octave cannot be assimilated to twelve fixed sounds, as has been attempted in the tempered scale. They determine the space in which the notes move but can in no way be taken for the notes themselves . . ." (1995, p. 7). When playing live music on a variable-pitch instrument like voice or violin, the music therapist can adjust their tones within the space of a note to be responsive to client's energetic needs.

When using recordings, the methods and equipment for sound reproduction will need to provide a full spectrum of sound. Specific performances of recorded music will be considered when planning sessions. John Diamond (1981) has found that his measurement of music's impact on life force is altered with different performances of the same music. This is a factor that music therapists do not always consider, though Dr. Helen Bonny's (1978) work is a notable exception.

Music Therapy Research Based on Complexity Science

Music therapy research will also change. Under the new theory, music therapy research will ". . . seek understanding rather than singular, exclusive 'causes.' Its aim would be illumination more than the ability to predict and control" (Harman, 1994b, p. 377). Research will become more phenomenological, demonstrating relationships between factors (music as one factor and decreased agitation in Alzheimer's patients another) without being required to prove that one factor *caused* the other. Phenomenology involves the study of direct experience. It would strive ". . . not to explain the world as if from outside, but to give voice to the world from our experienced situation *within* it, recalling us to our participation in the here-and-now . . ." (Abram, 1996, p. 47). Since complexity science tells us it is impossible to predict and replicate a complex system, research methods to discover, clarify, and understand events will be used (Denney, 2002). In these methods, direct experience and involvement of the researcher are paramount (Kenny, 1989).

Music therapy research will emphasize practical rather than theoretical understanding of the processes involved. The call for empirical research that predicts the therapeutic benefits of music therapy interventions for a specific therapeutic context will prove to be extremely difficult if not impossible. Practical research or research applicable for implementation can be divided into four types: exploration (researching understudied areas), demonstration (exploring in greater depth the positive results from exploration research), analysis of factors (using statistical methods to identify factor causally related to outcomes), and application/implementation (involving effectiveness of an intervention [Green, 1997]).

Like all research in complexity science, music therapy research will be dependent on the context or existing conditions present. Strictly controlled empirical studies will have a place and will bring important information but will not be the only verification recognized. Emphasis will be placed on effectiveness research. This acknowledges the importance of the environment, client's mood, intention of the therapist, musical elements, and so on. These factors are the elements of context and are the very things traditional experimental design eliminates or controls. The current trend toward qualitative and phenomenological research in music therapy is an important step toward this more inclusive research agenda (Aigen, 1995c; Forinash, 1995; Kenny, 1989; Wheeler, 1995).

The wholeness model of music therapy will require the asking of new and different research questions. "Nature is much like a Zen master who waits until the student asks the right question; only then is the student ready to hear the answer. The question is the first step toward wisdom" (Shepherd, 1993, p. 63). To discover the great potential of music therapy, more "what" than "why" research questions will be asked: What happens when Alzheimer's patients participate in drumming? versus Why does it happen? There are a number of possible research questions in wholeness science. "Is there sustained agreement between expected or desirable results and actual result?" "Does music therapy work?" "Can we demonstrate that it works?" "What do we seeing happening?" "What does this result imply?" "What are the consequences of this idea?" "What would it mean to my beliefs about music therapy?" (Shepherd, 1993). Ultimately, since we are decreasing the importance of proof as a standard, an aesthetic judgment may be needed. Is the explanation beautiful? Is it pleasing? I first became interested in complexity science theory because I found it so deeply satisfying. To me, this model is beautiful in its ability to explain so much of the previously "unexplainable." This is certainly a different approach than trying to prove what is right and wrong. "We gain unbounded ability to ask the questions but must sacrifice our absolute confidence in our answers" (Levenson, 1994, p. 311).

In the new wholeness paradigm a cooperative, interdisciplinary research approach will be critical. The old assumption affirmed that the world was made of parts that could be studied independently. This fragmentary research must yield to broader questions because many areas of inquiry are too broad for a single branch of science (Scott, 1995). Surely, this is true when we study music as therapy. Music therapy knowledge will advance through interdisciplinary investigation with many possible research collaborators, including composers, music educators, acousticians, biomusicologists, and ethnomusicologists. We share a common interest in music but bring different perspectives on the subject. Research collaboration with physiologists, neurologists, biochemists, and osteopathic and allopathic physicians will bring new discoveries to medical music therapy. As wholeness in music is explored, exciting and groundbreaking research will result in collaboration with engineers, complexity scientists, physicists, and mathematicians.

New research approaches based on experimental research from complexity science will need to be developed for music therapy. Complexity science has its own body of research methods and tools for quantification of data distinct from the statistical analysis of empirical science. Both descriptive and inferential statistics of the empirical method rely on global trends involving many subjects. They deal with structural relations, not with the ability to analyze *processes*. Traditional statistics ". . . seem better suited to static situations and are only awkwardly applied to processes" (Combs & Winkler, 1995, p. 52).

The analytical tools of complexity science mathematically show what factors are compounding and creating a certain effect. They shift analysis toward nonlinear representation so that irregularities in "messy" systems are acknowledged and not ignored as "experimental errors." In the mathematical equations of complexity science, individual differences are regarded as essential to the complex processes being researched. There is a shift away from group-oriented procedures and to a new emphasis on individual differences. The mathematical formulas used in complexity science research represent events in a qualitative fashion. These forms of mathematical analysis do not allow for prediction but do show the overall shape of highly complex, temporal events, like music (Combs & Winkler, 1995).

Many of the mathematical methods of complexity science determine *fractal dimension estimates*. These estimates determine if a process is regulated by complex, nonlinear influences. A smooth, linear function like a sine wave would score low on a test for fractal dimensionality. This would indicate a lack of deterministic chaos. A nonlinear event like a volcano eruption would score high for fractal dimensionality (Brown & Combs, 1995).

A number of specific mathematical approaches exist to test for fractal dimensionality. For example, the Lyapunov exponent of dynamical systems ". . . measures the rate of divergence of points on arbitrarily close trajectories providing an estimate of the chaotic dependence on initial conditions" (Johnson & Dooley, 1996, p. 54). A positive Lyapunov exponent shows that a system does have sensitive dependence on initial conditions and is influenced by deterministic chaos (Goertzel, 1995). Boolean algebraic techniques are also used. They simultaneously consider the many variables typical of a complex, moving system. These methods provide an understanding of the stability, phase transitions, and possible evolution of complex systems. These calculations give rise to Karnough maps, a visual plotting of the evolution of the complex system (Lemay et al., 1996). Another modeling tool is kinetic logic. It shows distinct dynamical patterns and possible attractors in the dynamical system (Kupper & Hoffman, 1996). Computer programs for personal computers can provide these calculations (Sarraille & Di Falco, 1992; Schaffer, Truty, & Fulmer, 1988). Another measure of complexity is the Verhulst's nonlinear differential equation. It is an algebraic expansion that shows what factors are compounding and creating a certain effect (Blackerly, 1998).

Analytical tools from complexity science were developed to analyze long, continuous runs of stable measurements as occur in flow turbulence measurements and fractal projections. However, these mathematical tools for evaluating continuous data in dynamical systems are not entirely applicable for research on discontinuous and shorter-duration phenomena like psychological processes and music therapy interventions (Lemay et al., 1996). When the mathematical analysis of complex systems in physics is applied to psychology, social systems, or a therapy intervention, the phenomenon under study may not meet the exacting mathematical criteria or technical properties of dynamical systems (Goertzel, 1995). This occurs because living systems are, in fact, more complex than processes in physics. Each variable in a living system increases the number of points that have to be tracked. Also, the long, uninterrupted runs of stable measurements needed for analysis are not possible in living systems. Even with these limitations, the most important contribution of complexity science to the life sciences may not be in theory but in these research methodologies (Rapp, 1993).

Various researchers have successfully applied modified forms of complexity science analysis to biological and psychological processes. Scheier and Tschacher (1996) used a method of surrogate data and nonlinear forecasting to assess the presence of nonlinearity and determinism in psychological data. The method of surrogate data serves the purpose of seeing whether certain classes of models for data can be rejected. "This involves generating many surrogate data sets satisfying the null hypothesis, and computing a statistic (such as the forecast error) for each" (Scheier & Tschacher, 1996, p. 29). This rigorous quantitative method is good for distinguishing chaos from various random processes even in short and irregular data sets. Kupper and Hoffman (1996) used a Boolean modeling approach in determining the presence of attractors in the dynamics of psychosis. They specifically used kinetic logic, which is a descriptive technique on an intermediate level between a purely qualitative approach and a description using true nonlinear differential equations.

Combs and Winkler (1995) suggest that the best research on human processes might be to use both a chaotic systems analysis and empirical, statistical analysis on the same data or experiment. The two approaches would complement each other and give a truer picture of the phenomenon under study. Music therapy research will benefit greatly from this combined approach. For example, kinetic logic modeling tools can be used to show what does or does not create a new attractor, such as a new behavior or change in symptom. In music therapy research, this could be used to show if music therapy in general is having an impact or, even, if a certain element of the music used in a music therapy intervention is adding to the effect. This modeling could show whether music therapy is or is not a factor in the complex system. Empirical research methods are already widely applied to music therapy processes. By adding analytical approaches from complexity science, a truer picture of the impact of music therapy on human functioning may emerge.

Music therapy research in complexity science will require new directions and research tools. First, extended data collection must occur. Useful data for this kind of research will need to be collected over a period of six months to a year. The data must be analyzed so that an in-depth map of factors influencing the system can be made. The mapping will begin to reveal attractors that are occurring. Analysis of the data will allow for the recognition and labeling of bifurcation points and the possible influence of a music therapy intervention (Wheeler, 2003). As a construct of complexity science, it will be important to take an "I don't know" approach to determining what factors are actually affecting the complex process under investigation (Masterpasqua

& Perna, 1997). Research will have to acknowledge that there is always missing information when dealing with a complex system (Briggs & Peat, 1999).

An effective music therapy practitioner and researcher will need to use all aspects of knowledge acquisition: the objective, the subjective, and the collective wisdom from human culture (Wilber, 1996). An understanding of the complexity and wholeness of the processes involved in music therapy requires data from hard logic, phenomenology, and intuition. Investigation into music therapy will require

> . . . a balancing act that at once clings to the best that science has to offer while all the time holding a reverence for traditional wisdom, knowing that the truths of science change daily while traditional wisdom is so deeply steeped in metaphor that its foundations are often obscure. (Combs, 1995, p. 14)

The music therapist in this new model of wholeness science must be both a scientist with systematic approaches to knowledge acquisition and an artist who relies on intuition, creativity, and spirituality (Faiver et al., 2001).

Now that a new theory of music therapy is proposed, where does that take us? What does all this mean for our relationship with music? First, I hope that it will change our opinions about music. Music is usually seen only as entertainment, a pleasant diversion, while music making is only for a talented few and those who can afford lessons. Music education is considered a frill and easy to eliminate when budgets get tight. Music will be available to everyone in schools because we realize music is fundamental to mental, emotional, and spiritual growth. I hope this new model will help us realize that music is basic human behavior. It is an important tool for bettering our lives and our community. Music will again have a valued place in society. Music making will be for everyone. The "hows" and "whys" of using music will shift. Musicians, songwriters, and composers will see the function of their music differently. They will become more aware of the positive and negative impact music may have on their audiences and produce music accordingly. But most important, we will all use music more in our daily lives. Music will again become a tool for personal and societal well-being.

Music as a Path to Knowledge

> One day as the Buddha sat in meditation under the bodhi tree, a barge floated past on the nearby river. From the distance, he heard the sounds of the stringed lute, for the barge carried a music teacher and his pupil. As the Buddha sat in quiet contemplation, he overheard the teacher say, "Remember, a string too slack makes not a sound, a string too tight breaks, only a string stretched just right makes beautiful music."

"Ah," murmured the Buddha. "The middle way is the best way in all things—not too much, not too little." And from a simple act of teaching music came a great truth, a great knowing. (based on May, 1991)

Investigation into the complexity of music and its effects on human functioning will bring many changes to music therapy. There is a vast amount of general knowledge that can be discovered by first studying music itself as an energetic phenomenon and then studying the human response to this event. The interaction of these two immensely complex dynamical systems—music and human functioning—may indeed be a "map" to the discovery of new insights, truths, and even wisdom about how our world works. An example will illustrate this point. Most of our current knowledge of human brain functioning comes from vision research (Scott, 1995). What information about auditory processing we have comes primarily from animal research, especially bird studies (Wallin, 1991). What human auditory processing information we have is based on single and pure tone research. Imagine what we could learn about human brain functioning if we studied how our brains perceive a complex musical input like a simple song, a barbershop quartet, or an African drumming ensemble. Imagine how much more we would learn if we could understand the processing involved in playing that music. Current scientific neurology tells us that, based on their knowledge, what a piano player does (psychomotor coordination, perception, motor feedback, etc.) to play a simple two-handed piece of music is impossible (Wilson, 1986). This shows the limits of the current scientific investigation and illustrates how studying the human behavior of music can lead to new knowledge. This book has reviewed research that reveals a great deal about how the brain works. As Wallin, Merker, and Brown (2000) note, "It is time to take music seriously as an essential and abundant source of information about human nature, human evolution, and human cultural history" (p. 6).

The historical investigation of music and its place in human culture in chapter 1 showed how much of our knowledge began with or was inspired by studying music and, particularly, instrument construction. McClain (1976) cites mathematical evidence that the study of music, particularly tone, provided the sum of human knowledge in the ancient world—mathematics, science, large musical structures, and the myths of deities and creation itself. Knowledge was learned from and communicated through music. "Music was therefore justly considered by the ancients as the key to all sciences and arts—the link between metaphysics and physics through which the universal laws and their applications could be understood" (Daniélou, 1995, p. 1). Over the centuries, many scientific and technological discoveries were the result of musical investigation. Medieval man sought knowledge of universal laws through intense study of acoustics. Much of our modern technology came from the building and refining of musical instruments where sound production became the ultimate test of success. "Modern physics, economics, manufacturing systems, robotics, and computing would not be where they are today without mechanical and information processes originally tried and tested in musical applications" (Maconie, 1990, p. i). Even basic telecommunications owes a basic debt to musical acoustics.

> The principle of information transmission employing a modulated carrier frequency (telephone, morse code, radio, television, digital audio) can be traced back to musical precursors in monotone plainchant and the combination of melody and drone accompaniment, the static element (monotone pitch, drone) acting as the carrier, and the dynamic element (text, melody) the message. (Maconie, 1990, p. 171)

Studying the uniquely human behavior of music will push knowledge to a new level and bring us ". . . face to face with something that is buried at the foundations of human existence" (Briggs & Peat, 1989, p. 110). We have an abundance of facts, as a result of science and empirical research, about music's effects on people, about health and healing, about the nature of our universe. But true knowledge is not made up of isolated, unconnected facts; knowledge itself is part of a dynamic whole. This whole provides an awareness of the basic essence of all things. As the British composer Ralph Vaughn Williams stated, "Music will enable you to see past facts to the very essence of things in a way which science cannot do" (quoted in Diamond, 1981, p. 73). Throughout history, music has stood in for the universe as a whole. Pythagoras did it when he built a cosmos on the scaffolding of the scale (Levenson, 1994). Music is now ready to stand in for our new universe of complexity, especially as it relates to health. In this way, music and science are truly closely related. "It makes sense that music and science should resemble each other, for both tackle the same kind of task, resolving some image of human experience into an abstract form that can be communicated from one human being to another" (Levenson, 1994, p. 312). Philosopher Arthur Schopenhouer stated, "Assuming that an absolutely correct and complete explanation of music, accounting for all the details, were to be conceptualized . . . that would also be a satisfactory . . . explanation of the world—in other words, a true philosophy" (quoted in Berendt, 1988, p. 84). Music contains everything we need to know—complexity processing, reductionistic evidence, and all aspects of human functioning, including perception and cognition, emotions, motor functioning, and spirit.

> Music is so ubiquitous and so important that human culture just would not be human culture without it. . . . And so we have no choice but to listen to music; not simply to listen to music but to *listen* to music, to what it is telling us about ourselves. (Wallin, Merker, & Brown, 2000, p. 483)

Our expanded vision brings us to this new philosophy of our universe—music becomes the answer, not just a cause of one effect or another.

Complexity science is pushing our understanding of what is possible. In fact, the point of people immersing themselves in complexity is to liberate their vision and expand knowledge into wisdom (Briggs & Peat, 1989). Wisdom is the knowledge of what is true, coupled with just judgment as to action. It is deep understanding and practical skills relating to the fundamental issues of life (Walsh, 2002). It is an ". . . ineffable knowing born of direct experience, a kind of *intuitive pragmatism* that works to the extent it takes account of the whole. It is inclusive and integrative and involves empathy and compassion" (deQuincey, 2000, p. 10). The study of music and its impact on human functioning will lead the way into this new wisdom by plunging us into its complexity, thus expanding our vision of what is possible. Wisdom is contained in the vibration, in the complexity (Rael, 1993). The word *wise* used as a verb means "to show the way to, to direct the course." Directing our course into wisdom, providing us with a means to move to the next level of knowledge just as it did in Pythagoras's time, may be music's ultimate purpose. We have wondered for centuries, "Why have music at all?" It has no survival benefit we can determine, no evolutionary advantage. Yet every human culture has had music. Why? Perhaps it truly is a gift programmed into our brain and central nervous system that set us on the road to knowledge. And if music is about multiple levels of deep relationship, of experience in all aspects of human functioning, of the fundamental way the world works, then, perhaps, we are hearing the mind of God when we listen to an Indian raga or a Brahms symphony. Music is the implicate order of the universe made manifest. It can now be our vehicle to true wisdom. Music is every aspect of human endeavor. It is cognitive perception and deep emotional expression, social conflict resolution and underlying principles of culture, and emergent entity and human internal imagination. It is, indeed, the map to knowledge of our world and ourselves. The tool we need to learn about ourselves and our world has been in our hands all along. We play it every day.

Bibliography

Abaronov, Y., & Vardi, M. (1980). Meaning of an individual "Feynaman path." *Physical Review Digest, 21* (8), 2235–2240.

Abraham, N. G., Albano, A. M., Passamante, E. A., Rapp, P. E., & Gilmore, R. (1993). *Complexity and chaos*, vol. 2. Singapore: World Science.

Abraham, R. (1994). *Chaos, Gaia, eros.* San Francisco: HarperSanFrancisco.

Abram, D. (1996). *The spell of the sensuous.* New York: Vintage Books.

Abrams, R. L., & Lind, R. C. (1978). Degenerate four-wave mixing in absorbing media. *Optical Letters, 2,* 94.

Abramson, H. (Ed.). (1967). *The use of LSD in psychotherapy and alcoholism.* New York: Bobbs-Merrill.

Achterberg, J. (1985). *Imagery in healing.* Boston: Shambhala.

Achterberg, J., Kenner, C., & Lawlis, G. F. (1982, March). Biofeedback, imagery, and relaxation: Pain and stress interventions for severely burned patients. Paper presented at the Bio-feedback Society of America, Chicago.

Adams, D. (1987). *Dirk Gently's holistic detective agency.* New York: Pocket Books.

Ader, R., & Cohen, N. (1975). Behaviorally conditioned immunosupression. *Psychosomatic Medicine, 37,* 333–340.

Ader, R., Felter, D. L., & Cohen, N. (Eds.). (1990). *Psychoneuroimmunology,* 2d ed. San Diego: Academic Press.

Adey, W. R. (1981). Tissue interactions with non-ionizing electromagnetic fields. *Physiological Review, 61,* 435.

Adey, W. R., & Lawrence, A. F. (1984). *Nonlinear electrodynamics in biological systems.* New York: Plenum Press.

Aharonov, Y., & Vardi, M. (1980). Meaning of an individual "Feynman path." *Physical Review Digest, 21* (8), 2235–2240.

Aigen, K. (1995a). Aesthetic foundation of clinical theory. In C. Kenny (Ed.), *Listening, playing, creating: Essays on the power of sound* (pp. 233–257). Albany: State University of New York Press.

Aigen, K. (1995b). Cognitive and affective processes in music therapy with individuals with developmental delays: A preliminary model for contemporary Nordoff-Robbins practice. *Music Therapy, 13* (1), 13–46.

Aigen, K. (1995c). Principles of qualitative research. In B. L. Wheeler (Ed.), *Music therapy research* (pp. 283–312). Phoenixville, PA: Barcelona Publishers.

Aihara, K., Matsumoto, G., & Ikegaya, Y. (1984). Periodic and non-periodic responses of a periodically forced Hodgkin-Huxley oscillator. *Journal of Theoretical Biology, 109* (2), 249–269.

Ainslie, P. (1995). Chaos, psychology, and spirituality. In R. Robertson & A. Combs (Eds.), *Chaos theory in psychology and the life sciences* (pp. 309–317). Mahwah, NJ: Laurence Erlbaum Associates, Inc.

Akanatsu, K., Alforink, C., Koebel, C., Luce, D., Milgrin-Luterman, J., & Thompson, A. R. (2000). *The current status of medical music therapy.* Unpublished MS, Michigan State University.

Albanese, C. L. (1992). *America: Religions and religion.* Belmont, CA: Wadsworth.

Alcoholics Anonymous. (1976). *The big book,* 3d ed. New York: Alcoholics Anonymous World Services, Inc.

Aldridge, D. (1995). Spirituality, hope and music therapy in palliative care. *The Arts in Psychotherapy, 22* (2), 103–109.

Aldridge, D. (1996). *Music therapy research and practice in medicine.* London: Jessica Kingsley Publishers, Ltd.

Aldridge, D. (1998). Life as jazz: Hope, meaning and music therapy in the treatment of life-threatening illness. *Advances in Mind–Body Medicine, 14,* 271–282.

Alexander, D. M., & Globus, G. G. (1996). Edge-of-chaos dynamics in recursively organized neural systems. In E. MacCormac & M. I. Stamenov (Eds.), *Fractals of brain, fractals of mind* (pp. 32–73). Philadelphia: John Benjamins North America.

Alkon, D. (1992). *Memory's voice.* New York: HarperCollins.

Allen, M., Cleary, S. F., & Hawkridge, F. M. (1992). *Charge and field effects in biosystems,* vols. 1–3. Boston: Birkhäusen.

Almaas, A. A. (1986a). *Essence: The Diamond approach to inner realization.* York Beach, ME: Samuel Weiser.

Almaas, A. A. (1986b). *The void: A psychodynamic investigation of the relationship between mind and space.* Berkeley, CA: Diamond Books.

Almaas, A. A. (1987). *Diamond hearts, bk. 1: Elements of the real man.* Berkeley, CA: Diamond Books.

Almaas, A. A. (1988a). *Diamond book 2: The freedom to be.* Berkeley, CA: Diamond Books.

Almaas, A. A. (1988b). *The pearl beyond price: Integration of personality into being: An object relations approach.* Berkeley, CA: Diamond Books.

Almaas, A. A. (1996). *The point of existence: Transformations of narcissism.* Berkeley, CA: Diamond Books.

Alperson, P. (1994). *What is music? An introduction to the philosophy of music*. University Park: State University of Pennsylvania Press.

Altschuler, I. M. (1954). The past, present, and future of music therapy. In E. Podolsky (Ed.), *Music therapy* (pp. 24–36). New York: Philosophical Library.

Alvin, J. (1975). *Music therapy*. London: Hutchinson.

Alvin, J. (1978). *Music therapy for the autistic child*. New York: Oxford University Press.

Amir, D. (1995). Music therapy. In C. Kenny (Ed.), *Listening, playing, creating: Essays on the power of sound* (pp. 51–57). Albany: State University of New York Press.

Amir, D. S. (1996). Music therapy—holistic model. *Music Therapy, 14* (1), 44–60.

Amunts, K., Schlaug, G., Jaenche, L., Steinmetz, H., Schleicher, A., & Zilles, K. (1996). Hand motor skills covary with size of motor cortex: A macrostructural adaptation? *NeuroImage, 3,* 5365.

Anderson, C. M., & Mandell, A. J. (1996). Fractal time and the foundations of consciousness. In E. MacCormac & M. I. Stamenov (Eds.), *Fractals of brain, fractals of mind* (pp. 76–126). Philadelphia: John Benjamins North America.

Anderson, J. A. (1995). *An introduction to neural networks*. Cambridge, MA: MIT Press.

Anderson, P. W. (1972). More is different: Broken symmetry and the nature of the hierarchical structure of science. *Science, 177,* 393–396.

Andress, B. (1980). *Music experiences in early childhood*. New York: Holt, Rinehart & Winston.

Andrews, T. (1993). *Sacred sounds*. St. Paul, MN: Llewellyn Publications.

Ansdell, G. (1990). Limitations and potential—A report on a music therapy group for clients referred from a counseling service. *Journal of British Music Therapy, 4* (1).

Ansdell, G. (1995). *Music for life: Aspects of creative music therapy with adult clients*. London: Jessica Kingsley Publishers, Ltd.

Anshel, A., & Kipper, D. A. (1988). The influence of group singing on trust and cooperation. *Journal of Music Therapy, 25* (3), 145–155.

Apel, W. (1969). *Harvard dictionary of music*, 2d ed. Cambridge, MA: Belknap Press.

Arezzo, J. (1997, November). The influence of music on neurological function. Paper presented at the National Association for Music Therapy Annual Conference, Los Angeles.

Aristotle. (1936). *On the soul, parva naturalia, on breath*. W. S. Hett (Trans.). Cambridge, MA: Harvard University Press.

Aristotle. (1958). *Politics*. E. Barker (Trans.). London: Oxford University Press.

Armstrong, T. (1993). *Seven kinds of smart*. New York: Penguin Group.

Arnheim, R. (1969). *Visual thinking*. Berkeley: University of California Press.

Arnold, M. (1975). Music therapy in a transactional analysis setting. *Journal of Music Therapy, 12* (3), 104–120.

Artress, L. (1995). *Walking a sacred path*. New York: Riverhead Books.

Ashbrook, J. (1993). *Brain, culture, and the human spirit: Essays from an emergent evolutionary perspective*. Lanham, MD: University Press of America.

Assagioli, R. (1965). *Psychosynthesis: A collection of basic writings*. New York: Viking.

Assagioli, R. (1991). *Transpersonal development: The dimension beyond psychosynthesis.* London: Crucible.

Aston, J. A., Harkness, E., & Ernst, E. (2000, June). The efficacy of "distant healing": A systematic review of randomized trials. *Annals of Internal Medicine*, 903–910.

Auer, D., Jones, R., Rupprecht, R., & Kraft, E. (1996). Does motor skill influence the cortical activation pattern in musicians: An FMRI study. *NeuroImage, 3*, 537.

Augustin, P., & Hains, A. A. (1996). Effect of music on ambulatory surgery patients preoperative anxiety. *AORN Journal, 63* (4), 750, 753–758.

Austin, D. S. (1996). The role of improvised music in psychodynamic music therapy with adults. *Music Therapy, 14* (1), 29–43.

Ax, A. F. (1957). Physiological differentiation between fear and anger in humans. *Psychosomatic Medicine, 15*, 433–442.

Ayres, A. J. (1979). *Sensory integration and the child.* Los Angeles: Western Psychological Services.

Baars, B. J. (1997). *In the theater of consciousness.* New York: Oxford University Press.

Babloyantz, A. (1989). Estimation of correlation dimensions from single and multi-channel recordings. In E. Basar & T. H. Bullock (Eds.), *Brain dynamics* (pp. 122–130). Berlin: Springer-Verlag.

Backus, J. (1969). *The acoustical foundations of music*, 2d ed. New York: Norton.

Bak, P., & Chen, K. (1991). Self-organized criticality. *Scientific American, 264* (1), 46–52.

Baker, F. A. (2000). Modifying the Melodic Intonation Therapy program for adults with severe non-fluent aphasia. *Music Therapy Perspectives, 18*, 110–114.

Baker, L. W. (1991). The use of music and relaxation techniques to reduce pain of burn patients during daily debridement. In C. Maranto (Ed.), *Applications of music in medicine* (pp. 85–121). Washington, DC: National Association for Music Therapy.

Baron, A., & Cerella, J. (1993). Laboratory tests of the disuse account of cognitive decline. In J. Cerella, J. Rybach, W. Hoyer, & M. L. Commons (Eds.), *Adult information processing: Limits on loss* (pp. 176–203). New York: Academic Press.

Barrie, J. M., Freeman, W. J., & Lenhart, M. D. (1996). Spatiotemporal analysis of prepyriform, visual, auditory and somesthetic surface EEGs in trained rabbits. *Journal of Neurophysiology, 76*, 520–539.

Barry, D. T. (1991). Muscle sounds from evoked twitches in the hand. *Archives of Physical Medical Rehabilitation, 72*, 573.

Bartlett, D., Kaufman, D., & Smeltekop, R. (1993). The effects of music listening and perceived sensory experiences on the immune system as measured by Interlaukin-1 and cortisol. *Journal of Music Therapy, 30* (4), 194–209.

Basar, E. (1989). Chaotic dynamics and resonance phenomena in brain function: Progress, perspectives and thoughts. In E. Basar & T. H. Bullock (Eds.), *Brain dynamics* (pp. 1–30). Berlin: Springer-Verlag.

Basar, E., & Bullock, T. H. (Eds.). (1989). *Brain dynamics.* Berlin: Springer-Verlag.

Basti, G., & Perrone, A. (1989). On the cognitive function of deterministic chaos in neural networks. In *International Joint Conference on Neural Networks*, vol. 1 (pp. 657–663). San Diego: IEEE.

Bateson, G. (1972). *Steps to an ecology of mind*. New York: Ballantine Books.

Bateson, G. (1979). *Mind and nature*. New York: E. P. Dutton.

Bateson, G., & Bateson, M. C. (1988). *Angels fear: Towards an epistemology of the sacred*. New York: Bantam Books.

Beaulieu, J. (1987). *Music and sound in the healing arts*. Barrytown, NY: Station Hill Press.

Beck, A. J. (1976). *Cognitive therapy and the emotional disorders*. New York: Meridan.

Becker, R. O., & Marino, A. A. (1982). *Electromagnetism and life*. Albany: State University of New York Press.

Becker, R. O., & Selden, G. (1985). *The body electric*. New York: William Morrow & Co.

Beebe, B., Gerstonan, L., Carson, B., Dolins, M., Zigman, A., Rosensweig, H., Faughey, K., & Korman, M. (1982). Rhythmic communication in the mother–infant dyad. In M. Davis (Ed.), *Interaction rhythms* (pp. 79–100). New York: Human Sciences Press.

Beebe, B., Jaffe, J., Feldstein, S., Mays, K., & Alson, D. (1985). Interpersonal timing: The application of an adult dialogue model to mother–infant vocal and kinetic interactions. In T. F. Field & N. Fox (Eds.), *Social perception in infants* (pp. 217–247). Norwood, NJ: Ablex.

Beebe, B., Lachman, F., & Jaffe, J. (1997). Mother–infant interaction structures and presymbolic self and object representations. *Psychoanalytic Dialogues*, 7, 133–182.

Bellamy, T., & Sontag, E. (1973). Use of contingent music to increase assembly line production rates of retarded students in a simulated sheltered workshop. *Journal of Music Therapy*, 10 (4), 125–136.

Benor, D. J. (1990). Survey of spiritual healing research. *Complimentary Medical Research*, 4 (1), 9–33.

Benor, D. J. (1992). *Healing research: Holistic energy medicine and spirituality*, vol. 2. London: Helix Editions, Ltd.

Benson, H. (1975). *The relaxation response*. New York: William Morrow.

Benson, H. (1996). *Timeless healing: The power and biology of belief*. New York: Scribner.

Bentov, I. (1976). Micromotion of the body as a factor in the development of the nervous system. In L. Sammella (Ed.), *Kundalini: Psychosis or transcendence?* San Francisco: H. S. Dakin Co.

Benward, B., & White, G. (1997). *Music in theory and practice*, vol. 1. Madison, WI: Brown & Benchmark.

Benzon, W. (2001). *Beethoven's anvil: Music in mind and culture*. New York: Basic Books.

Berendt, J. E. (1983). *Nada Brahma: The world is sound*. Rochester, VT: Destiny Books.

Berendt, J. E. (1988). *The third ear*. Longmead, England: Element Books, Ltd.

Berger, D. (2002). *Music therapy, sensory integration and the autistic child*. London: Jessica Kingsley Publishers Ltd.

Bergin, A. E. (1983). Religiosity and mental health: A critical reevaluation and meta-analysis. *Professional Psychology: Research and Practice*, 14, 170–184.

Bergstrom, M. (1967). An analysis of the information-carrying system of the brain. *Synthesis, 17*, 425.

Berlyne, D. E. (1971). *Aesthetics and psychobiology.* New York: Appleton-Century-Croft.

Berne, E. (1961). *Transactional analysis in psychotherapy.* New York: Grove Press.

Bernieri, F., & Rosenthal, R. (1991). Interpersonal coordination, behavior matching, and interpersonal synchrony. In R. Feldman & B. Rime (Eds.), *Fundamentals of nonverbal behavior* (pp. 401–432). Cambridge, MA: Cambridge University Press.

Bianchi, E. (1985). *Aging as a spiritual journey.* New York: Crossroads.

Bitcon, C. (1976). *Alike and different: Clinical and educational uses of Orff-Schulwerk.* Santa Ana, CA: Rosha Press.

Bittman, B. (2000, November). Music therapy and psychoneuroimmunology: Integrative medicine for the mind, body, and spirit. Paper presented at the American Music Therapy Association Annual Conference, St. Louis, MO.

Bittman, B., Berk, L. S., Felten, D., Westengard, J., Simonton, O. C., Pappas, J., & Ninehouser, M. (2001). Composite effects of group drumming music therapy on modulation of neuroendocrine-immune parameters in normal subjects. *Alternative Therapies in Health and Medicine, 7* (1), 38–47.

Black, S. (1997, January). The musical mind. *The American School Board Journal*, 20–22.

Blackerly, R. (1998). *Application of chaos theory to psychology models.* Austin, TX: Performance Strategies Publications.

Blackeslee, T. R. (1980). *The right brain.* New York: Anchor/Doubleday.

Blacking, J. (1973). *How musical is man?* Seattle: University of Washington Press.

Blum, T. (Ed.). (1993). *Prenatal perception, learning and bonding.* Seattle: Leonardo.

Boettcher, W. S., Hahn, S. S., & Shaw, G. L. (1994). Mathematics and music: A search for insight into higher brain function. *Leonardo Music Journal, 4*, 53–58.

Bohm, D. (1980). *Wholeness and the implicate order.* London: ARK Paperbacks.

Boller, F., & Grafman, J. (Eds.). (1988). *Handbook of neuropsychology*, vol. 8. New York: Elsevier.

Bonny, H. (1978). *The role of taped music programs in the GIM process.* Baltimore: ICM Books.

Bonny, H. (1988). Forward. In L. Summer, *Imagery and music in the institutional setting* (p. ix). St. Louis, MO: MMB Music, Inc.

Bonny, H. (2001). Music and spirituality. *Music Therapy Perspectives, 19* (1), 59–62.

Bonny, H. L., & Savary, L. M. (1990). *Music and your mind*, 2d ed. Barrytown, NY: Station Hill Press.

Booth, L. (1995). A new understanding of spirituality. In R. J. Kus (Ed.), *Spirituality and chemical dependency* (pp. 9–17). New York: Haworth.

Borchgrevink, H. M. (1982). Prosody and musical rhythm are controlled by the speech hemisphere. In M. Clynes (Ed.), *Music, mind, and brain* (pp. 151–170). New York: Plenum Press.

Borczon, R. (1997). *Music therapy: Group vignettes.* Gilsum, NH: Barcelona Press.

Bordier, N. (2001). The power of personal stories. *Noetic Sciences Review, 56,* 21–23.

Borling, J., & Scartelli, J. (1987). The effects of sequenced versus simultaneous EMG biofeedback and sedative music on frontalis relaxation training. *Journal of Music Therapy, 23* (3), 157–165.

Borling, J. E. (1981). The effects of sedative music on alpha rhythms and focused attention in high-creative and low-creative subjects. *Journal of Music Therapy, 18* (2), 101–108.

Borysenko, J. (1998). The science of bodymind and spirit. *Bridges, 9* (3), 1, 4–7, 16.

Bower, T. G. R. (1977). *Primer of infant development.* San Francisco: Freeman.

Bowers, J. (1998). Effects of an intergenerational choir for community-based seniors and college students on age-related attitudes. *Journal of Music Therapy, 35* (1), 2–18.

Boxberger, R. (1962). Historical basis for the use of music in therapy. In E. H. Schneider (Ed.), *Music therapy 1961* (pp. 125–166). Lawrence, KS: Allen Press.

Boxberger, R. (1963). History of NAMT, Inc. In E. H. Schneider (Ed.), *Music therapy 1962* (pp. 133–197). Lawrence, KS: National Association for Music Therapy.

Boxill, E. (1985). *Music therapy for developmentally disabled.* Austin, TX: Pro-ed.

Boyle, M. E. (1989). Comatose and head injured patients: Applications for music in treatment. In M. H. M. Lee (Ed.), *Rehabilitation, music and human well-being* (pp. 137–148). St. Louis, MO: MMB Music, Inc.

Bregman, A. S. (1990). *Auditory scene analysis: The perceptual organization of sound.* Cambridge, MA: A Bradford Book.

Brewer, C., & Campbell, D. (1990). *Rhythms of learning.* Tucson: Zephyr Press.

Briggs, J., & Peat, F. D. (1989). *Turbulent mirror.* New York: Harper & Row.

Briggs, J., & Peat, F. D. (1999). *Seven life lessons of chaos: Spiritual wisdom from the science of change.* New York: HarperCollins Publishers.

Bright, R. (1972). *Music in geriatric care.* New York: St. Martin's Press.

Broderson, A. (Ed.). (n.d.). *Alfred Schutz: Collected papers II. Studies in social theory.* The Hague.

Brophy, T. M. (1999). *The mechanism demands a mysticism: An exploration of spirit, matter and physics.* Blue Hill, ME: Medicine Bear Publishing.

Broucek, M. (1987). Beyond healing to "whole-ing": A voice for the deinstitutionalization of music therapy. *Music Therapy, 6* (2), 50–58.

Brown, S. (2000). The "musilanguage" model of music evolution. In N. L Wallin, B. Merker, & S. Brown (Eds.), *The origins of music* (pp. 271–300). Cambridge, MA: MIT Press.

Brown, S., Merker, B., & Wallin, N. L. (2000). An introduction to evolutionary musicology. In N. L Wallin, B. Merker, & S. Brown (Eds.), *The origins of music* (pp. 3–24). Cambridge, MA: MIT Press.

Brown, T. L., & Combs, A. (1995). Constraint, complexity, and chaos: A methodological follow-up on the nostril cycle. In R. Robertson & A. Combs (Eds.), *Chaos theory in psychology and the life sciences* (pp. 61–64). Mahwah, NJ: Lawrence Erlbaum Associates, Inc.

Bruga, M. A., & Severtsen, B. (1984). Evaluating the effects of music on electro-encephalogram patterns of normal subjects. *Journal of Neurosurgical Nursing, 16* (2), 96–100.

Bruhn, K., Cohen, D., Fletcher, R., McKinney, C., Smith, D. S., & Tims, F. C. (1996, November). Music making and wellness: Strategic alliances between music therapy and the music product industry. Paper presented at the 1996 Joint Conference of NAMT & AAMT, Nashville.

Bruscia, K. E. (1987). *Improvisational models of music therapy.* Springfield, MO: Charles C. Thomas.

Bruscia, K. E. (1991a). Embracing life with AIDS: Psychotherapy through Guided Imagery and Music (GIM). In K. E. Bruscia (Ed.), *Case studies in music therapy* (pp. 581–602). Phoenixville, PA: Barcelona Publishers.

Bruscia, K. E. (1992). Visits from the other side: Healing persons with AIDS through Guided Imagery and Music. In D. Campbell (Ed.), *Music and miracles* (pp. 195–207). Wheaton, IL: Theosophical Publishing House.

Bruscia, K. E. (1995). Modes of consciousness. In C. Kenny (Ed.), *Listening, playing, creating: Essays on the power of sound* (pp. 165–196). Albany: State University of New York Press.

Bruscia, K. E. (1998a). *Defining music therapy,* 2d ed. Gilsum, NH: Barcelona Publishers.

Bruscia, K. E. (1998b). An introduction to music psychotherapy. In K. Bruscia (Ed.), *The dynamics of music psychotherapy* (pp. 1–15). Gilsum, NH: Barcelona Publishers.

Bruscia, K. E. (1998c). The many dimensions of transference. In K. Bruscia (Ed.), *The dynamics of music psychotherapy* (pp. 17–33). Gilsum, NH: Barcelona Publishers.

Bruscia, K. E. (1998d). Preface. In K. Bruscia (Ed.), *The dynamics of music psychotherapy* (pp. xxi–xiv). Gilsum, NH: Barcelona Publishers.

Bruscia, K. E. (1998e). The signs of countertrransference. In K. Bruscia (Ed.), *The dynamics of music psychotherapy* (pp. 71–91). Gilsum, NH: Barcelona Publishers.

Bruscia, K. E. (1998f). Understanding countertransference. In K. Bruscia (Ed.), *The dynamics of music psychotherapy* (pp. 51–70). Gilsum, NH: Barcelona Publishers.

Bruscia, K. E. (Ed.). (1991b). *Case studies in music therapy.* Phoenixville, PA: Barcelona Publishers.

Bruscia, K. E. (Ed.). (1998g). *The dynamics of music psychotherapy.* Gilsum, NH: Barcelona Publishers.

Bryant, D. R. (1987). A cognitive approach to therapy through music. *Journal of Music Therapy, 24* (1), 27–34.

Bullard, B. (1993). Language learning and superlearning. In R. Russell (Ed.), *Using the whole brain* (pp. 123–126). Norfolk, VA: Hampton Roads Publishing Co.

Bullowa, M. (1979). *Before speech.* Cambridge, MA: Cambridge University Press.

Bunt, L. (1994). *Music therapy: An art beyond words.* New York: Routledge.

Burford, B. (1988). Action cycles: Rhythmic actions for engagement with children and young adults with profound mental handicap. *European Journal of Special Needs Education, 3,* 189–208.

Burke, J., & Ornstein, R. (1995). *The axemaker's gift*. New York: G. P. Putnam's Sons.

Burr, H. S. (1944). The meaning of bioelectric potentials. *Yale Journal of Biological Medicine*, 16, 353.

Burr, H. S. (1972). *Blueprint for immortality: The electric patterns of life*. Essex, England: Neville Spearman Publishers.

Burrows, D. (1995). Sound and meaning. In C. Kenny (Ed.), *Listening, playing, creating: Essays on the power of sound* (pp. 119–128). Albany: State University of New York Press.

Bush, C. A. (1995). *Healing imagery and music*. Portland, OR: Rudra Press.

Butz, M. R. (1993). Practical application from chaos theory to the psychotherapeutic process, a basic consideration of dynamics. *Psychological Reports*, 73, 543–554.

Buzsaki, G., Llinas, R., Singer, W., Bertoz, A., & Christen, Y. (Eds.). (1994). *Temporal coding in the brain*. Berlin: Springer-Verlag.

Byerly, C. L. (1967). A school curriculum for prevention and remediation of deviancy. In D. Schrieber (Ed.), *Profile of the school dropout* (pp. 275–312). New York: Vintage Books.

Byrd, R. C. (1988). Positive therapeutic effects of intercessory prayer in a coronary care unit population. *Southern Medical Journal*, 81 (7), 826–829.

Cahill, L., Prins, B., Weber, M., & McGaugh, J. L. (1994). Beta-adrenegic activation and memory for emotional events. *Nature*, 371, 702–704.

Caine, J. (1991). The effects of music on the selected stress behaviors, weight, caloric and formula intake, and length of hospital stay of premature and low birth weight neonates in a newborn intensive care unit. *Journal of Music Therapy*, 28 (4), 180–192.

Callanan, M., & Kelley, P. (1992). *Final gifts: Understanding the special awareness, needs, and communication of the dying*. New York: Bantam Books.

Campbell, D. (1983). *Introduction to the musical brain*. St. Louis, MO: Magnamusic-Baton, Inc.

Campbell, D. (1990). *Healing yourself with your own voice* (cassette recording). Boulder: True Recordings.

Campbell, D. (1991a). *Curative aspects of tone and breath*. Boulder: Institute for Music, Health, and Education.

Campbell, D. (1997). *The Mozart effect*. New York: Avon Books.

Campbell, D. (2000). *The Mozart effect for children*. New York: HarperCollins Publishers.

Campbell, D. (Ed.). (1991b). *Music physician for times to come*. Wheaton, IL: Quest Books.

Campbell, D. (Ed.). (1992). *Music and miracles*. Wheaton, IL: Quest Books.

Campbell, D. K. (1996). Coherent structures amidst chaos: Solitons, fronts, and vortices. In D. E. Herbert (Ed.), *Chaos and the changing nature of science and medicine: An introduction* (pp. 115–131). Woodbury, NY: American Institute of Physics.

Campbell, J. (1968). *The hero with a thousand faces*, 2d ed. Princeton, NJ: Princeton University Press.

Canadian Association for Music Therapy. (n.d.). About music therapy (pamphlet). Canadian Association for Music Therapy.

Cannon, W. B. (1932). *The wisdom of the body*. New York: W. W. Norton & Co.

Capra, F. (1975). *The Tao of physics*. Toronto: Bantam Books.

Capra, F. (1983). *The turning point*. London: Fontana.

Carlson, N. P. (1992). *Foundations of physiological psychology*. Boston: Allyn & Bacon.

Carrington, P. (1987). Managing meditation in clinical practice. In M. West (Ed.), *The psychology of meditation*. Oxford: Clarendon Press.

Carroccio, D. F., & Carroccio, B. B. (1972). Toward a technology of music therapy. *Journal of Music Therapy, 9* (2), 51–55.

Carstens, C., Huskins, E., & Hounshell, G. (1995). Listening to Mozart may not enhance performance on the Revised Minnesota Paper Form Board Test. *Psychological Reports, 77* (1), 111–114.

Carterette, E. C., & Kendall, R. A. (1995). Convergent research methods in music cognition. In R. Steinberg (Ed.), *Music and the mind machine: The psychophysiology and psychopathology of the sense of music* (pp. 3–18). Berlin: Springer-Verlag.

Cartwright, J., & Huckaby, G. (1972). Intensive preschool language program. *Journal of Music Therapy, 9* (4), 137–146.

Cassette, M. D. (1976). The influence of a music therapy activity upon peer acceptance, group cohesiveness, and interpersonal relationships of adult psychiatric patients. *Journal of Music Therapy, 13* (2), 66–76.

Cassity, M. D. (1981). The influence of a socially valued skill on peer acceptance in music therapy group. *Journal of Music Therapy, 18* (3), 148–154.

Castro-Caldas, A., Petersson, K. M., Reis, A., Stone-Elander, S., & Ingovor, M. (1998). Learning to read and write during childhood influences the functional organization of the adult brain. *Brain, 121*, 1053–1063.

Ceci, S. J., & Liker, J. K. (1986). A day at the races: A study of IQ, expertise and cognitive complexity. *Journal of Experimental Psychology, 115*, 255–266.

Cerella, J., Ryback, J., Hoyer, W., & Commons, M. L. (Eds.). (1993). *Adult information processing: Limits on loss*. New York: Academic Press.

Cervantes, J. M., & Ramirez, O. (1992). Spirituality and family dynamics in psychotherapy with Latino children. In A. Vargas & J. D. Koss-Chioino (Eds.), *Working with culture: Psychotherapeutic interventions with ethnic minority children and adolescents* (pp. 103–128). San Francisco: Jossey-Bass.

Chalmers, D. J. (1996). *The conscious mind*. New York: Oxford University Press.

Chan, A., Ho, Y-C., & Cheung, M-C. (1998). Music training improves verbal memory. *Nature, 396* (6707), 128.

Chandler, E. (1999). Spirituality. *Physical, Psychosocial and Pastoral Care of the Dying, 14* (3–4), 63–74.

Chen, W., Kato, T., Zhu, X-H., Adrian, G., & Ugurbil, K. (1996). Functional mapping of human brain during music imagery processing. *NeuroImage, 3*, 5205.

Childre, D. L. (1991). *Heart zones*. Boulder Creek, CA: Planetary Publications.

Childre, D. L. (1994). *Freeze frame: Fast action stress relief.* Boulder Creek, CA: Planetary Publications.

Childs, C. (1997). Deep seeing. *Noetic Sciences Review, 44,* 18–24.

Chomsky, N. (1966). *Cartesian linguistics.* New York: Harper & Row.

Chomsky, N. (1968). *Death and modern man.* New York: Harcourt Brace & World.

Chomsky, N. (1980). *Rules and representation.* New York: Columbia University Press.

Chopra, D. (1990). *Perfect health.* New York: Harmony Books.

Christie-Murray, D. (1988). *Reincarnation: Ancient beliefs and modern evidence.* Garden City, NY: Avery.

Churchland, P., & Sejenowski, T. J. (1998). *The computational brain.* Cambridge, MA: MIT Press.

Claeys, M. S., Miller, A. C., Dalloul-Rampersad, R., & Kollar, M. (1989). The role of music and music therapy in the rehabilitation of traumatically brain injured clients. *Music Therapy Perspectives, 6,* 71–77.

Clair, A. A. (1996). *Therapeutic uses of music with older adults.* Baltimore: Health Professions Press.

Clair, A. A., & Bernstein, B. (1990a). A comparison of singing, vibrotactile and non-vibrotactile instrumental playing responses in severely regressed persons with dementia of the Alzheimer's type. *Journal of Music Therapy, 27* (3), 119–125.

Clair, A. A., & Bernstein, B. (1990b). A preliminary study of music therapy programming for severely regressed persons with Alzheimer's type dementia. *Journal of Applied Gerontology, 9,* 299–311.

Clair, A. A., Bernstein, B., & Johnson, G. (1995). Rhythm characteristics in persons diagnosed with dementia, including those with probable Alzheimer's type. *Journal of Music Therapy, 32,* 113–131.

Clark, M., McCorkle, R., & Williams, S. (1981). Music therapy–assisted labor and delivery. *Journal of Music Therapy, 18* (2), 88–100.

Clark, M. S. (1998–1999). The Bonny method of Guided Imagery and Music and spiritual development. *Journal of the Association for Music and Imagery, 6,* 55–62.

Clendon-Wallen, J. (1991). The use of music therapy to influence the self-confidence of adolescents who are sexually abused. *Music Therapy Perspectives, 9,* 73–81.

Clynes, M. (1977). *Sentics: The touch of emotions.* Garden City, NY: Anchor Books, Doubleday.

Clynes, M. (Ed.). (1982). *Music, mind, and brain: The neuropsychology of music.* New York: Plenum Press.

Clynes, M., & Nettheim, N. (1982). The living quality of music. In M. Clynes (Ed.), *Music, mind, and brain: The neuropsychology of music* (pp. 47–81). New York: Plenum Press.

Clynes, M., & Walker, J. (1982). Neurobiologic functions of rhythm, time, and pulse. In M. Clynes (Ed.), *Music, mind, and brain* (pp. 171–216). New York: Plenum Press.

Coffman, D. D., & Adamek, M. S. (1999). The contributions of wind band participation to quality of life of senior adults. *Music Therapy Perspectives, 17* (1), 27–31.

Cofrancesco, E. M. (1985). The effect of music therapy on hand grasp strength and functional task performance in stroke patients. *Journal of Music Therapy, 22* (3), 129–145.

Cohen, H., Rossignol, S., & Grillner, S. (1988). *Neural control of rhythmic movements in vertebrates.* New York: Wiley.

Cohen, N. S. (1992). The effect of singing instruction on the speech production of neurologically impaired persons. *Journal of Music Therapy, 29* (2), 87–102.

Cohen, N. S. (1993). The application of singing and rhythmic instruction as a therapeutic intervention for persons with neurogenic communication disorders. *Journal of Music Therapy, 30* (2), 81–99.

Cohen, N. S. (1995). The effect of musical cues on the nonpurposive speech of persons with aphasia. *Journal of Music Therapy, 32* (1), 46–57.

Cohn, R. (1974). Theme centered model. In J. B. P. Shaffer & M. D. Galinsky (Eds.), *Group therapy and sensitivity training* (pp. 242–264). Englewood Cliffs, NJ: Prentice-Hall.

Collinge, W. (1998). *Subtle energy.* New York: Warner Books, Inc.

Colwell, C. M. (1994). Therapeutic applications of music in the whole language kindergarten. *Journal of Music Therapy, 31* (4), 238–247.

Combs, A. (1995). *The radiance of being: Complexity, chaos and the evolution of consciousness.* St. Paul, MN: Paragon House.

Combs, A., & Winkler, M. (1995). The nostril cycle: A study in the methodology of chaos science. In R. Robertson & A. Combs (Eds.), *Chaos theory in psychology and the life sciences* (pp. 51–60). Mahwah, NJ: Lawrence Erlbaum Associates, Inc.

Commons, M. L., Armon, C., Kohlberg, L., Richards, F. A., Grotzer, T. A., & Sinnott, J. D. (Eds.). (1990). *Adult development, vol. 2: Models and methods in the study of adolescent and adult thought.* New York: Praeger.

Commons, M. L., Richard, F. A., & Arnon, C. (Eds.). (1984). *Beyond formal operations: Late adolescent and adult cognitive development.* New York: Praeger.

Cook, C. M., & Persinger, M. (1997). Experimental induction of "sense presence" in normal subjects and an exceptional subject. *Perceptual Motor Skills, 85,* 683.

Cook, J. E. (1991). Correlated activity in the CNS: A role on every timescale? *Trends in Neuroscience, 14* (9), 347–401.

Cook, M., & Freethy, M. (1973). Use of music as a positive reinforcer to eliminate complaining behavior. *Journal of Music Therapy, 10* (4), 213–216.

Cook, N. (1990). *Music, imagination, and culture.* New York: Oxford University Press.

Cook, P. M. (1997). *Shaman, jhankri and nele: Music healers of indigenous cultures.* Roslyn, NY: Ellipsis Arts.

Cook, P. R. (Ed.). (1999). *Music, cognition, and computerized sound.* Cambridge, MA: MIT Press.

Cook-Greuter, S. R. (1990). Maps for living: Ego-development stages from symbiosis to conscious universal embeddedness. In M. L. Commons, C. Armon, L. Kohlberg, F. A. Richards, T. A. Grotzer, & J. D. Sinnott (Eds.), *Adult development, vol. 2: Models and methods in the study of adolescent and adult thought* (pp. 79–104). New York: Praeger.

Copland, A. (1952). *Music and imagination*. Cambridge, MA: Harvard University Press.

Cordobes, T. K. (1997). Group songwriting as a method for developing group cohesion for HIV-seropositive adult patients with depression. *Journal of Music Therapy, 34* (1), 46–67.

Corrick, J. A. (1983). *The human brain: Mind and matter*. New York: Arco Publishing, Inc.

Cousineau, P. (Ed.). (1994). *Soul*. San Francisco: HarperSanFrancisco.

Cowan, D. S. (1991). Music therapy in the surgical arena. *Music Therapy Perspectives, 9*, 42–45.

Cowan, J. C. (1991, June 22). The projection and reception of electroholomorphic fields by the brain: A proposed mechanism. Presentation at International Society for the Study of Subtle Energies and Energy Medicine Conference, Boulder.

Cowan, T. (1996). *Shamanism as a spiritual practice for daily life*. Freedom, CA: Crossing Press.

Crandall, J. (1995). Floors of music. In C. Kenny (Ed.), *Listening, playing, creating: Essays on the power of sound* (pp. 77 80). Albany: State University of New York Press.

Critchley, M. (1977). Experiences during musical perception. In M. Critchley & R. A. Henson (Eds.), *Music and the brain* (pp. 217–232). London: William Heinemann Medical Books Ltd.

Critchley, M., & Henson, R. A. (Eds.). (1977). *Music and the brain: Studies in the neurology of music*. Springfield, IL: Charles C. Thomas Publishers.

Crowe, B. J. (1987). Stimulating creativity in the mentally retarded through music experiences. *The Arts in Psychotherapy, 14*, 237–241.

Crowe, B. J. (1991a). Music: The ultimate physician. In D. Campbell (Ed.), *Music physician for times to come* (pp. 111 120). Wheaton, IL: Quest Books.

Crowe, B. J. (1991b). Testimony. *U.S. Special Committee on Aging Hearing testimony: Forever young: Music and aging*. Washington, DC: U.S. Government Printing Office.

Crowe, B. J. (1992). The profession of music therapy in the United States. *Open Ear* (Spring), 2–5. Bainbridge, WA: Open Ear Center.

Crowe, B. J., & Scovel, M. (1996). An overview of sound healing practices: Implications for the profession of music therapy. *Music Therapy Perspectives, 14* (1), 21–29.

Csikszentmihalyi, M. (1993). *The evolving self: A psychology for the third millenium*. New York: HarperCollins.

Cuthbert, B., Kristeller, J. L., Simons, R., & Lang, P. J. (1981). Strategies of arousal control: Biofeedback, meditation, and motivation. *Journal of Experimental Psychology: General, 110*, 518–546.

Cutietta, R., Hamann, D., & Walker, L. M. (1995). *Spin-offs: The extra musical advantages of a musical education*. United Musical Instruments USA, Inc.

Dacher, E. (1997). Healing: What matters in healthcare. *Noetic Sciences Review, 42*, 49–51.

Damasio, A. R. (1989). The brain binds entities and events in multiregional activation from convergence zones. *Neural Computation, 1,* 123–132.

Damasio, A. R. (1994). *Descartes' error: Emotion, reason, and the human brain.* New York: G. P. Putnam's Sons.

Damasio, A. R. (1999). *The feeling of what happens: Body and emotion in the making of consciousness.* New York: Harcourt Brace & Co.

Damasio, A. R., & Damasio, H. (1977). Musical faculty and cerebral dominance. In M. Critchley (Ed.), *Music and the brain* (pp. 141–155). London: William Heinemann Medical Books Ltd.

Daniélou, A. (1995). *Music and the power of sound: The influence of tuning and interval on consciousness.* Rochester, VT: Inner Traditions.

Darrow, A-A. (1984). A comparison of rhythmic responsiveness in normal and hearing impaired children and an investigation of the relationship of rhythmic responsiveness to the suprasegmental aspects of speech perception. *Journal of Music Therapy, 21* (2), 48–66.

Darrow, A-A., & Goll, H. (1989). The effect of vibrotactile stimuli via the Somatron on the identification of rhythmic concepts by hearing impaired children. *Journal of Music Therapy, 26* (3), 115–124.

Darwin, C. (1871). *The descent of man and selection in relation to sex.* London: Murray.

Davidson, J. (1976). The physiology of meditation and mystical states of consciousness. *Perspectives in Biology and Medicine* (Spring), 345–379.

Davidson, J., & Davidson, R. (1980). *The psychobiology of consciousness.* New York: Plenum Press.

Davis, J. (1999). *The Diamond approach: An introduction to the teachings of A. A. Almaas.* Boston: Shambhala.

Davis, M. (Ed.). (1982). *Interaction rhythms.* New York: Human Sciences Press.

Denney, M. (2002). Walking the quantum talk. *Noetic Sciences Review, 60,* 19–23.

deQuincey, C. (1998). Engaging presence. *Noetic Sciences Review, 45,* 24–27.

deQuincey, C. (2000). Consciousness: Truth or wisdom? *Noetic Sciences Review, 51,* 10–13, 44–46.

deQuincey, C. (2002). *Radical nature: Rediscovering the soul of matter.* Montpelier, VT: Invisible Cities Press.

Deutsch, D. (Ed.). (1982). *Psychology of music.* Orlando: Academic Press.

Dewey, J. (1934). *Art as experience.* New York: Minton, Balch, & Co.

Dewey, J. (1958). *Experience and nature.* New York: Dover.

Dewey, J. (1963). *Experience and education.* New York: Collier Books.

Diamond, J. (1981). *The life energies in music,* vol. 1. New York: Archaeus Press.

Diamond, J. (1983). *The life energies in music,* vol. 2. Valley Cottage, NY: Archaeus Press.

Diamond, J. (1985). *Life energy.* New York: Paragon House.

Dilts, R., & McDonald, R. (1997). *Tools of the spirit.* Capitola, CA: Meta Publications.

Dissanayake, E. (2000). Antecedents of the temporal arts in early mother–infant interaction. In N. L Wallin, B. Merker, & S. Brown (Eds.), *The origins of music* (pp. 389–440). Cambridge, MA: MIT Press.

Ditto, W. L. (1996). Applications of chaos in biology and medicine. In D. E. Herbert (Ed.), *Chaos and the changing nature of science and medicine: An introduction* (pp. 175–200). Woodbury, NY: American Institute of Physics.

Doka, K. J. (1993). The spiritual needs of the dying. In K. J. Doka & J. D. Morgan (Eds.), *Death and spirituality* (pp. 143–150). Amityville, NY: Baywood.

Doka, K. J., & Morgan, J. D. (Eds.). (1993). *Death and spirituality*. Amityville, NY: Baywood.

Doore, G. (Ed.). (1988). *Shaman's path: Healing, personal growth, and empowerment.* Boston: Shambhala Publications Inc.

Dorrow, L. G. (1976). Televised music lessons as educational reinforcement for correct mathematical responses with the educably mentally retarded. *Journal of Music Therapy, 23* (2), 77–86.

Dossey, L. (1989). *Recovering the soul.* New York: Bantam Books.

Dossey, L. (1992). Modern medicine and the relationship between mind and matter. In B. Rubik (Ed.), *The interrelationship between mind and matter* (pp. 149–168). Philadelphia: Center for Frontier Sciences.

Dostalek, C., Faber, J., Krasa, H., Roldam, F., & Vele, F. (1979). Meditational yoga exercises in EEG and EMG. *Ceskoslovenska Psychologies, 23,* 61–65.

Douglas, D. (1985). *Accent on rhythm.* St. Louis, MO: MMB Music.

Drake, C. (1993). Reproduction of musical rhythms by children, adult musicians and adult nonmusicians. *Perceptual Psychophysiology, 53* (1), 25–33.

Dvorkin, J. M. (1998). Transference and countertransference in group improvisation therapy. In K. Bruscia (Ed.), *The dynamics of music psychotherapy* (pp. 287–298). Gilsum, NH: Barcelona Publishers.

Eagle, C. T., Jr. (1991). Steps to a theory of quantum therapy. *Music Therapy Perspectives, 9,* 56–60.

Eagle, C. T., Jr. (1996). An introductory perspective on music psychology. In D. A. Hodges (Ed.), *Handbook of music psychology,* 2d ed. (pp. 1–28). San Antonio, TX: Institute for Music Research Press.

Eccles, J. C. (1989). *Evolution of the brain: Creation of the self.* New York: Routledge.

Eckman, J. P., & Ruelle, D. (1992). Fundamental limitations for estimating dimensions and Lyapunov exponents in dynamical systems. *Physica, 560,* 185–187.

Edelman, G. M. (1987). *Neural Darwinism: The theory of neuronal group selection.* New York: Basic Books.

Edelman, G. M. (1989). *The remembered past.* New York: Basic Books, Inc.

Edelman, G. M. (1992). *Bright air, brilliant fire: On the matter of the mind.* New York: Basic Books.

Edelman, G. M., & Mountcastle, V. B. (1978). *The mindful brain.* Cambridge, MA: MIT Press.

Edgerton, C. L. (1994). The effect of improvisational music therapy on the communicative behaviors of autistic children. *Journal of Music Therapy, 31* (1), 31–62.

Edie, J. M. (1973). Introduction. In M. Merleau-Ponty, *Consciousness and the acquisition of language* (pp. xi–xxxii). Evanston, IL: Northwestern University Press.

Edwards, E. (1981). *Music education for the deaf*. Waterford, ME: Merriam Eddy Co.

Ehrlich, D. (1997). *Inside the music*. Boston: Shambhala.

Eidson, C. E., Jr. (1989). The effect of behavioral music therapy on the generalizations of interpersonal skills form sessions to the classroom by emotionally handicapped middle school students. *Journal of Music Therapy, 26* (4), 206–221.

Eisenstein, S. R. (1974). The effect of contingent guitar lessons on reading behavior. *Journal of Music Therapy, 11* (3), 138–146.

Ekman, P. (1992). An argument for the basic emotions. *Cognition and Emotion, 6,* 175.

Eliade, M. (1964). *Shamanism: Archaic techniques of ecstasy*. Princeton, NJ: Princeton University Press.

Elliott, C. A. (1986). Rhythmic phenomena—Why the fascination? In J. R. Evans & M. Clynes (Eds.), *Rhythm in psychological, linguistic and musical processes* (pp. 2–12). Springfield, IL: Charles C. Thomas.

Ellis, A. (1975). *Reason and emotion in psychotherapy*. Secaucus, NJ: L. Stuart..

Ellis, A., & Grieger, R. (1977). *Handbook of rational emotive therapy*. New York: Human Sciences.

Engler, J. (1986). Therapeutic aims in psychotherapy and meditation: Developmental stages in the representation of self. In K. Wilbur, J. Engler, & D. P. Brown (Eds.), *Transformations of consciousness* (pp. 17–51). Boston: Shambhala.

Erickson, E. (1959). *Identity and the life cycle*. New York: International University Press.

Erickson, E. (1963). *Childhood and society,* 2d ed. New York: W. W. Norton & Co.

Erickson, E., Erickson, J., & Kivnick, H. (1986). *Vital involvement in old age*. New York: W. W. Norton & Co.

Estes, C. P. (1992). *Women who run with the wolves*. New York: Ballantine Books.

Evans, J. R., & Clynes, M. (Eds.). (1986). *Rhythm in psychological, linguistic and musical processes*. Springfield, IL: Charles C. Thomas.

Eyster, J. M., & Prokofsky, E. W. (1977). Soft modes and structure of the DNA double helix. *Physical Review of Letters, 38* (7), 371–373.

Fadiman, J. (1980). The transpersonal stance. In R. N. Walsh & F. Vaughan (Eds.), *Beyond ego: Transpersonal dimensions in psychology* (pp. 175–181). Los Angeles: Jeremy P. Tarcher.

Fahrion, S. L., Wirkus, M., & Pooley, P. (1992). EEG amplitude, brain mapping, and synchrony in and between a bioenergy practitioner and client during healing. *Subtle Energies, 3* (1), 19–32.

Faiver, C., Ingersoll, R. E., O'Brien, E., & McNally, C. (2001). *Explorations in counseling and spirituality*. Belmont, CA: Wadsworth/Thomson Learning.

Falk, D. (2000). Hominid brain evolution and the origins of music. In N. L Wallin, B. Merker, & S. Brown (Eds.), *The origins of music* (pp. 197–216). Cambridge, MA: MIT Press.

Farnsworth, P. (1981). *The social psychology of music*. Ames: Iowa State University Press.

Fawzy, F. I., Fawzy, N. W, & Hyun, C. S. (1993). Malignant melanoma: Effects of an early structured psychiatric intervention, coping, and affective state on the recurrence and survival six years later. *Archives of General Psychiatry, 50,* 681–689.

Feder, S., Karmel, R. L., & Pollock, G. H. (Eds.). (1993). *Psychoanalytic explorations in music*. Madison, WI: International Universities.

Feigenbaum, M. (1993). The transition to chaos. In J. Holt (Ed.), *Chaos: The new science* (pp. 45–54). Lanham, MD: University Press of America, Inc.

Feld, S. (1994). Left-up-over-sounding. In C. Keil & S. Feld (Eds.), *Music grooves* (pp. 109–156). Chicago: University of Chicago Press.

Feld, S., & Fox, A. A. (1994). Music and language. *Annual Review of Anthropology*, 23, 25–53.

Feldman, R., & Rime, B. (Eds.). (1991). *Fundamentals of nonverbal behavior*. Cambridge, MA: Cambridge University Press.

Felton, D. L., Felton, S. Y., & Carlson, S. L. (1985). Noradrenergic synaptic enervation of lymphoid tissue. *Journal of Immunology*, 135 (2), 755–763.

Fernandez, M. (1997). Acoustics and universal movement. In T. Wigram & C. Dileo (Eds.), *Music vibration* (pp. 27–35). Cherry Hill, NJ: Jeffrey Books.

Feynman, R., Leighton, R. B., & Sands, M. (1963). *The Feynman lectures on physics*. Reading, MA: Addison-Wesley Publishing Co.

Ficken, T. (1976). The use of songwriting in a psychiatric setting. *Journal of Music Therapy*, 13 (4), 163–172.

Field, T. F., & Fox, N. (Eds.). (1985). *Social perception in infants*. Norwood, NJ: Ablex.

Fifer, W. P., & Moon, C. M. (1994). The role of mother's voice in the organization of brain functions in the newborn. *Acta Paediatrica*, 83, 86–93.

Fingarette, H. (1963). *The self in transformation: Psychoanalysis, philosophy, and the life of the spirit*. New York: Harper & Row.

Fink, R. A., & Bettle, J. (1996). *Chaotic cognition: Principles and applications*. Mahwah, NJ: Lawrence Erlbaum Associates.

Fiske, H. E. (1993). *Music cognition and aesthetic attitudes*. Lewiston, ID: Edwin Mellen Press.

Fitzpatrick, J., & Whall, A. L. (1989). *Conceptual models of nursing*, 2d ed. Norwalk, CT: Appleton & Lange.

Flatischler, R. (1992a). *The forgotten power of rhythm*. Mendocino, CA: LifeRhythm.

Flatischler, R. (1992b). The influence of musical rhythmicity in internal rhythmical events. In R. Spintge & R. Droh (Eds.), *Music medicine* (pp. 241–248). St. Louis, MO: MMB Music, Inc.

Forinash, M. (1995). Phenomenological research. In B. L. Wheeler (Ed.), *Music therapy research* (pp. 367–388). Phoenixville, PA: Barcelona Publishers.

Forward, W., & Wolpert, A. (Eds.). (1993). *Chaos, rhythm and flow in nature*. Edinburgh: Floris Books.

Fox, M. (1981). *Whee, we wee all the way home: A guide to sensual, prophetic spirituality*. Santa Fe: Bear & Co.

Fox, M. (1995, April). Keynote address. Paper presented at the Awakening the Spirit Conference, New York.

Fraisse, P. (1982). Rhythm and tempo. In D. Deutsch (Ed.), *The psychology of music* (pp. 149–180). Orlando: Academic Press.

Frame, M. W. (2003). *Integrating religion and spirituality into counseling*. Pacific Grove, CA: Brooks/Cole-Thomson Learning.

Frame, M. W., & Williams, C. B. (1996). Counseling African Americans: Integrating spirituality in therapy. *Counseling and Values, 41*, 16–28.

Franklin, P. (1985). *The idea of music: Schoenberg and others*. London: Macmillan.

Frayer, D. W., & Nicolay, C. (2000). Fossil evidence of the origin of speech sounds. In N. L Wallin, B. Merker, & S. Brown (Eds.), *The origins of music* (pp. 217–234). Cambridge, MA: MIT Press

Freeman, A. (2001a). God as an emergent property. In A. Freeman (Ed.), *The emergence of consciousness* (pp. 147–159). Thorventon, England: Imprint Academic.

Freeman, A. (Ed.). (2001b). *The emergence of consciousness*. Thorventon, England: Imprint Academic.

Freeman, W. (1992). Tutorial on neurobiology: From single neurons to brain chaos. *International Journal of Bifurcation and Chaos, 2* (3), 451–482.

Freeman, W. (1998). The neurobiology of multimodal sensory integration. *Integrative Physiological and Behavioral Science, 33*, 12–17.

Freeman, W. (2000). A neurobiological role of music in social bonding. In N. L Wallin, B. Merker, & S. Brown (Eds.), *The origins of music* (pp. 411–424). Cambridge, MA: MIT Press.

Freeman, W. J., & Barrie, J. M. (1994). Chaotic oscillations and the genesis of meaning in the cerebral cortex. In G. Buzsaki, R. Llinas, W. Singer, A. Bertoz, & Y. Christen (Eds.), *Temporal coding in the brain* (pp. 13–37). Berlin: Springer-Verlag.

Freud, S. (1920). *A general introduction to psychoanalysis*. New York: Square Press.

Fried, R. (1990). Integrating music in breathing training and relaxation: I & II. *Biofeedback and Self-Regulation, 15* (2), 161–178.

Friedlander, L. H. (1994). Group music psychotherapy in an inpatient psychiatric setting for children: A developmental approach. *Music Therapy Perspectives, 12* (2), 92–97.

Frohlich, H. (1977). Coherent excitation in biological systems. *Biophysics, 22*, 743–744.

Frohlich, H. (1986). Coherent excitation in active biological systems. In F. Gatmann & H. Keyzer (Eds.), *Modern biochemistry*. New York: Plenum Press.

Fry, D. (1971). *Some effects of music*. Monograph Series No. 9. Tunbridge Wells, England: Institute for Cultural Research.

Fuhada, E., & Inoue, S. (1985). *Bioelectrical repair and growth*. Lancaster, England: MPP Press, Ltd.

Fukuyama, M. A., & Sevig, T. D. (1999). *Integrating spirituality into multicultural counseling*. London: Sage.

Furman, C. E. (Ed.). (1988). *Effectiveness of music therapy procedures: Documentation of research and clinical practice*. Washington, DC: National Association for Music Therapy.

Furman, C. E. (Ed.). (2000). *Effectiveness of music therapy procedures: Documentation of research and clinical practice*. Silver Spring, MD: American Music Therapy Association.

Gabrielsson, A. (1995). Expressive intention and performance. In R. Steinberg (Ed.), *Music and the mind machine: The psychophysiology and psychopathology of the sense of music* (pp. 35–47). Berlin: Springer-Verlag.

Gagnon, T. A., & Rein, G. (1990). The biological significance of water structured with non-Hertzian time reversed waves. *Journal of US Psychotronics Association, 4*, 26.

Gallo, F. P. (1999). *Energy psychology: Explorations at the interface of energy, cognition, behavior, and health.* Boca Raton, FL: CRC Press LLC.

Galloway, H., & Kraus, T. (1982). Melodic Intonation Therapy with language delayed apraxic children. *Journal of Music Therapy, 19* (2), 102–113.

Gardner, H. (1983). *Frames of mind: The theory of multiple intelligences.* New York: Basic Books.

Gartner, J., Larson, D. B., & Allen, G. D. (1991). Religious commitment and mental health: A review of empirical literature. *Journal of Psychology and Theology, 19*, 6–25.

Garwood, E. C. (1988). The effects of contingent music in combination with a bell pad on enuresis of a mentally retarded adult. *Journal of Music Therapy, 25* (2), 103–109.

Gaston, E. T. (1968a). Man and music. In E. T. Gaston (Ed.), *Music in therapy* (pp. 7–29). New York: Macmillan.

Gaston, E. T. (Ed.). (1968b). *Music in therapy.* New York: Macmillan.

Gatmann, F., & Keyzer, H. (Eds.). (1986). *Modern biochemistry.* New York: Plenum Press.

Geissmann, T. (2000). Gibbon songs and human music. In N. L Wallin, B. Merker, & S. Brown (Eds.), *The origins of music* (pp. 103–123). Cambridge, MA: MIT Press.

George, L. K., Larson, D. B., Koenig, H. G., & McCullough, M. E. (2000). Spirituality and health: What we know, what we need to know. *Journal of Social and Clinical Psychology, 19* (1), 102–116.

Gerber, R. (1988). *Vibrational medicine.* Santa Fe: Bear & Co.

Geringer, J. M., & Breen, T. (1975). The role of dynamics in musical expression. *Journal of Music Therapy, 12* (1), 19–29.

Geschwind, N. (1965). Disconnection syndrome in animals and man. *Brain, 88:* 237–94, 585–644.

Gfeller, K. (1983). Musical mnemonics as an aid to retention with normal and learning disabled students. *Journal of Music Therapy, 20* (4), 179–189.

Gfeller, K. (1988). Musical components and styles preferred by young adults for aerobic fitness activity. *Journal of Music Therapy, 25* (1), 28–43.

Gfeller, K. (1990a). The function of aesthetic stimuli in the therapeutic process. In R. Unkefer (Ed.), *Music therapy in the treatment of adults with mental disorders* (pp. 70–81). New York: Schirmer Books.

Gfeller, K. (1990b). Music as communication. In R. Unkefer (Ed.), *Music therapy in the treatment of adults with mental disorders* (pp. 50–62). New York: Schirmer Books.

Gfeller, K., & Hanson, N. (Eds.). (1995). *Music therapy programming for individuals with Alzheimer's disease and related disorders.* Washington, DC: Department of Health and Human Services.

Gibson, J. (1966). *The senses considered as perceptual systems*. Boston: Houghton Mifflin.

Gignoux, J. H. (2002). Going deeper. *Noetic Sciences Review, 61*, 27–29.

Gilbert, J. P. (1977). Music therapy perspectives on death and dying. *Journal of Music Therapy, 14* (4), 165–171.

Gilchrist, M. (1972). *The psychology of creativity*. London: Melbourne University Press.

Gillespie, B. (1999a). Haptics. In P. R. Cook (Ed.), *Music, cognition, and computerized sound* (pp. 229–245). Cambridge, MA: MIT Press.

Gillespie, B. (1999b). Haptics in manipulation. In P. R. Cook (Ed.), *Music, cognition, and computerized sound* (pp. 247–260). Cambridge, MA: MIT Press.

Gilmor, T. M., Madaule, P., & Thompson, B. (Eds.) (1989). *About the Tomatis method*. Toronto: Listening Centre Press.

Gleick, J. (1987). *Chaos*. New York: Penguin Books.

Gleick, J. (1993). Chaos and beyond. In J. Holte (Ed.), *Chaos: The new science* (pp. 119–127). Lanham, MD: University Press of America, Inc.

Globus, G. G. (1992). Towards a noncomputational cognitive neuroscience. *Journal of Cognitive Neuroscience, 4* (4), 299–310.

Godwin, J. (Ed.). (1987). *Music, mysticism and magic*. New York: Arkana.

Godwin, J. (Ed.). (1989). *Cosmic music*. Rochester, VT: Inner Traditions International.

Godwin, J. (Ed.). (1993). *The harmony of the spheres: A sourcebook of the Pythagorean tradition in music*. Rochester, VT: Inner Traditions International.

Goertzel, B. (1994). *Chaotic logic: Language, mind and reality from the perspective of complex systems science*. New York: Plenum.

Goertzel, B. (1995). A cognitive law of motion. In R. Robertson & A. Combs (Eds.), *Chaos theory in psychology and the life sciences* (pp. 135–153). Mahwah, NJ: Lawrence Erlbaum Associates, Inc.

Goldberger, A. L., Bhargava, V., West, B. J., & Mandell, A. (1985). On a mechanism of cardiac electrical stability: The fractal hypothesis. *Biophysics Journal, 48*, 525–528.

Goldberger, A. L., Kobalter, K., & Bhargava, V. (1986). 1/f-like scaling in normal neutrophil dynamics: Implications for hematologic monitoring. *IEEE Transactions Biomedical Engineering, 33*, 874–876.

Goldberger, A. L., & West, B. J. (1987). Fractals in physiology and medicine. *Yale Journal of Biological Medicine, 60*, 421–435.

Goldberger, A. L., West, B. J., & Rigney, D. R. (1990). Chaos and fractals in human physiology. *Scientific American, 262*, 42–29.

Goldberger, G. L. (1992). Applications of chaos to physiology and medicine. In J. M. Kim & J. Stringer (Eds.), *Applied chaos* (pp. 321–331). New York: John Wiley & Sons, Inc.

Goldman, J. (1992). *Healing sounds: The power of harmonics*. Rockport, MA: Element Books.

Goldstein, A. (1990). Thrills in response to music. *Physiological Psychology, 8*, 126–129.

Goldstein, S. L. (1990). A songwriting assessment for hopelessness in depressed adolescents: A review of the literature and a pilot study. *The Arts in Psychotherapy, 17*
(2), 117–124.

Goleman, D. (1995). *Emotional intelligence.* New York: Bantam Books.

Goodwin, B. C. (1994). *How the leopard got its spots: The evolution of complexity.* New
York: Charles Scribner's Sons.

Goodwyn, S., & Acredolo, L. (2000). *Baby minds: Brain building games your baby will
love.* New York: Bantam Books.

Gorder, W. D. (1980). Divergent production abilities as constructs of musical creativity. *Journal of Research in Music Education, 28,* 43–42.

Gordon, J. (1996). *Manifesto for a new medicine.* Reading, MA: Addison-Wesley Publishing Co., Inc.

Goswami, A. (2001). Quantum yoga. *Noetic Sciences Review, 56,* 26–31.

Gowan, J. C. (1978). *New directions in creativity research.* New York: Harper & Row.

Graham, R. (1975). *Music for the exceptional child.* Reston, VA: Music Educators National Conference.

Green, E. (1997). ISSSEEM's challenge: Observations on the science of subtle energy. *Bridges, 8* (3), 4–7.

Green, E., & Green, A. (1989). *Beyond biofeedback.* New York: Knoll Publishing Co.

Green, E. E., Parks, P. A., Guzer, P. M., Fahrion, S. L., & Coyne, L. (1991). Anomalous electrostatic phenomena in exceptional subjects. *Subtle Energy, 2* (3),
69–94.

Green, J., & Shellenberger, R. (1993). The subtle energy of love. *Subtle Energy, 4* (1),
31–55.

Greer, R. D. (1976). Music instruction as behavior modification. *Journal of Music
Therapy, 13* (3), 130–141.

Greer, S., & Morris, T. (1975). Psychological attributes of women who develop breast
cancer: A controlled study. *Journal of Psychosomatic Research, 19,* 147–153.

Gregory, R. L. (Ed.). (1987). *The Oxford companion to the mind.* Oxford: Oxford University Press.

Gregson, R. A. M. (1996). N-dimensional nonlinear psychophysics. In E. MacCormac & M. I. Stamenov (Eds.), *Fractals of brain, fractals of mind* (pp. 155–178).
Philadelphia: John Benjamins North America.

Grof, C., & Grof, S. (1993). Addiction as spiritual emergency. In R. Walsh & F.
Walsh (Eds.), *Paths beyond ego* (pp. 137–146). Los Angeles: Jeremy P. Tarcher, Inc.

Grof, S. (1975). *Realms of the human unconscious.* New York: Viking.

Grossman, N. (2002). Who's afraid of life after death? *Noetic Sciences Review, 61,*
30–35, 46.

Grosso, M. (1992). *Soulmaking.* Charlottesville, VA: Hampton Roads Publishing Co.,
Inc.

Grout, D. J. (1960). *A history of Western music.* New York: W. W. Norton & Co.

Guck, M. A. (1997). Two types of metaphoric transference. In J. Robinson (Ed.),
Music and meaning (pp. 201–212). Ithaca, NY: Cornell University Press.

Guidano, V. F. (1987). *Complexity of the self: A developmental approach to psychopathology and therapy.* New York: Guilford.

Guidano, V. F., & Liotti, G. (1983). *Cognitive processes and emotional disorders.* New York: Guilford.

Guilford, J. (1968). *Intelligence, creativity, and their educational implications.* San Diego: Robert R. Knapp.

Gutheil, E. A. (1952). *Music and your emotions.* New York: Liveright.

Guyton, A. C. (1979). *Physiology of the human body,* 5th ed. Philadelphia: W. B. Saunders Co.

Gyatso, T., Dalai Lama XIV. (1999). *Ethics for a new millennium.* New York: Riverhead Books.

Haaland, J. (1999). Mind and nonlocality. *Bridges, 10* (1), 13–18.

Haas, F., Distenfeld, S., & Axen, K. (1986). Effects of perceived musical rhythm on respiratory patterns. *Journal of Applied Physiology, 61,* 1185–1191.

Hado Music Corporation. (1996). *Hado music: A blending of science and music.* Thousand Oaks, CA: Hado Music Corporation.

Hale, S. E. (1995). *Song and silence: Voicing the soul.* Albuquerque: La Alameda Press.

Hall, R. V. (1983). *Managing behavior.* Austin, TX: Pro-ed.

Halpern, S. (1985). *Sound health.* New York: Harper & Row.

Hamel, P. M. (1976). *Through music to the self.* Boulder: Shambhala.

Hameroff, S. R. (1994). Quantum coherence in microtubules: A neural basis for emergent consciousness? *Journal of Consciousness Studies, 1,* 91–118.

Handel, P. H., & Chung, A. L. (Eds.). (1993). *Noise in physical systems and 1/f fluctuation.* St. Louis, MO: AIP Conference Proceedings 285.

Hanser, S. (1987). *Music therapist's handbook.* St. Louis, MO: Warren H. Green, Inc.

Hanser, S., Larson, S., & O'Connell, A. C. (1983). The effect of music on relaxation of expectant mothers during labor. *Journal of Music Therapy, 20* (2), 50–58.

Hanser, S. B. (1974). Group contingent music listening with a group of emotionally disturbed boys. *Journal of Music Therapy, 11* (4), 220–225.

Harding, C., & Ballard, K. D. (1982). The effectiveness of music as a stimulus and as a contingent reward in promoting the spontaneous speech of three physically handicapped preschoolers. *Journal of Music Therapy, 19* (2), 86–101.

Harman, W. (1994a). A re-examination of the metaphysical foundations of modern science: Why is it necessary? In W. Harman (Ed.), *New metaphysical foundation of modern science* (pp. 1–13). Sausalito, CA: Institute for Noetic Sciences.

Harman, W. (1994b). Toward a "science of wholeness." In W. Harman (Ed.), *New metaphysical foundation of modern science* (pp. 375–396). Sausalito, CA: Institute for Noetic Sciences.

Harman, W. (1997). Biology revisioned. *Noetic Sciences Review, 41,* 39–42.

Harman, W. (1998). What are noetic sciences? *Noetic Sciences Review, 47,* 32–33.

Harman, W. (Ed.). (1994c). *New metaphysical foundation of modern science.* Sausalito, CA: Institute for Noetic Sciences.

Harnard, S. (Ed.). (1987). *Categorical perception.* New York: Cambridge University Press.

Harner, M. (1982). *The way of the shaman*. New York: Bantam Books.

Harper, G., & Harper, H. (1977). Music, emotion, and autonomic function. In M. Critchley & R. Henson (Eds.), *Music and brain* (pp. 202–216). London: William Heinemann Medical Books Ltd.

Harrer, G., & Harrer, H. (1977). Music, emotion, and autonomic function. In M. Critchley & B. Henson (Eds.), *Music and the brain. Studies in the neurology of music* (pp. 202–216). Springfield, IL: Charles C. Thomas Publishers.

Hart, M., & Stevens, J. (1990). *Drumming at the edge of magic: A journey into the spirit of percussion*. San Francisco: HarperSanFrancisco.

Harvey, A. W. (1992). On developing a program in music medicine: A neurophysiological basis for music as therapy. In R. Spintge & R. Droh (Eds.), *Music medicine* (pp. 71–79). St. Louis, MO: MMB Music Inc.

Hauck, L. P., & Martin, P. L. (1970). Music as a reinforcer in patient-controlled duration of time-out. *Journal of Music Therapy, 7* (2), 43–53.

Hauser, M. C. (2000). Primate vocalization in emotion and thought. In N. L. Wallin, B. Merker, & S. Brown (Eds.), *The origins of music* (pp. 77–98). Cambridge, MA: MIT Press.

Hebb, D. (1952). *The organization of behavior*. New York: John Wiley & Sons.

Henderson, S. M. (1983). Effects of a music therapy program upon awareness of mood in music, groups cohesion, and self-esteem among hospitalized patients. *Journal of Music Therapy, 20* (1), 14–20.

Herbert, D. E. (1996). *Chaos and the changing nature of science: An introduction*. Woodbury, NY: American Institute of Physics.

Herman, J. L. (1992). *Trauma and recovery*. New York: Basic Books.

Hernandez-Peon, R. (1961). The efferent control of afferent signals entering the central nervous system. *Annals of New York Academy of Science, 89*, 866–882.

Hero, B. (1992). *Lambdoma unveiled*. Wells, ME: Strawberry Hill Farm Studios Press.

Hero, B. (1995). *The Lambdoma, resonant, harmonic scale*. Wells, ME: Strawberry Hill Farm Studios Press.

Herrmann, N. (1990). *The creative brain*. Lake Lure, NC: N. Herrmann.

Hesser, B. (1995). The power of sound. In C. Kenny (Ed.), *Listening, playing, creating: Essays on the power of sound* (pp. 43–50). Albany: State University of New York Press.

Hetlinger, E. (Ed.). (1989). *Springs of music*. Schurman Co., Inc.

Hibbard, C. (1999). Conscious intention in healing effects. *Bridges, 10* (4), 9–11.

Hibbard, C. (2002). Living in the question and not knowing: The integration of spiritual practice and social change. *Bridges, 13* (3), 4–6.

Higgins, K. M. (1997). Musical idiosyncrasy and perspectival listening. In J. Robinson (Ed.), *Music and meaning* (pp. 83–102). Ithaca, NY: Cornell University Press.

Hilliard, R. E. (2001). The effects of music therapy–based bereavement groups on mood and behavior of grieving children: A pilot study. *Journal of Music Therapy, 38* (4), 291–306.

Hillman, J. (1975). *Re-visioning psychology.* New York: Harper & Row.

Hinterkopf, E. (1994). Integrating spiritual experience in counseling. *Counseling and Values,* 38, 165–175.

Hodges, D. A. (1980a). Physiological responses to music. In D. A. Hodges (Ed.), *Handbook of music psychology* (pp. 393–400). Lawrence, KS: National Association for Music Therapy.

Hodges, D. A. (1996a). Neuromusical research: A review of the literature. In D. Hodges (Ed.), *Handbook of music psychology,* 2d ed. (pp. 197–284). San Antonio, TX: IMR Press.

Hodges, D. A. (Ed.). (1980b). *Handbook of music psychology.* Lawrence, KS: National Association for Music Therapy.

Hodges, D A. (Ed.). (1996b). *Handbook of music psychology,* 2d ed. San Antonio, TX: IMR Press.

Hoffman, J. (1995). *Rhythmic medicine.* Leawood, KS: Jamillan Press.

Holdrege, C. (2002). The dynamic heart and circulation. *In Context,* 7, 15–18.

Holland, J. (1994). Complexity made simple. *The Bulletin of the Santa Fe Institute,* 9 (3), 3–4.

Holte, J. (Ed.). (1993). *Chaos: The new science.* Lanham, MD: University Press of America, Inc.

Homans, P. (Ed.). (1968). *The dialogue between theology and psychology.* Chicago: University of Chicago Press.

Hood, M. (1971). *The ethnomusicologist.* New York: McGraw-Hill.

Hooper, J., & Teresi, D. (1986). *The three-pound universe.* New York: Macmillan.

Hoskins, C. (1988). Use of music to increase verbal response and improve expressive language abilities of preschool language delayed children. *Journal of Music Therapy,* 25 (2), 73–84.

Hubbard, T. L. (2002). Cognitive science and shamanism I: Webs of life and neural nets. *Shamanism,* 15 (1), 4–10.

Hudson, W. C. (1973). Music: A physiologic language. *Journal of Music Therapy,* 10 (3), 137–140.

Hughes, C. W. (1948). *The human side of music.* New York: Philosophical Library.

Hull, A. (1998). *Drum circle spirit: Facilitating human potential through rhythm.* Tempe, AZ: White Cliffs Media, Inc.

Humbert, E. (1988). *C.G. Jung: The fundamentals of theory and practice.* Wilmette, IL: Chiron Publications.

Hunt, H. T. (1995). *On the nature of consciousness: Cognitive, phenomenological, and transpersonal perspectives.* New Haven, CT: Yale University Press.

Hunt, V. V. (1996). *Infinite mind.* Malibu, CA: Malibu Publishing Co.

Hurt, C., Rice, R., McIntosh, G. C., & Thaut, M. H. (1998). Rhythmic auditory stimulation in gait training for patients with traumatic brain injury. *Journal of Music Therapy,* 35 (4), 228–241.

Hurt, C. P. (1996). Rhythmic auditory stimulation in gait training for patients with traumatic brain injury. Unpublished M.A. thesis, Colorado State University.

Husemann, A. (1994). *The harmony of the human body*. Edinburgh: Flores Books.

Husserl, E. (1960). *Cartesian meditations: An introduction to phenomenology*. D. Cairns (Trans.). The Hague: Martinus Nijhoff Publishers.

Husserl, E. (1965). *Phenomenology and the crisis of philosophy*. New York: Harper & Row.

Hutchinson, M. (1986). *Megabrain: New tools and techniques for brain growth and mind expansion*. New York: Ballantine.

Ikemi, Y., Nakagawa, S., Nakagawa, T., & Minezasu, S. (1975). Psychosomatic consideration on cancer patients who have made a narrow escape from death. *Dynamische Psychiatric, 31*, 77–92.

Imbertz, M. (2000). Innate competencies in musical communication. In N. L Wallin, B. Merker, & S. Brown (Eds.), *The origins of music* (pp. 449–462). Cambridge, MA: MIT Press.

Ingerman, S. (1991). *Soul retrieval*. San Francisco: HarperSanFrancisco.

Irwin, M., Daniels, M., Bloom, E. T., Smith, T. L., & Weiner, H. (1987). Life events, depressive symptoms and immune function. *American Journal of Psychiatry, 144*, 437–441.

Isenberg-Grzeda, C. (1995). The sound image. In C. Kenny (Ed.), *Listening, playing, creating: Essays on the power of sound* (pp. 135–149). Albany: State University of New York Press.

Iverson, J. (2000). The relationship between gesture and speech in congenitally blind and sighted language-learners. *Journal of Nonverbal Behavior, 24* (2), 105–131.

Jackendoff, R. (1987). *Consciousness and the computational mind*. Cambridge, MA: MIT Press.

Jackendoff, R., & Lerdahl, F. (1982). A grammatical parallel between music and language. In M. Clynes (Ed.), *Music, mind, and brain: The neuropsychology of music* (pp. 83–116). New York: Plenum Press.

Jackson, A. (1992). Energetic medicine: A new science of healing: Interview with Dr. Hiroshi Motoyama. *Share International Magazine, 11* (7), 5–7.

Jacobson, J. J., & Yamanski, W. S. (1994). A possible physical mechanism in the treatment of neurological disorders with externally applied pecotesla magnetic fields. *Subtle Energies, 5* (3), 239–252.

James, M. R. (1984). Sensory integration: A theory for therapy and research. *Journal of Music Therapy, 21* (2), 79–88.

James, M. R., & Freed, B. S. (1989). A sequential model for developing group cohesion in music therapy. *Music Therapy Perspectives, 7*, 28–34.

James, W. (1890). *The principles of psychology*. 2 vols. New York: Dover.

Janov, A. (1996). *Why you get sick and how you get well*. West Hollywood, CA: Dove Books.

Jantsch, E., & Waddington, C. H. (Eds.). (1976). *Evolution and consciousness: Human systems in transition*. Reading, MA: Addison-Wesley.

Jauregui, A. (2002). Nothing needs fixing. *Noetic Sciences Review, 61*, 22–25.

Jaynes, J. (1976). *Origin of consciousness in the break-down of the bicameral mind*. Boston: Houghton Mifflin.

Jenny, H. (1972). *Cymatics: Wave phenomena, vibrational effects, harmonic oscillations with their structure, kinetics and dynamics*, vol. 2. Basil, Germany: Basillius Presse.

Jensen, K. L. (2001). The effects of selected classical music on self-disclosure. *Journal of Music Therapy, 38* (1), 2–27.

Jibu, M., & Yasue, K. (1995). *Quantum brain dynamics and consciousness*. Philadelphia: John Benjamins North America.

Jing, L. S., Hui-Ju, S., Guo, W., & Maranto, C. D. (1991). Music and medicine in China: The effects of music electroacupuncture on cerebral hemiplegia. In C. D. Maranto (Ed.), *Applications of music in medicine* (pp. 191–199). Washington, DC: National Association for Music Therapy.

John, E. R., Harmony, T., Prechep, L. S., Valdez-Sosa, M., & Valdez-Sosa, P. A. (Eds.). (1990). *Machinery of the mind: Data, theory and speculations about higher brain functions*. Boston: Birkhauser.

Johnson, J. K., Cotman, C. W., Jasaki, C. S., & Shaw, G. L. (1998). Enhancement in spatial-temporal reasoning after a Mozart listening condition in Alzheimer's disease: A case-study. *Neurological Research, 20*, 666–672.

Johnson, T. L., & Dooley, K. J. (1996). Looking for chaos in time series data. In W. Sulis & A. Combs (Eds.), *Nonlinear dynamics in human behavior* (pp. 44–76). Singapore: World Scientific.

Johnston, V. S. (1999). *Why we feel: The science of human emotion*. Cambridge, MA: Perseus Books.

Jorgensen, E. (1997). *In search of music education*. Urbana: University of Illinois Press.

Jorgensen, H. (1974). The use of a contingent music activity to modify behaviors which interfere with learning. *Journal of Music Therapy, 11* (1), 41–46.

Jourdain, R. (1997). *Music, the brain, and ecstasy*. New York: Avon Books.

Jung, C. G. (1922). *On the relation of analytical psychology to poetry: The collected work of C. G. Jung*. London: Routledge.

Jung, C. G. (1933). *Modern man in search of soul*. New York: Harcourt.

Jung, C. G. (1969). *Structure and dynamics of the psyche*, vol. 8. Princeton, NJ: Princeton University Press.

Jung, C. G. (1987). Letter to Bill Wilson. *Parabola, 12* (2), 71.

Kabuto, M., Kageyama, T., & Netta, H. (1993). EEG power spectrum changes due to listening to pleasant music and their relation to relaxation effects. *Nippon Eiseigaku Zasshi, 48* (4), 807–818.

Kagan, J. (1984). *The nature of the child*. New York: Basic Books.

Kaptchuk, T., & Croucher, M. (1987). *The healing arts*. New York: Summit Books.

Karni, A., Tanner, D., Rubenstein, B. S., Askenasy, J. J. M., & Sage, D. (1994). Dependence on REM sleep for overnight learning of a perceptual skill. *Science, 265*, 679–682.

Karras, B. (1985). *Down memory lane*. Mt. Airy, MD: Eldersong.

Katsch, S., & Merle-Fishman, C. (1985). *The music within you*. New York: Simon & Schuster, Inc.

Kaufman, S. A. (1993). *Origins of order*. New York: Oxford University Press.

Kaznacheyev, V. P., Shurin, S. P., Mikhailova, L. P., & Ignatovish, N. V. (1979). Distant intercellular interactions in a system of two tissue cultures. In S. Krippner (Ed.), *Psychoenergetic systems: The interaction of consciousness, energy and matter* (pp. 223-226). New York: Gordon and Breach Science Publishers.

Keil, C. (1966). Motion and feeling through music. *Journal of Aesthetics and Art Criticism, 24* (3), 337–349.

Keil, C., & Feld, S. (Eds.). (1994). *Music grooves.* Chicago: University of Chicago Press.

Kelly, K. (1994). *Out of control.* Reading, MA: Addison-Wesley.

Kenny, C. B. (1982). *The mythic artery.* Atascadero, CA: Ridgeview Publishing Co.

Kenny, C. B. (1985). Music: A whole systems approach. *Music Therapy, 5* (1), 3–11.

Kenny, C. B. (1989). *The field of play: A guide for the theory and practice of music therapy.* Atascadero, CA: Ridgeview Publishing Co.

Kenny, C. B. (1998). Embracing complexity: The creation of a comprehensive research culture in music therapy. *Journal of Music Therapy, 35* (3), 201–217.

Kenny, C. B. (Ed.). (1995). *Listening, playing, creating: Essays on the power of sound.* Albany: State University of New York Press.

Kenyon, C. T. (1994). *Brain states.* Captain Cook, HI: United States Publishing.

Keyes, L. E. (1973). *Toning: The creative power of the voice.* Marina del Rey, CA: DeVorss & Co.

Khan, H. I. (1967). Chapter 56 in J. Godwin (Ed.), *Music, mysticism and magic: A sourcebook* (pp. 260–267). New York: Routledge & Kegan Paul.

Khan, H. I. (1983). *The music of life.* Santa Fe: Omega Press.

Khorran-Sefat, D., Dierks, T., & Hacker, H. (1996). Cerebellar activation during music listening. *NeuroImage, 3,* 5312.

Kierkegaard, S. (1941). *Fear and trembling* and *Sickness unto death.* W. Lowrie (Trans.). Princeton, NJ: Princeton University Press.

Kim, J. H., & Stringer, J. (Eds.). (1992). *Applied chaos.* New York: John Wiley & Sons.

King, C. (1996). Fractal neurodynamics and quantum chaos. In E. MacCormac & M. I. Stamenov (Eds.), *Fractals of brain, fractals of mind* (pp. 179–233). Philadelphia: John Benjamins North America.

King, P. (1990). *Music alone.* Ithaca, NY: Cornell University Press.

Koenig, H., McCullough, M. E., & Larson, D. B. (2001). *Handbook of religion and health.* New York: Oxford University Press.

Koepchen, H. P., Droh, R., Spintge, R., Abel, H-H., Klussendorf, D., & Koralewski, E. (1992). Physiological rhythmicity and music in medicine. In R. Spintge & R. Droh (Eds.), *Music medicine* (pp. 39–70). St. Louis, MO: MMB Music, Inc.

Koga, M., & Tims, F. (2001, October–November). The music making and wellness project. *American Music Teacher,* 18–22.

Koplowitz, H. (1984). Post-logical thinking. In M. L. Commons, F. A. Richard, & C. Armon (Eds.), *Beyond formal operations: Late adolescent and adult cognitive development* (pp. 272–296). New York: Praeger.

Kosslyn, S. M., & Koenig, O. (1995). *Wet mind: The new cognitive neuroscience*. New York: Free Press.

Krampe, R. T., & Ericsson, K. A. (1996). Maintaining excellence: Deliberate practice and elite performance in young and older pianists. *Journal of Experimental Psychology: General, 125* (4), 331–359.

Kreitler, H., & Kreitler, S. (1972). *Psychology of the arts*. Durham, NC: Duke University Press.

Krout, R. (1989). Contemporary guitar applications. *Music Therapy Perspectives, 17* (2), 51–53.

Krout, R. (1995). *Contemporary acoustic guitar skills for music leaders*. St. Louis, MO: MMB Music.

Krout, R. (2000). Hospice and palliative music therapy: A continuum of creative caring. In C. Furman (Ed.), *Effectiveness of music therapy procedures: Documentation of research and clinical practice*, 2d ed. (pp. 323–411). Silver Spring, MD: American Music Therapy Association.

Kuhn, T. (1970). *The structures of scientific revolutions*, 2d ed. Chicago: University of Chicago Press.

Kuhn, T. (1977). *The essential tension: Selected studies in scientific tradition and change*. Chicago: University of Chicago Press.

Kumar, A. M. (1997, November). Music and molecular neuroendocrinology. Paper presented at the American Music Therapy Association Annual Conference, Los Angeles.

Kumar, A. M., Tims, F., Cruess, D. G., Mintzer, M. T., Ironson, G., Loewenstein, D., Caltan, R., Fernandez, J. B., Eisdorfer, C., & Kumar, M. (1999). Music therapy increases serum melatonin levels in patients with Alzheimer's disease. *Alternative Therapies in Health and Medicine, 5* (6), 49–57.

Kunej, D., & Turk, I. (2000). New perspectives on the beginnings of music: Archeological and musicological analysis of a middle Paleolithic bone "flute." In N. L Wallin, B. Merker, & S. Brown (Eds.), *The origins of music* (pp. 235–270). Cambridge, MA: MIT Press.

Kupper, Z., & Hoffman, H. (1996). Logical attractors: A Boolean approach to the dynamics of psychosis. In W. Sulis & A. Combs (Eds.), *Nonlinear dynamics in human behavior* (pp. 296–315). Singapore: World Scientific.

Kus, R. J. (Ed.). (1995). *Spirituality and chemical dependency*. New York: Haworth.

Kwee, M. (1990). *Psychotherapy, meditation, and health*. London: EastWest Publications.

Lakes, P. S., & Saha, S. (1978). Propagation of acoustic energy in bone. *Instrumentation, 12*, 106.

Langer, E. J. (1989). *Mindfulness*. New York: Addison-Wesley.

Langer, S. (1942). *Philosophy in a new key*. Cambridge, MA: Harvard University Press.

Langer, S. (1953). *Feeling and form*. London: Routledge & Kegan Paul.

Langer, S. (1957). *Problems of art: Ten philosophical lectures*. New York: Charles Scribner & Sons.

Langner, F. (1967). Six years experience with LSD therapy. In H. Abramson (Ed.), *The use of LSD in psychotherapy and alcoholism*. New York: Bobbs-Merrill.

Larson, B. A. (1978). Use of the motorvator in improving gross-motor coordination, visual perception and IQ scores: A pilot study. *Journal of Music Therapy, 15* (3), 145–149.

Larter, R. (2002). Life lessons from the newest science. *Noetic Sciences Review, 59,* 22–27.

LaShan, L. L., & Gassman, M. L. (1958). Some observations on psychotherapy with patients with neoplastic disease. *American Journal of Psychotherapy, 12,* 723–734.

Laskow, L. (1992). *Healing with love.* San Francisco: HarperSanFrancisco.

Laskow, L. (1999). Healer intentions. *Bridges, 10* (3), 12–15.

Laszlo, E. (1987). *Evolution: The grand synthesis.* Boston: Shambhala.

Lathom, W. (1980). *The role of music therapy in the education of handicapped children and youth.* Washington, DC: National Association for Music Therapy.

Lawlis, F. (1996). *Transpersonal medicine: A new approach to healing body–mind–spirit.* Boston: Shambhala.

LeDoux, J. (1996). *The emotional brain.* New York: Simon & Schuster.

Lee, M. H. M. (Ed.). (1989). *Rehabilitation, music and human well-being.* St. Louis, MO: MMB, Inc.

Leeds, J. (2001). *The power of sound.* Rochester, VT: Healing Arts Press.

Lees, H. (Ed.). (1992). *Music education: Sharing musics of the world.* New Zealand: University of Canterbury.

Lehmann, D. (1990). Brain electric microstates and cognition: The atoms of thought. In E. R. John, T. Harmony, L. S. Prechep, M. Valdez-Sosa, & P. A. Valdez-Sosa (Eds.), *Machinery of the mind: Data, theory and speculations about higher brain functions* (pp. 209–225). Boston: Birkhauser.

Lehrman, R. L. (1990). *Physics the easy way,* 2d ed. Hauppauge, NY: Barron's Educational Series, Inc.

Lemay, P., Dauwaldeer, J-P., Pomini, V., & Bersier, M. (1996). Quality of life—A dynamic perspective. In W. Sulis & A. Combs (Eds.), *Nonlinear dynamics in human behavior* (pp. 276–295). Singapore: World Scientific.

Leng, X., & Shaw, G. L. (1990). Coding of musical structure and the Trion model of the cortex. *Music Perception, 8* (1), 149–162.

Leng, X., & Shaw, G. L. (1991). Toward a neural theory of higher brain function using music as a window. *Concepts in Neuroscience, 2* (2), 229–258.

Leonard, G. (1997). Living energy: Subtle fields, subtle healing. *Noetic Sciences Review, 43,* 8–15.

Leonard, L. (1990). *Witness to the fire.* Boston: Shambhala.

Lerdahl, R., & Jackendoff, R. (1983). *A generative theory of tonal music.* Cambridge, MA: MIT Press.

Levenson, T. (1994). *Measure for measure: A musical history of science.* New York: Simon & Schuster.

Levin, M. (1993). Current and potential applications of bioelectromagnetics in medicine. *Subtle Energy, 4* (1), 77–85.

Levine, M. (2002). *A mind at a time.* New York: Simon & Schuster.

Levinson, J. (1997). Music and negative emotion. In J. Robinson (Ed.), *Music and meaning* (pp. 215–241). Ithaca, NY: Cornell University Press.

Levitin, D. J. (1999). Memory for musical attributes. In P. R. Cook (Ed.), *Music, cognition, and computerized sound* (pp. 209–227). Cambridge, MA: MIT Press.

Lewin, R. (1992). *Complexity: Life at the edge of chaos.* New York: Macmillan.

Lewis, K. (1998–1999). The Bonny method of G.I.M.: Matrix for transpersonal experience. *Journal of the Association of Music and Imagery, 6,* 63–86.

Lewis, R., & Lewontin, R. (1985). *The dialectical biologist.* Cambridge, MA: Harvard University Press.

Lichtenberg, J. D. (1987). Infant studies and clinical work with adults. *Psychoanalytic Inquiry, 7,* 311–330.

Liebman, M. (1986). *Neuroanatomy made easy and understandable.* Rockville, MD: Freeman & Co.

Lincoln, Y. S., & Guba, E. S. (1985). *Naturalistic inquiry.* Beverly Hills: Sage Publications.

Lindberg, K. A. (1995). Songs of healing: Songwriting with an abused adolescent. *Music Therapy, 13* (1), 93–108.

Lipe, A. W. (2002). Beyond therapy: Music, spirituality, and health in human experience: A review of literature. *Journal of Music Therapy, 39* (3), 209–240.

Lipit, L. P., & Rovee-Collier, C. K. (Eds.). (1981). *Advances in infancy research,* vol. 1. Norwood, NJ: Ablex.

Lipsitz, L. A., & Goldberger, A. L. (1992). Loss of "complexity" and aging: Potential applications of fractals and chaos theory to senescense. *Journal of American Medical Association, 267,* 1806–1809.

Lipton, B. (2001). Insight into cellular "consciousness." *Bridges, 12* (1), 1, 4–6.

Litvak, S., & Senzee, A. W. (1986). *Toward a new brain.* Englewood Cliffs, NJ: Prentice Hall.

Lloyd, R. (1987). *Explorations in psychoneuroimmunology.* Orlando: Grune & Stratton.

Locke, J. L. (1993). *The child's path to spoken language.* Cambridge, MA: Harvard University Press.

Loewy, J. V. (1995). The musical stages of speech: A developmental model of preverbal sound making. *Music Therapy, 13* (1), 47–73.

Loewy, J. V. (Ed.). (1997). *Music therapy and pediatric pain.* Cherry Hill, NJ: Jeffrey Books.

Lomax, A. (1968). *Folk song style and culture.* New Brunswick, NJ: Transaction Books.

Longtin, A. (1993). Nonlinear forecasting of spike train from sensory neurons. In N. B. Abraham, A. M. Albano, E. A. Passamante, P. E. Rapp, & R. Gilmore (Eds.), *Complexity and chaos* (pp. 167–183). Singapore: World Scientific.

Lorch, C. A., Lorch, V., Diefendorf, A. O., & Earl, P. W. (1994). Effect of stimulative and sedative music on systolic blood pressure, heart rate, and respiratory rate in premature infants. *Journal of Music Therapy, 31* (2), 105–118.

Lowen, S. B., & Teich, M. C. (1993). Fractal auditory-nerve firing patterns may derive from fractal switching in sensory hair-cell ion channels. In P. H. Handel & A.

L. Chung (Eds.), *Noise in physical systems and 1/f fluctuation* (pp. 745–748). St. Louis, MO: AIP Conference Proceedings 285.

Luce, D. (2001). Cognitive therapy and music therapy. *Music Therapy Perspectives, 19* (2), 96–103.

Lundin, R. (1953). *An objective psychology of music.* New York: Ronald Press.

Lutz, C. A. (1998). *Unnatural emotions.* Chicago: University of Chicago Press.

MacCormac, E. R. (1996). Fractal thinking. In E. MacCormac & M. I. Stamenov (Eds.), *Fractals of brain, fractals of mind* (pp. 127–154). Philadelphia: John Benjamins North America.

MacCormac, E. R., & Stamenov, M. I. (Eds.). (1996). *Fractals of brain, fractals of mind.* Philadelphia: John Benjamins North America.

MacCurdy, J. T. (1925). *The psychology of emotion.* New York: Harcourt, Brace, & Co.

Mackey, M. C., & Glass, L. (1977). Oscillation and chaos in physiological control systems. *Science, 197,* 287–289.

MacLean, P. D. (1973). *A triune concept of the brain and behavior.* Toronto: University of Toronto Press.

MacLean, P. D. (1990). *The triune brain in evolution: Role in paleocerebral functions.* New York: Plenum.

Maconie, R. (1990). *The concept of music.* Oxford: Clarendon Press.

Maconie, R. (1997). *The science of music.* Oxford: Clarendon Press.

Madsen, C. K., Cotter, V., & Madsen, C. H. (1968). A behavioral approach to music therapy. *Journal of Music Therapy, 5* (3), 69–71.

Madsen, C. K., Dorrow, L .G., Moore, R. S., & Wonble, J. V. (1978). Effect of music via television as reinforcement for correct mathematics. *Journal of Research in Music Education, 24,* 51–59.

Madsen, C. K., & Forsythe, J. L. (1973). The effect of contingent music listening on increases of mathematical response. *Journal of Research in Music Education, 21,* 176–181.

Madsen, C. K., & Madsen, C. H., Jr. (1968). Music as a behavior modification technique with a juvenile delinquent. *Journal of Music Therapy, 5* (3), 72–76.

Madsen, C. K., Moore, R. S., Wagner, M. J., & Yarbough, C. (1975). A comparison of music as reinforcement for correct mathematical responses versus music as reinforcement for attentiveness. *Journal of Music Therapy, 22* (2), 84–95.

Madsen, C. K., Standley, J. M., & Gregory, D. (1991). The effect of a vibrotactile device, Somatron, on physiological and psychological response: Musicians vs. nonmusicians. *Journal of Music Therapy, 28* (1), 120–134.

Madsen, S. A. (1991). The effect of music paired with and without gestures on the learning and transfer of new vocabulary: Experimenter-derived nonsense words. *Journal of Music Therapy, 28* (4), 222–230.

Mahlberg, M. (1973). Music therapy in the treatment of an autistic child. *Journal of Music Therapy, 10* (4), 184–188.

Mahler, M. (1968). *On human symbiosis and the vicissitudes of individuation.* New York: International University Press.

Makeig, S. (1982). Affective versus analytic perception of musical intervals. In M. Clynes (Ed.), *Music, mind, and brain* (pp. 227–250). New York: Plenum Press.

Malone, A. B. (1996). The effects of live music on the distress of pediatric patients receiving intravenous starts, venipunctures, injections, and heel sticks. *Journal of Music Therapy, 33* (1), 19–33.

Maman, F. (1997). *The role of music in the twenty-first century.* Redondo Beach, CA: Tama-Do Press.

Manchester, R. A. (1988). Medical aspects of music development. *Psychomusicology, 7,* 147–151.

Mandelbrot, B. B. (1982). *The fractal geometry of nature.* New York: W. H. Freeman.

Mandelbrot, B. B. (1993). Fractals. In J. Holt (Ed.), *Chaos: The new science* (pp. 1–34). Lanham, MD: University Press of America, Inc.

Mandell, A. J. (1983). From intermittency to transitivity in neurobiological flow. *American Journal of Physiology, 245* (14), R484–R494.

Mandell, S. E. (1988). Music therapy: A personal peri-surgical experience. *Music Therapy Perspectives, 5,* 109–110.

Mandell, S. E. (1996). Music for wellness: Music therapy for stress management in a rehabilitation program. *Music Therapy Perspectives, 14* (1), 38–43.

Mandler, G. (1984). *Mind and body.* New York: Norton.

Mankin, L., Wellman, M., & Owen, A. (1979). *Prelude to musicianship.* New York: Holt, Rinehart, & Winston.

Maranto, C. D. (1992). A comprehensive definition of music therapy with an integrative model for music medicine. In R. Spintge & R. Droh (Eds.), *Music medicine* (pp. 19–29). St. Louis, MO: MMB Music, Inc.

Maranto, C. D. (1996). A cognitive model of music in medicine. In R. R. Pratt & R. Spintge (Eds.), *Music medicine,* vol. 2 (pp. 327–332). St. Louis, MO: MMB Music, Inc.

Maranto, C. D. (Ed.). (1991). *Applications of music in medicine.* Washington, DC: National Association for Music Therapy.

Maranto, C. D., & Scartelli, J. (1992). Music in the treatment of immune-related disorders. In R. Spintge & R. Droh (Eds.), *Music medicine* (pp. 142–153). St. Louis, MO: MMB Music, Inc.

Martin, J. A. (1991). Music therapy at the end of life. In K. E. Bruscia (Ed.), *Case studies in music therapy* (pp. 617–632). Phoenixville, PA: Barcelona Publishers.

Martin, J. E., & Carlson, C. R. (1988). Spirituality dimensions of health psychology. In W. R. Miller & J. E. Martin (Eds.), *Behavior therapy and religion* (pp. 57–110). Newbury Park, CA: Sage.

Marteniuk, R. G. (1976). *Information processing in motor skills.* New York: Holt, Rinehart, & Winston.

Maslow, A. (1970). *Religion, values and peak experiences.* New York: Viking Penguin.

Maslow, A. (1971). *The farther reaches of human nature.* New York: Viking.

Maslow, A. (1982). *Toward a psychology of being,* 2d ed. New York: Van Nostrand Reinhold.

Maslow, A. (1987). *Motivation and personality*, rev. ed. R. Pranger, J. Fadiman, C. McReynolds, & R. Cox (Eds.). New York: Harper & Row.

Masterpasqua, F., & Perna, P. (Eds.). (1997). *The psychological meaning of chaos*. Washington, DC: American Psychological Association.

Mathews, M. (1999). The auditory brain. In P. R. Cook (Ed.), *Music, cognition, and computerized sound* (pp. 11–20). Cambridge, MA: MIT Press.

Mathews, P. C., & Strogatz, S. H. (1990). Phase diagram for the collective behavior of limit-cycle oscillators. *Physics Review Letter, 65,* 1701–1704.

Mathieu, W. A. (1991). *The listening book*. Boston: Shambhala.

Maturana, H. R., & Varela, F. J. (1980). *Autopoiesis and cognition: The realization of the living*. Boston: D. Reidel.

Maturana, H. R., & Varela, F. J. (1987). *The tree of knowledge: The biological roots of human understanding*. Boston: Shambhala.

Maturana, H. R., & Varela, F. J. (1992). *The tree of life*. Boston: Shambhala.

Matzke, D. (2001). Supercomputer suggests supermind. *Bridges, 12* (1), 7–11.

Maultsby, M. (1972). Combining music therapy and rational behavior therapy. *Journal of Music Therapy, 14* (2), 89–97.

Maxfield, M. (1994). The journey of the drum. *ReVision, 16* (4), 157–163.

May, G. G. (1977). *Simply sane*. New York: Crossroad Publishing Co.

May, G. G. (1982). *Care of mind, care of spirit*. New York: HarperSanFrancisco.

May, G. G. (1988). *Addiction and grace*. San Francisco: Harper & Row.

May, G. G. (1991). *The awakened heart: Living beyond addictions*. San Francisco: HarperSanFrancisco.

Mazziotta, J. C., Phelps, M. E., Carson, R. E., & Kuhl, D. E. (1982). Topographic mapping of human cerebral metabolism: Auditory stimulation. *Neurology, 32,* 921–937.

Mazzola, G. (1995). Neuronal response in limbic and neocortical structures during perception of consonance and dissonance. In R. Steinberg (Ed.), *Music and the mind machine: The psychophysiology and psychopathology of the sense of music* (pp. 89–97). Berlin: Springer-Verlag.

McAdams, S., & Bigand, E. (Eds.). (1993). *Thinking in sound: The cognitive psychology of human audition*. Oxford: Oxford University Press.

McCarthy, T. (1978). *The critical theory of Jürgen Habermas*. Cambridge, MA: MIT Press.

McCarty, B. C., McElfresh, C. T., Rice, S. V., & Wilson, S. J. (1976). The effect of contingent background music on inappropriate bus behavior. *Journal of Music Therapy, 15* (3), 150–156.

McClain, E. G. (1976). *The myth of invariance: The origin of the gods, mathematics, and music from the Rg Veda to Plato*. York Beach, ME: Nicolas-Hays, Inc.

McClellan, R. (1988). *The healing forces of music*. Rockport, MA: Element Books.

McCraty, R., Atkinson, M., & Rein, G. (1993). ECG spectra: The measurement of coherent and incoherent frequencies and their relationship to mental and emotional states. *Proceedings of the Third Annual Conference ISSSEEM*, Monterey, CA, 44–48.

McCraty, R., Atkinson, M., & Tiller, W. A. (1993). New electrophysiological correlates associated with intentional heart focus. *Subtle Energy, 4* (3), 251–268.

McCraty, R., Atkinson, M., & Tiller, W. A. (1995). The effects of emotions on short-
term power spectrum analysis of heart rate variability. *American Journal of Cardiol-
ogy, 76,* 1089.

McCulloch, W. S., & Pitts, W. H. (1943). A logical calculus of the ideas immanent
in nervous activities. *Bulletin of Mathematical Biophysics, 5,* 115–133.

McElwain, J. (1979). The effect of spontaneous and analytical listening on the
evoked cortical activity in the left and right hemispheres of musicians and nonmusicians. *Journal of Music Therapy, 26* (4), 180–189.

McGaugh, J. (1989). Involvement of hormonal and neuromodular systems in the regulation of memory storage. *Annual Review of Neuroscience, 12,* 255–287.

McGaugh, J. (1990). Significance and remembrance: The role of neuromodulatory
systems. *Psychological Science, 15,* 15–25.

McGaugh, J. (1994, October 20). Stress hormones hike emotional memories. *Nature,
146,* 262.

McGaugh, J. L., Bermudez-Rattoni, F., & Prado-Acala, R. A. (Eds.). (1995). *Plasticity in the central nervous system: Learning and memory.* Hillsdale, NJ: Erlbaum.

McGaugh, J. L., Cahill, L., Parent, M. B., Mesches, M. H., Coleman-Mesches, K., &
Solinas, J. A. (1995). Involvement of the amygdala in the regulation of memory
storage. In J. L. McGaugh, F. Bernudez-Rattoni, & R. A. Prado-Alcada (Eds.),
Plasticity in the central nervous system: Learning and memory (pp. 17–40). Hillsdale,
NJ: Erlbaum.

McGrann, J. V., Shaw, G. L., Shenoy, K. V., Leng, X., & Mathews, R. B. (1993).
Computation by symmetry operations in a structured model of brain. Recognition
of rotational invariance and time reversal. *Physics Review, 49* (6), 5830–5839.

McGuire, M. (1988). *Ritual healing in suburban America.* New Brunswick, NJ: Rutgers
University Press.

McIntosh, G. C., Brown, S. H., Rice, R. R., & Thaut, M. H. (1997). Rhythmic au-
ditory-motor facilitation of gait patterns in patients with Parkinson's disease. *Journal of Neurology, Neurosurgery, and Psychiatry, 62,* 22–26.

McKee, G., Humphreys, B., & McAdam, D. W. (1973). Scaled internalization of alpha activity during linguistic and musical tasks. *Psychophysiology, 10,* 441–443.

McKinney, C. H., Antoni, M. H., Kumar, M., Tims, F. C., & McCabe, P. M. (1997a).
Effects of Guided Imagery and Music (GIM) therapy on mood and cortisol in
healthy adults. *Health Psychology, 16* (4), 390–400.

McKinney, C. H., Tims, F. C., Kumar, A. M., & Kumar, M. (1997b). The effects of
selected classical music and spontaneous imagery on plasma beta-endorphin in
healthy adults. *Journal of Behavioral Medicine, 20* (1), 85–99.

McMullen, P. (1980). Music as perceived stimulus object and affective response: An
alternative theoretical framework. In D. A. Hodges (Ed.), *Handbook of music psychology* (pp. 183–193). Lawrence, KS: National Association for Music Therapy.

McNiff, S. (1992). *Art as medicine.* Boston: Shambhala.

Mehler, J., & Fox, R. (Eds.). (1985). *Neonate cognition: Beyond the blooming buzzing confusion*. Hillsdale, NJ: Erlbaum.

Meijer, P. H. E., Mountain, R. D., & Soulen, R. J., Jr. (Eds.). (1981). *Sixth International Conference on Noise in Physical Systems*. National Bureau of Standards Special Publication, 614. Washington, DC: National Bureau of Standards.

Melzak, R., & Wall, P. D. (1965). Pain mechanism: A new theory. *Science, 150*, 971–979.

Menuhin, Y., & Davis, C. (1979). *The music of man*. New York: Simon & Shuster.

Merker, B. (2000). Synchronous chorusing and human origins. In N. L Wallin, B. Merker, & S. Brown (Eds.), *The origins of music* (pp. 315–327). Cambridge, MA: MIT Press.

Merleau-Ponty, M. (1962). *Phenomenology of perception*. C. Smith (Trans.). London: Routledge & Kegan Paul.

Merleau-Ponty, M. (1964). *The primacy of perception and other essays*. Evanston, IL: Northwestern University Press.

Merleau-Ponty, M. (1973). *Consciousness and the acquisition of language*. Evanston, IL: Northwestern University Press.

Merriam, A. P. (1964). *The anthropology of music*. Evanston, IL: Northwestern University Press.

Metias, M. H. (1985). *Creativity in art, religion, and culture*. Amsterdam, the Netherlands: Rodopi, BV.

Metzler, R. K., & Berman, T. (1991). Selected effects of sedative music on the anxiety of bronchoscopy patients. In C. D. Maranto (Ed.), *Applications of music in medicine* (pp. 163–178). Washington, DC: National Association for Music Therapy.

Metzner, R. (1994). Addiction and transcendence as altered states of consciousness. *Journal of Transpersonal Psychology, 26* (1), 1–17.

Meyer, L. (1956). *Emotion and meaning in music*. Chicago: University of Chicago Press.

Meyer, L. (1967). *Music, the arts, and ideas: Patterns and predictions in twentieth-century culture*. Chicago: University of Chicago Press.

Michel, D. (1976). *Music therapy: An introduction to therapy and special education through music*. Springfield, IL: Charles C. Thomas.

Michel, D. E., & Jones, J. L. (1991). *Music for developing speech and language skills in children*. St. Louis, MO: MMB Music, Inc.

Michel, D. E., & May, N. H. (1974). The development of music therapy procedures with speech and language disorders. *Journal of Music Therapy, 11* (3), 74–80.

Michel, D. E., Parker, P., Giokas, D., & Werner, J. (1982). Music therapy and remedial reading: Six studies testing specialized hemispheric processing. *Journal of Music Therapy, 19* (4), 219–229.

Miller, G. (2000). Evolution of human music through sexual selection. In N. L Wallin, B. Merker, & S. Brown (Eds.), *The origins of music* (pp. 329–360). Cambridge, MA: MIT Press.

Miller, W. R., & Martin, J. E. (Eds.). (1988). *Behavior therapy and religion*. Newbury Park, CA: Sage.

Miluk-Kolassa, B., Matejek, M., & Stupnicki, R. (1996). The effects of music listening on changes in selected physiological parameters in adult pre-surgical patients. *Journal of Music Therapy, 33* (3), 208–218.

Miluk-Kolassa, B., Obminski, Z., Stupnicki, R., & Golec, L. (1994). Effects of music treatment on salivary cortisol in patients exposed to pre-surgical stress. *Experimental and Clinical Endocrinology, 102* (2), 118–120.

Minson, R. (1992). A sonic birth. In D. Campbell (Ed.), *Music and miracles* (pp. 89–97). Wheaton, IL: Quest Books.

Modell, A. H. (1990). *Other times, other realities: Towards a theory of psychoanalytic treatment.* Cambridge, MA: Harvard University Press.

Molino, J. (2000). Toward an evolutionary theory of music and language. In N. L Wallin, B. Merker, & S. Brown (Eds.), *The origins of music* (pp. 165–176). Cambridge, MA: MIT Press.

Moore, J. C. (1988). *Neuroanatomy simplified.* Mexico: Centro de Aprendizaje de Cuernayaca.

Moore, T. (1992). *Care of the soul.* New York: HarperCollins.

Moreno, J. J. (1999). *Acting your inner music: Music therapy and psychodrama.* St. Louis, MO: MMB Music, Inc.

Morris, S. E. (1993). Recapturing the intuitive in therapy and education. In R. Russell (Ed.), *Using the whole brain: Integrating the right and left brain with Hemi-Sync sound patterns* (pp. 139–147). Norfolk, VA: Hampton Roads Publishing Co.

Morton, L. L., Kershner, J. R., & Siegel, L. S. (1990). The potential for therapeutic applications of music on problems related to memory and attention. *Journal of Music Therapy, 27* (4), 195–208.

Moses, H. G. (2000). Music as a self-organizing stream of energetic information. *Bridges, 11* (2), 15–16.

Mountcastle, V. B. (1978). An organizing principle for cerebral function: The unit module and the distributed system. In G. M. Edelman & V. B. Mountcastle (Eds.), *The mindful brain* (pp. 7–50). Cambridge, MA: MIT Press.

Mountcastle, V. B. (1997). The columnar organization of the neocortex. *Brain, 120,* 701–722.

Mpitsos, G. J., Burton, R. M., Jr., Creech, H. C., & Sonila, S. O. (1988). Evidence for chaos in spike trains of neurons that generate rhythm motor patterns. *Research Bulletin, 21,* 529–538.

Munro, S. (1984). *Music therapy in palliative/hospice care.* St. Louis, MO: MMB Music, Inc.

Munro, S., & Mount, B. (1978). Music therapy in palliative care. *Canadian Medical Association Journal, 119* (9), 1029–1034.

Musha, T. (1981). 1-f fluctuation in biological systems. In P. H. E. Meijer, R. D. Mountain, & R. J. Soulen Jr. (Eds.), *Sixth International Conference on Noise in Physical Systems* (pp. 143–146). National Bureau of Standards Special Publication, 614. Washington, DC: National Bureau of Standards.

Myss, C. (1996). *Anatomy of the spirit.* New York: Crown Publishers.

Nagler, J. C., & Lee, M. H. M. (1989). Music therapy using computer music technology. In M. H. M. Lee (Ed.), *Rehabilitation, music and human well-being* (pp. 226–241). St. Louis, MO: MMB Music, Inc.

Nakada, T., Fujii, Y., Suzuki, K., & Kwell, I. L. (1998). "Musical brain" revealed by Highfield (3 tesla) functional MRI. *NeuroReport, 9,* 3853–3856.

National Association for Music Therapy. (1960). *A career in music therapy* (pamphlet). Lawrence, KS: National Association for Music Therapy.

National Association for Music Therapy. (1983). Standards of clinical practice. *Music Therapy Perspectives, 1* (2), 13–16.

National Association for Music Therapy. (1994). *NAMT member sourcebook 1994.* Silver Spring, MD: National Association for Music Therapy.

Nauta, W. J. H., & Feirtag, M. (1986). *Fundamental neuroanatomy.* New York: W. H. Freeman & Co.

Needleman, J. (1975). *A sense of the cosmos.* New York: E. P. Dutton.

Neher, A. (1961). Auditory driving observed with scalp electrodes in normal subjects. *Electroencephalography and Clinical Neurophysiology, 13,* 449–451.

Neher, A. (1962). A physiological explanation of unusual behavior in ceremonies involving drums. *Human Biology, 34* (2), 151–160.

Nelson, D. I., Anderson, V. G., & Gonzales, A. D. (1984). Music activities as therapy for children with autism and other pervasive developmental disorders. *Journal of Music Therapy, 21* (3), 100–116.

Nettl, B. (1956a). Aspects of primitive and folk music relevant to music therapy. In E. T. Gaston (Ed.), *Music therapy 1955* (pp. 36–39). Lawrence, KS: National Association for Music Therapy.

Nettl, B. (1956b). *Music in primitive culture.* Cambridge, MA: Harvard University Press.

Nettl, B., & Bohlman, P. V. (Eds.). (1991). *Comparative musicology and the anthropology of music.* Chicago: University of Chicago Press.

Neumann, E. (1956). *The psyche and the transformation of the reality planes in spring.* Dallas: Spring Publications.

Newberg, A., d'Aquil, E., & Rause, V. (2001). *Why God won't go away.* New York: Ballantine Books.

Newman, J., Rosenbach, J. H., Burns, K., Latimer, B. C., Motocha, H. R., & Vogt, E. R. (1995). An experimental list of the "Mozart effect": Does listening to his music improve spatial ability? *Perceptual and Motor Skills, 81* (3), 1379–1387.

Newton, N. (1996). *Foundations of understanding.* Philadelphia: John Benjamins.

Ngugi, T. (1993). *Moving the center: The struggle for cultural freedoms.* London: James Currey, Ltd.

Nicosia, G. J. (1994). The quantitative analysis of electroencephalography representing a localized psychogenic amnesia and its resolution by eye movement desensitization and reprocessing psychotherapy. Paper presented at International EMDR Conference, Sunnyvale, CA.

Nocera, S. (1979). *Reaching the special learner through music.* Morristown, NJ: Silver-Burdett.

Nordenström, B. E. W. (1983). *Biologically closed electric circuits*. Stockholm: Nordic Medical Publications.

Nordoff, P., & Robbins, C. (1971). *Music therapy for handicapped children*. New York: St. Martin's Press.

Nordoff, P., & Robbins, C. (1977). *Creative music therapy*. New York: John Day Co.

Norris, P. (2000). Clinical work on the new frontier using elements of the map. *Bridges, 11* (4), 4–5.

Noy, P. (1993). How music conveys emotion. In S. Feder, R. L. Karmel, & G. H. Pollock (Eds.), *Psychoanalytic explorations in music* (pp. 125–149). Madison, WI: International Universities.

O'Connell, D. F., & Alexander, C. N. (1994). *Self-recovery: Treating addictions using transcendent meditation and Maharishi Ayur-Veda*. New York: Haworth Press.

O'Donohue, J. (1997). *Anam Cara: A book of Celtic wisdom*. New York: HarperCollins.

Offer, D. (2000, June). The psychological world of the aging baby boomers. *Journal of American Academy of Child and Adolescent Psychiatry*.

Ogden, P. (1996). Hakomi integrative somatics: Hands-on psychotherapy. *Bridges, 7* (1), 4–7, 16.

Ohno, S. (1988). On periodicities governing the construction of genes and proteins. *Anim Genet, 19* (4), 305–316.

Ohno, S., & Ohno, M. (1986). The all pervasive principle of repetitious recurrence governs not only coding sequence construction but also human endeavor in musical composition. *Immunogenetics, 24*, 71–78.

Olariu, S., & Popescu, J. (1985). The quantum effect of electromagnetic fluxes. *Review of Modern Physics, 57*, 339.

Olds, C. (1984). *Fetal response to music*. Wickford, England: Runwell Hospital.

Olds, J. (1962). Hypothalamic substrates of reward. *Physiological Review, 42*, 554–604.

O'Loughlin, P. (1995). Meetings with unsounded voice. In C. Kenny (Ed.), *Listening, playing, creating: Essays on the power of sound* (pp. 161–164). Albany: State University of New York Press.

Ornish, D. (1998). *Love and survival*. New York: HarperCollins.

Ornstein, R. (1986). *Multimind*. Boston: Houghton Mifflin.

Ornstein, R. (1991). *The evolution of consciousness: The origins of the way we think*. New York: Simon & Schuster.

Ornstein, R., & Sobel, D. (1987). *The healing brain*. New York: Simon & Schuster.

Ornstein, R., & Thompson, R. (1984). *The amazing brain*. Boston: Houghton Mifflin.

Oshman, D. T. (1996, October). Acupuncture and related methods. *Journal of Bodywork and Movement Therapies*, 40–43.

Ott, E., Grebogi, C., & Yorke, J. A. (1990). Controlling chaos. *Physical Review Letters, 64* (11), 1194–1196.

Otto, R. ([1923] 1958). *The idea of the holy*. J. Harvey (Trans.). London: Oxford University Press.

Oubre, A. (1997). *Instinct and revelation: Reflections on the origins of numinous perception*. Amsterdam: Gordon & Breach.

Oudshoorn, N. (1966). A natural order of things? Reproductive sciences and the politics of othering. In G. Robertson, M. Marsh, L. Tichner, J. Bird, B. Curtis, & T. Putnam (Eds.), *Future natural*. London: Routledge.

Overy, K. (2000). Dyslexia, temporal processing and music: The potential of music as an early learning aid for dyslexic children. *Journal for Research in Psychology of Music and Music Education*, 28, 218–229.

Pal'tsev, Y. I., & El'ner, A. M. (1967). Change in the functional state of the segmental apparatus of the spinal cord under influence of sound stimuli and its role in voluntary movement. *Biophysics*, 12, 1219–1226.

Panneton, R. K. (1985). Prenatal auditory experience with melodies: Effects on postnatal auditory preferences in human newborns. Ph.D. dissertation, University of North Carolina.

Papousek, H., & Papousek, M. (1981). Musical elements in the infant's vocalization: Their significance for communication, cognition, and creativity. In L. P. Lipsit, & C. K. Rovee-Collier (Eds.), *Advances in infancy research*, vol. 1 (pp. 163–224). Norwood, NJ: Ablex.

Parker, A. (1998). *How to choose music to support physiological and emotional processes: A neuro-psychological approach*. Unpublished MS, Prescott College.

Parkhurst, S. J. (1998). Mi, my self and E.I.: Effects of vibroacoustic music on symptom reduction of patients with environmental illness. *Dissertation Abstracts International*, 59 (10), 5296B (University Microfilms No. AAG9910831).

Pearson, E. N. (1957). *Space, time and self*. Wheaton, IL: Theosophical Publishing House.

Peat, F. D. (1992a). A science of harmony and gentle center. In B. Rubik (Ed.), *The interrelationship between mind and matter* (pp. 191–206). Philadelphia: Center for Frontier Sciences.

Peat, F. D. (1992b). Towards a process theory of healing: Energy, activity, and global form. *Subtle Energies*, 3 (2), 1–40.

Peat, F. D. (1995). Chaos: The geometrization of thought. In R. Robertson, & A. Combs (Eds.), *Chaos theory in psychology and the life sciences* (pp. 359–372). Mahwah, NJ: Lawrence Erlbaum Associates, Inc.

Peay, P. (1999). Beyond the ego. *Common Boundary*, 17 (6), 18–25.

Pecci, E. F. (1997). Foreword in W. A. Tiller, *Science and human transformation: Subtle energies, intentionality and consciousness* (pp. xiii–xix). Walnut Creek, CA: Pavior Publishing.

Peitgen, H-O. (1993). The causality principle, deterministic law and chaos. In J. Holt (Ed.), *Chaos: The new science* (pp. 35–44). Lanham, MD: University Press of America, Inc.

Peitgen, H-O., & Saupe, S. (1989). *The science of fractal images*. Berlin: Springer-Verlag.

Pellionisz, A. J. (1989). Neural geometry: The need of researching association of covariant and contravariant coordinates that organize a cognitive space by relating multisensory-multimotor representations. In *International Joint Conference on Neural Networks*, vol. 1 (pp. 711–715). San Diego: IEEE.

Pennebaker, J. W., Keicolt-Glaser, J. K., & Glaser, R. (1988). Disclosure of traumas and immune function: Health implications for psychotherapy. *Journal of Consulting and Clinical Psychology, 56,* 239–245.

Penrose, R. (1989). *The emperor's new mind: Concerning computers, minds, and the laws of physics.* New York: Oxford University Press.

Pepper, D. M. (1982). Nonlinear optical phase conjunction. *Optical Engineer, 21,* 155.

Peretz, I. (1993). Auditory agnosia: A functional analysis. In S. McAdams & E. Bigand (Eds.), *Thinking in sound: The cognitive psychology of human audition* (pp. 199–230). Oxford: Oxford University Press.

Peretz, I., & Morais, J. (1993). Specificity for music. In F. Boller & J. Grafman (Eds.), *Handbook of neuropsychology,* vol. 8 (pp. 373–390). New York: Elsevier.

Pert, C. (1997). *Molecules of emotion: Why we feel the way we feel.* New York: Scribner.

Pert, C., Ruff, M., Weber, R. J., & Herkenham, M. (1985). Neuropeptides and their receptors: A psychosomatic network. *Journal of Immunology, 135* (2), 820–826.

Peters, J. (1987). *Music therapy: An introduction.* Springfield, IL: Charles C. Thomas Publishers, Ltd.

Peters, J. (2000). *Music therapy: An introduction,* 2d ed. Springfield, IL: Charles C. Thomas Publishers, Ltd.

Piaget, J. (1977). *The essential Piaget.* New York: Basic Books.

Piaget, J. (1980). *Adaptation and intelligence.* Chicago: University of Chicago Press.

Pickover, C. A. (1994). *Chaos in wonderland.* New York: St. Martin's Press.

Picone, M., Goldberger, Z., Schlaug, G., Bly, B. M., Tnagaraj, V., Edelman, R. R., & Warach, S. (1997). Neuroanatomical correlates of absolute pitch. *Cognitive Neuroscience Society Abstracts,* 88.

Pierce, J. (1999). Passive nonlinearities in acoustics. In P. R. Cook (Ed.), *Music, cognition, and computerized sound* (pp. 277–284). Cambridge, MA: MIT Press.

Pinker, S. (1997). *How the mind works.* New York: W. W. Norton & Co., Inc.

Plach, T. (1980). *The creative use of music in group therapy.* Springfield, IL: Charles C. Thomas.

Podolsky, E. (Ed.). (1954). *Music therapy.* New York: Philosophical Library.

Polk, C., & Postow, E. (1986). *CRC handbook of biological effects of electromagnetic fields.* Boca Raton, FL: CRC Press.

Polkinghorne, J. (1993). Chaos and cosmos: A theological approach. In J. Holt (Ed.), *Chaos: The new science* (pp. 105–118). Lanham, MD: University Press of America.

Pollack, N., & Namazi, K. (1992). The effect of music participation on the social behavior of Alzheimer's disease patients. *Journal of Music Therapy, 29* (1), 54–62.

Ponath, L. H., & Bitcon, C. H. (1972). A behavioral analysis of Orff-Schulwerk. *Journal of Music Therapy, 9* (2), 56–63.

Popp, F-A., & Becker, G. (1989). *Electromagnetic bio-information.* Munich: Urban & Schwarzenberg.

Popper, K. (1982). *Quantum theory and the schism in physics.* Totowa, NJ: Rowman & Littlefield.

Popper, K. (1983). *Realism and the aim of science.* London: Hutchinson.

Popper, K., & Eccles, J. (1977). *The self and its brain*. Berlin: Springer International.

Prassas, S. G., Thaut, M. H., McIntosh, G. G., & Rice, R. R. (1997). Effects of auditory rhythmic cueing on gait kinematic parameters in hemiparetic stroke patients. *Gait and Posture, 6,* 218–223.

Pratt, C. C. ([1931] 1968). *The meaning of music,* 2d ed. New York: Johnson Reprint Corp.

Preisler, A., Gallasch, E., & Schulter, G. (1989). Hemisphere asymmetry and the processing of harmonies in music. *International Journal of Neuroscience, 47,* 131–140.

Pressman, M. (2002). Exploring the invisible realm with spiritual psychotherapy. *Bridges, 12* (4), 11–15, 18.

Presti, G. M. (1984). A levels system approach to music therapy with severely behaviorally handicapped children in the public school system. *Journal of Music Therapy, 21* (3), 117–125.

Pribram, K. H. (1982). What the fuss is all about. In K. Wilber (Ed.), *The holographic paradigm and other paradoxes* (pp. 27–34). Boulder: Shambhala.

Pribram, K. H. (1991). *Brain and perception: Holonomy and structure in figural processing*. Hillsdale, NJ: Lawrence Erlbaum.

Prickett, C. A., & Moore, R. S. (1991). The use of music to aid memory of Alzheimer's patients. *Journal of Music Therapy, 28* (2), 101–110.

Priestley, M. (1975). *Music therapy in action*. St. Louis, MO: Magnamusic-Baton.

Priestley, M. (1994). *Essays on analytical music therapy*. Gilsum, NH: Barcelona Publishers.

Prigogine, I. (1993). Time, dynamics and chaos: Integrating Poincaré's "non-integrable systems." In J. Holt (Ed.), *Chaos: The new science* (pp. 55–88). Lanham, MD: University Press of America.

Prigogine, I., & Stengers, L. (1984). *Order out of chaos: Man's new dialogue with nature*. New York: Bantam.

Prince, R. (1982). Shamans and endorphins: Hypothesis for a synthesis. *Ethos, 10* (4).

Proust, M. (1981). *Remembrance of things past,* vol. 3. London: Chatto & Windus.

Puharich, H. K. (1984). Method and means of shielding a person from the polluting effects of ELF magnetic waves and other environmental pollution. U.S. Patent no. 616-183.

Purves, D., Augustine, G. J., Fitzpatrick, D., Katz, L. C., LaMantia, A-S., & McNamara, J. O. (1997). *Neuroscience*. Sunderland, MA: Sinauer Associates, Inc.

Putnam, F. W. (1989). The psychophysiologic investigation of multiple personality disorder. *Psychiatric Clinics of North America, 7* (1), 31–39.

Quinn, J. F. (1989). On healing, wholeness, and the healing effect. *Health Care, 1010,* 552–556.

Quinn, J. F. (1998). Caring and healing: A nursing model for an integrative health care system. *Bridges, 9* (2), 1, 4–7, 19.

Rabin, B. S., Cohn, S., Ganguli, R., Lysle, D. J., & Cunnick, J. E. (1989). Bidirectional interaction between the central nervous system and the immune system. *Critical Reviews in Immunology, 9* (4), 279–312.

Radcliffe-Brown, A. R. (1948). *The Andaman islanders*. New York: Free Press.

Radocy, R. E., & Boyle, J. D. (1997). *The psychological foundations of musical behavior*, 3d ed. Springfield, IL: Charles C. Thomas.

Rael, J. (1993). *Being and vibration*. Tulsa, OK: Council Oak Books.

Rao, K. R. (1992). Meditation and mind/matter interface. In B. Rubik (Ed.), *The interrelationship between mind and matter* (pp. 111–142). Philadelphia: Center for Frontier Sciences.

Rapp, P. (1993). Chaos in neuroscience: Cautionary tales from the frontier. *Biologist, 40* (2), 89–94.

Rapp, P. E., Zimmerman, I. O., Albano, A. M., de Guzman, C., & Greenbaum, N. N. (1985). Dynamics of spontaneous neural activity in the simian motor cortex: The dimensions of chaotic neurons. *Physics Letters, 110A*, 335–338.

Rauscher, E. A., & Rubik, B. A. (1983). Human volitional effects on a model bacterial system. *Psi Research, 2*, 38.

Rauscher, F. H., Robinson, K. D., & Jens, J. J. (1998). Improved maze learning through early music exposure in rats. *Neurological Research, 20*, 427–432.

Rauscher, F. H., Shaw, G., & Ky, N. (1995). Listening to Mozart enhances spatial-temporal reasoning: Towards a neurophysiological basis. *Neuroscience Letters, 125*, 44–47.

Reich, W. (1949). *Character analysis*. New York: Noonday Press.

Reid, B. L. (1989). On the nature of growth based on experiments designed to reveal a structure for laboratory space. *Medical Hypothesis, 29*, 127.

Reid, D. H., Hill, B. K., Rawers, R. J., & Montegar, C. A. (1975). The use of contingent music in teaching social skills to a nonverbal, hyperactive boy. *Journal of Music Therapy, 12* (1), 2–18.

Reimer, B. (1989). *A philosophy of music education*. Englewood Cliffs, NJ: Prentice Hall.

Rein, G. (1978). An exosomatic effect on neurotransmitter metabolism in mice. Paper presented at the Second International S.P.R. Conference, Cambridge University.

Rein, G. (1986). A psychokinetic effect on neurotransmitter metabolism: Alterations in the degradative enzyme MAO. *Research in Parapsychology*, 77.

Rein, G. (1988). Biological interactions with scalar energy–cellular mechanisms of action. *Proceedings of 7th International Association of Psychotronics Research*.

Rein, G. (1989). The effect of non-Hertzian scalar waves on the immune system. *Journal of U.S. Psychotronics Association, 1* (2), 15.

Rein, G. (1991). Utilization of a cell culture bioassay for measuring quantum field generated from a modified caduceus coil. *Proceedings of 26th Intersociety Energy Conversion Engineering Conference, 4*, 440.

Rein, G. (1992). The scientific basis for healing with subtle energy. In L. Laskow, *Healing with love* (pp. 279–391). San Francisco: HarperSanFrancisco.

Rein, G. (n.d.). *Quantum biology*. Miller Place, NY: G. Rein.

Rein, G., & Korins, K. (1987, June). Inhibition of neurotransmitter uptake in neuronal cells by pulsed EM fields. *Proceedings of the 9th Bioelectromagnetic Society*.

Rein, G., & McCraty, R. (1993a). Local and non-local effects of coherent heart frequencies on conformational changes of DNA. *Proceedings of the Joint USPA/IAPR Psychotronics Conference*, Milwaukee.

Rein, G., & McCraty, R. (1993b). Modulation of DNA by coherent heart frequencies. *Proceedings of Third Annual Conference of ISSSEEM*, Boulder.

Remen, R. N. (1997). Initiation. *Noetic Sciences Review*, 44, 10 17.

Remen, R. N. (1998). On defining spirit. *Noetic Sciences Review*, 47, 64.

Restak, R. M. (1979). *The brain: The last frontier*. Garden City, NY: Doubleday.

Restak, R. M. (1986). *The infant mind*. Garden City, NY: Doubleday.

Reuer, B., & Crowe, B. J. (1995). *Best practice in music therapy: Utilizing group percussion strategies for promoting volunteerism in the well older adult*. San Diego: University Center on Aging.

Richards, T. L., Lappin, M. S., Acosta-Urquidi, J., Kraft, G. H., Heide, A. C., Lawrie, F. W., Merrill, G. B., & Cunningham, C. A. (1997). Double blind study of pulsing magnetic field effects on multiple sclerosis. *The Journal of Alternative and Complementary Medicine*, 3 (1), 21–29.

Richardson, K. (2000). *The making of intelligence*. New York: Columbia University Press.

Richman, B. (1993). On the evolution of speech: Singing as the middle term. *Journal of Current Anthropology*, 34, 721–722.

Richman, B. (2000). On rhythm, repetition, and meaning. In N. L Wallin, B. Merker, & S. Brown (Eds.), *The origins of music* (pp. 301–314). Cambridge, MA: MIT Press.

Rider, M. (1977). The relationship between auditory and visual perception on tasks employing Piaget's concept of conservation. *Journal of Music Therapy*, 14 (3), 126–138.

Rider, M. (1981). The assessment of cognitive functioning level through musical perception. *Journal of Music Therapy*, 18 (3), 110 119.

Rider, M. (1985). Entrainment mechanisms are involved in pain reduction, muscle relaxation, and music-mediated imagery. *Journal of Music Therapy*, 22 (4), 183–192.

Rider, M. (1992). Mental shifts and resonance: Necessities for healing? *ReVision*, 14 (3), 149–157.

Rider, M. (1997). *The rhythmic language of health and disease*. St. Louis, MO: MMB Music, Inc.

Rider, M., Achterberg, J., Lawlis, G. F., Goven, A., Toledo, R., & Butler, J. R. (1990). Effect of immune system imagery on secretory IgA. *Biofeedback and Self-Regulation*, 15, 317–333.

Rider, M., Mickey, C., Weldon, C., & Hawkinson, R. (1991). The effects of toning, listening, and singing on psychophysiological responses. In C. Maranto (Ed.), *Applications of music in medicine* (pp. 73–84). Washington, DC: National Association for Music Therapy.

Rider, M. S., Floyd, J. W., & Kirkpatrick, J. (1985). The effect of music, imagery, and relaxation on adrenal cortico-steroids and the re-entrainment of circadian rhythms. *Journal of Music Therapy*, 22 (1), 46–58.

Rider, M. S., & Weldin, C. (1990). Imagery, improvisation, and immunity. *Arts in Psychotherapy, 17* (3), 211–216.

Riego, E., Silva, A., & De la Fuente, J. (1995). The sound of the DNA language. *Biological Research, 28* (3), 197–204.

Rimoldi, H. (1951). Personal tempo. *Abnormal Social Psychology, 42,* 283–303.

Robb, S. L. (1996). Techniques in song writing: Restoring emotional and physical well-being in adolescents who have been traumatically injured. *Music Therapy Perspectives, 14,* 30–37.

Robb, S. L. (2000). The effect of therapeutic music interventions on the behavior of hospitalized children in isolation: Developing a contextual support model of music therapy. *Journal of Music Therapy, 37* (2), 118–146.

Robb, S. L., Nichols, R. J., Rutan, R. L., Bishop, B. L., & Parker, J. C. (1995). The effects of music assisted relaxation on preoperative anxiety. *Journal of Music Therapy, 32* (1), 2–21.

Robbins, T. (1998). The pharmacology of thought and emotion. In S. Rose (Ed.), *From brains to consciousness* (pp. 33–52). Princeton, NJ: Princeton University Press.

Robertson, G., Marsh, M., Tichner, L., Bird, J., Curtis, B., & Putnam, T. (Eds.). (1966). *Future natural.* London: Routledge.

Robertson, I. H. (1999). *Mind sculpture: Unlocking your brain's potential.* London: Bantam Press.

Robertson, R., & Combs, A. (Eds.). (1995). *Chaos theory in psychology and the life sciences.* Mahwah, NJ: Laurence Erlbaum Associates.

Robinson, J. (Ed.). (1997). *Music and meaning.* Ithaca, NY: Cornell University Press.

Roederer, J. G. (1982). Physical and neuropsycholgical foundations of music. In M. Clynes (Ed.), *Music, mind, and brain* (pp. 37–46). New York: Plenum Press.

Roehmann, F. L., & Wilson, F. R. (1988). *The biology of music making: Proceedings of the 1984 Denver Conference.* St. Louis, MO: MMB, Inc.

Rogers, A., & Flemming, P. (1981). Rhythm and melody in speech therapy for the neurologically impaired. *Music Therapy, 1,* 33–38.

Rogers, L. (1976). Human EEG response to certain rhythmic pattern stimuli, with possible relation to EEG lateral asymmetry measures and EEG correlates of chanting. Ph.D. dissertation, Department of Physiology, University of California, Los Angeles.

Rogers, L., & Walters, D. (1981). Methods for finding single generators, with application to auditory driving of human EEG by complex stimuli. *Journal of Neuroscience Methods, 4,* 257–265.

Rogers, W. R. (1968). Order and chaos in psychopathology and ontology. In P. Homans (Ed.), *The dialogue between theology and psychology: A challenge to traditional correlations of order to mental health and ultimate reality, and of chaos to mental illness and alienation* (pp. 249–262). Chicago: University of Chicago Press.

Roof, W. C. (1999). *Spiritual marketplace.* Princeton, NJ: Princeton University Press.

Root-Bernstein, R. S. (1989). *Discovering.* Cambridge, MA: Harvard University Press.

Rose, S. (1998a). Brain, mind and the world. In S. Rose (Ed.), *From brains to consciousness* (pp. 1–17). Princeton, NJ: Princeton University Press.

Rose, S. (1998b). *Lifelines: Biology beyond determinism*. New York: Oxford University Press.

Rose, S. (Ed.). (1998c). *From brains to consciousness*. Princeton: Princeton University Press.

Roskam, K. S. (1993). *Feeling the sound: The influence of music on behavior*. San Francisco: San Francisco Press.

Rossi, E. L. (1986). *The psychobiology of mind–body healing*. New York: W. W. Norton & Co.

Rossignol, S. (1971). Reaction of spinal motor neurons to musical sound. *Proceedings XXV International Physics Congress IX*, abstract 48.

Rossignol, S., & Melville-Jones, G. (1976). Audio-spinal influences in man studied by the H-reflex and its possible role in rhythmic movement synchronized to sound. *Electroencephalagraphy and Clinical Neurophysiology, 41*, 83–92.

Rothstein, E. (1995). *Emblems of mind*. New York: Avon Books.

Rubik, B. (1993). Energy medicine: A challenge for science. *Noetic Sciences Review, 28*, 311–318.

Rubik, B. (Ed.). (1992). *The interrelationship between mind and matter*. Philadelphia: Center for Frontier Science.

Rudhyar, D. (1982). *The magic of tone and the art of music*. Boulder: Shambhala Publications.

Rudolph, G. (1988). *Dreamsinging*. Unpublished MS, Human Relations Institute, San Francisco.

Rugenstein, L. (1996). Wilber's spectrum model of transpersonal psychology and its application to music therapy. *Music Therapy, 14* (1), 9–28.

Ruggieri, V., & Milizia, M. (1982). Rhythmic reproduction, arousal, and chosen time. *Perceptual Motor Skills, 54*, 527–537.

Russell, R. (Ed.). (1993). *Using the whole brain: Integrating the right and left brain with Hemi-Sync sound patterns*. Norfolk, VA: Hampton Roads Publishing Co.

Ruud, E. (1978). *Music therapy and its relationship to current treatment theories*. St. Louis, MO: Magnamusic-Baton, Inc.

Ruud, E. (1995). Improvisation as a liminal experience: Jazz and music therapy as modern "rites de passage." In C. Kenny (Ed.), *Listening, playing, creating: Essays on the power of sound* (pp. 91–117). Albany: State University of New York Press.

Ruud, E. (1998a). *Music therapy: Improvisation, communication, and culture*. Gilsum, NH: Barcelona Publishers.

Ruud, E. (1998b). Science as metacritique. *Journal of Music Therapy, 35* (3), 218–224.

Ruud, E. (Ed.). (1986). *Music and health*. Oslo: Norsk Musikforiag A/S.

Sacks, C. (1948). *Our musical heritage*. New York: Prentice Hall.

Sacks, C. (1953). *Rhythm and tempo: A study in music history*. New York: Norton & Co.

Sacks, O. (1985). *The man who mistook his wife for a hat*. New York: Summit Books.

Sacks, O. (1990). *Awakenings*. New York: HarperCollins.

Sacks, O. (1998). Music and the brain. In C. M. Tomaino (Ed.), *Clinical applications of music in neurologic rehabilitation* (pp. 1–18). St. Louis, MO: MMB Music, Inc.

Sadigh, M. (1993). Insight-oriented psychotherapy. In R. Russell (Ed.), *Using the whole brain: Integrating the right and left brain with Hemi-Sync sound patterns* (pp. 176–179). Norfolk, VA: Hampton Roads Publishing Co.

Sadigh, M., & Kozicky, P. W. (1993). The effects of Hemi-Sync on electrocortical activity. In R. Russell (Ed.), *Using the whole brain: Integrating the right and left brain with Hemi-Sync sound patterns* (pp. 217–226). Norfolk, VA: Hampton Roads Publishing Co.

Safranek, M., Koshland, G., & Raymond, G. (1982). Effect of auditory rhythm on muscle activity. *Perceptual Motor Skills, 46*, 883–894.

Sahtouris, E. (2002). Globalization: An evolutionary leap? *Noetic Sciences Review, 58*, 17, 21.

Sammella, L. (Ed.). (1976). *Kundalini: Psychosis or transcendence?* San Francisco: H. S. Dakin Co.

Sandyk, R. (1992). Magnetic fields in the therapy of Parkinsonism. *International Journal of Neuroscience, 66*, 209–235.

Sanford, J. A. (1987). *The kingdom within*, rev. ed. San Francisco: Harper & Row.

Saperston, B. (1973). The use of music in establishing communication with an autistic mentally retarded boy. *Journal of Music Therapy, 10* (4), 184–188.

Sardello, R. (1995). *Love and the soul*. New York: HarperCollins.

Sarraille, J., & Di Falco, P. (1992). *Fd3 fractal factory software*. Department of Philosophy and Cognitive Studies, 80 West Vista Avenue, Turlock, CA, 95381.

Saver, J., & Rabin, J. (1997). The neural substrates of religious experience. *Journal of Neuropsychiatry, 9*, 498.

Scarantino, B. A. (1987). *Music power*. New York: Dodd, Mead & Co.

Scartelli, J. (1984). The effect of EMG biofeedback and sedative music, EMG biofeedback only, and sedative music only on frontalis muscle relaxation ability. *Journal of Music Therapy, 21* (2), 67–78.

Scartelli, J. (1991). A rationale for subcortical involvement in human response to music. In C. D. Maranto (Ed.), *Applications of music in medicine* (pp. 30–40). Washington, DC: National Association for Music Therapy.

Scartelli, J. (1992). Music therapy and psychoneuroimmunology. In R. Spintge & R. Droh (Eds.), *Music medicine* (pp. 137–141). St. Louis, MO: MMB Music, Inc.

Scartelli, J., & Borling, J. (1986). The effects of sequenced versus simultaneous and sedative music on frontalis relaxation training. *Journal of Music Therapy, 23* (3), 157–165.

Schachter, H. M. (1993). Fear, cancer, and Hemi-Sync: A new departure. In R. Russell (Ed.), *Using the whole brain: Integrating the right and left brain with Hemi-Sync sound patterns* (pp. 56–64). Norfolk, VA: Hampton Roads Publishing Co.

Schaffer, W., Truty, G., & Fulmer, S. (1988). *Dynamical systems software*. PO Box 35241, Tucson, AZ, 85740.

Scheiby, B. B. (1998). The role of musical transference in analytical music therapy. In K. Bruscia (Ed.), *The dynamics of music psychotherapy* (pp. 213–247). Gilsum, NH: Barcelona Publishers.

Scheier, C., & Tschacher, W. (1996). Appropriate algorithms for nonlinear time series analysis in psychology. In W. Sulis & A. Combs (Eds.), *Nonlinear dynamics in human behavior* (pp. 27–43). Singapore: World Scientific.

Scherer, K., & Ekman, P. (Eds.). (1984). *Approaches to emotion.* Hillsdale, NJ: Erlbaum.

Scherg, H. (1987). Psychosocial factors and disease bias in breast cancer patients. *Psychosomatic Medicine, 49,* 302–312.

Schlaug, G., Janche, L., Huang, Y., Staiger, J. F., & Steinmetz, H. (1995a). Increased corpus callosum size in musicians. *Neuropsychology, 33,* 1047–1055.

Schlaug, G., Janche, L., Huang, Y., & Steinmetz, H. (1995b). In vivo evidence of structural brain asymmetry in musicians. *Science, 267,* 699–701.

Schlitz, M., Taylor, E., & Lewis, N. (1998). Toward a noetic model of medicine. *Noetic Sciences Review, 47,* 44–52.

Schneck, D. J. (1997). A paradigm for the physiology of human adaptation. In D. J. Schneck & J. K. Schneck (Eds.), *Music in human adaptation* (pp. 1–22). Blacksburg: Virginia Polytechnic Institute and State University.

Schneck, D. J., & Schneck, J. K. (Eds.). (1997). *Music in human adaptation.* Blacksburg: Virginia Polytechnic Institute and State University.

Schneider, C. (2001). Early childhood brain development and the potential for violence. *Bridges, 12* (2), 10–12.

Schneider, E. H. (Ed.). (1962). *Music therapy 1961.* Lawrence, KS: Allen Press.

Schneider, E. H. (Ed.). (1963). *Music therapy 1962.* Lawrence, KS: Allen Press.

Schoen, Max (Ed.). (1927). *The effects of music.* New York: Harcourt, Brace.

Schoner, G., & Kelso, J. A. S. (1989). Dynamic pattern generation in behavioral and neural system. In K. L. Kelmer & D. E. Koshland Jr. (Eds.), *Molecules to models: Advances in neuroscience* (pp. 311–324). Washington, DC: American Association of the Advancement of Science.

Schoor, J. A. (1993). Music and pattern change in chronic pain. *Advanced Nursing Science, 15* (33), 27–36.

Schore, A. N. (1994). *Affect regulation and the origin of the self: The neurobiology of emotional development.* Hillsdale, NH: Erlbaum.

Schreiber, D. (Ed.). (1967). *Profile of the school dropout.* New York: Vintage Books.

Schroeder-Sheker, T. (1993). Music for dying: A personal account of the new field of musical thanantology—History, theories, and clinical narratives. *ADVANCES, The Journal of Mind–Body Health, 9* (1) (Winter), 36–48.

Schullion, P. M., & Schoen, M. (Eds.). (1948). *Music and medicine.* New York: Schuman.

Schunk, H. A. (1999). The effect of singing paired with signing on receptive vocabulary skills of elementary ESL students. *Journal of Music Therapy, 34* (2), 119–124.

Schutz, A. (n.d.). Making music together: A study in social relationships. In A. Broderson (Ed.), *Alfred Schutz: Collected papers II. Studies in social theory* (pp. 159–178). The Hague.

Schwartz, G. E., Nelson, L., Russik, L. G., & Allen, J. J. B. (1996). Electrostatic body-motion registration and the human antenna-receiver effect: A new method for investigating interpersonal dynamical energy system interactions. *Subtle Energy, 7* (2), 149–184.

Schwartz, G. E., Russik, L. G., & Beltran, J. (1995). Interpersonal hand-energy registration: Evidence for implicit performance and perception. *Subtle Energy, 6* (3), 183–200.

Schwartz, T. (1996). Foreword in K. Wilber, *A brief history of everything* (pp. xi–xiv). Boston: Shambhala.

Scott, A. (1995). *Stairway to the mind.* New York: Springer-Verlag.

Sears, W. (1958). The effect of music on muscle tonus. In E. T. Gaston (Ed.), *Music therapy 1957* (pp. 199–205). Lawrence, KS: McGraw-Hill.

Sears, W. (1968). Processes in music therapy. In E. T. Gaston (Ed.), *Music in therapy* (pp. 30–46). New York: Macmillan.

Seeger, A. (1987). *Why Suza sing.* Cambridge: Cambridge University Press.

Sekeles, C. (1996). *Music: Motion and emotion.* St. Louis, MO: MMB Music Inc.

Seki, H. (1983). Influence of music on memory and education, and the application of its underlying principles to acupuncture. *International Journal of Acupuncture and Electro-therapeutics Research, 8,* 1–16.

Selman, R., & Byrne, D. (1974). A structural analysis of levels of role-taking in middle childhood. *Child Development, 45* (3), 803–806.

Selye, H. (1978). *The stress of life.* New York: McGraw-Hill.

Sergent, J. (1993). Mapping the musician brain. *Human Brain Mapping, 1,* 20–38.

Sergent, J., Zuck, E., Terriats, S., & McDonald, B. (1992). Distributed neural network underlying musical sight-reading and keyboard performance. *Science, 257,* 106–109.

Sessions, R. (1971). *The musical experience of composer, performer, listener.* Princeton, NJ: Princeton University Press.

Shaffer, J. B. P., & Galinsky, M. D. (Eds.). (1974). *Group therapy and sensitivity training.* Englewood Cliffs, NJ: Prentice Hall.

Shafranske, E. P., & Gorsuch, R. L. (1984). Factors associated with the perception of spirituality in psychotherapy. *Journal of Transpersonal Psychology, 16,* 231–241.

Shafranske, E. P., & Maloney, H. N. (1990). Clinical psychologists' religious and spiritual orientation and their practice of psychotherapy. *Psychotherapy, 27,* 72–78.

Shainberg, D. (1973). *The transforming self.* New York: Intercontinental Medical Books.

Shapiro, D. (1990). Meditation, self-control, and control by benevolent other: Issues of content and context. In M. Kwee (Ed.), *Psychotherapy, meditation, and health.* London: EastWest Publications.

Shaw, G. (1999, March). Music as brain builder. *Science, 283,* 2007.

Shaw, G. (2000). *Keeping Mozart in mind.* San Diego: Academic Press.

Shaw, G. L., & Ky, K. N. (1995). Listening to Mozart enhances spatial-temporal reasoning: Towards a neurophysiological basis. *Neuroscience Letters, 185,* 44–47.

Shepard, R. (1999). Cognitive psychology and music. In P. R. Cook (Ed.), *Music, cognition, and computerized sound* (pp. 21–36). Cambridge, MA: MIT Press.

Shephard, R. (1978). Externalization of mental images and the act of creation. In B. S. Randhawa & W. E. Coffman (Eds.), *Visual learning, thinking and communication* (pp. 133–189). San Diego: Academic Press.

Shepherd, L. J. (1993). *Lifting the veil: The feminine face of science.* Boston: Shambhala.

Shetler, D. J. (1990). The inquiry into prenatal musical experience. In F. R. Wilson & F. L. Roehmann (Eds.), *Music and child development* (pp. 44–62). St. Louis, MO: MMB, Inc.

Shi-Jing, L., Hui-Ju, S., Guo, W., & Maranto, C. D. (1991). Music and medicine in China: The effects of music electro-acupuncture on cerebral hemiplegia. In C. Maranto (Ed.), *Applications of music in medicine* (pp. 191–199). Washington, DC: National Association for Music Therapy.

Shulman, H. (1997). *Living at the edge of chaos: Complex systems in culture and psyche.* Zurich: Daimon Verlag.

Shumacher, J. E. (1992). *Religion and mental health.* New York: Oxford University Press.

Shweder, R. A. (1992). *Thinking through culture: Expeditions in cultural psychology* Cambridge, MA: Harvard University Press.

Siegel, B. S. (1986). *Love, medicine and miracles.* New York: Harper & Row.

Siegel, R. K. (1977, October). Hallucinations. *Scientific American, 53–78.*

Siegmeister, E. (1965). *Harmony and melody,* vol. 1. Belmont, CA: Wadsworth Publishing Co., Inc.

Singer, W. (1998). Consciousness from a neurobiological perspective. In S. Rose (Ed.), *From brains to consciousness* (pp. 228–245). Princeton: Princeton University Press.

Skaggs, R. (1997). *Finishing strong: Treating chemical addictions with music and imagery.* St. Louis, MO: MMB Music, Inc.

Skarda, C. A., & Freeman, W. J. (1987). How brains make chaos in order to make sense of the world. *Behavioral and Brain Science, 10,* 161–195.

Skarda, C. A., & Freeman, W. J. (1990). Chaos and the new science of the brain. *Concepts in Neuroscience, 1* (2), 275–285.

Skille, O. (1991). *Vibroacoustic therapy: Manual and reports.* Levanger, Norway: ISUA Publications.

Skille, O. (1992). Vibroacoustic research 1980–1991. In R. Spintge & R. Droh (Eds.), *Music medicine* (pp. 249–266). St. Louis, MO: Magna Music Baton.

Sloboda, J. A. (1985). *The musical mind: The cognitive psychology of music.* Oxford: Clarendon Press.

Slotoroff, C. (1994). Drumming techniques for assertiveness and anger management in short-term psychiatric setting for adult and adolescent survivors of trauma. *Journal of Music Therapy, 12* (2), 111–116.

Smale, S. (1992). What is chaos? In J. Holt (Ed.), *Chaos: The new science* (pp. 89–104). Lanham, MD: University Press of America.

Small, J. (1982). *Transformers: The therapists of the future.* Marina del Rey, CA: DeVorss & Co.

Smith, C. W., & Best, S. (1990). *Electromagnetic man: Health and hazard in the electrical environment.* London: J. M. Dent & Sons, Ltd.

Smith, H. (1989). *Beyond the post-modern mind,* 2d ed. Wheaton, IL: Theosophical Publishing House.

Smith, O. W. (1957). Relationship of rhythm discrimination to motor rhythm performance. *Journal of Applied Psychology, 41,* 365–369.

Smith, W. B. (1964). *The new science.* Ontario: Fern-Graphic.

Smolensky, P. (1988). On the proper treatment of connectionism. *Behavior and Brain Sciences, 11,* 1–74.

Smoll, F., & Schulz, R. (1978). Relationship among measures of preferred tempo and motor rhythm. *Physical Therapy, 62,* 161–168.

Solomon, A. L. (1981). Music in special education before 1930: Hearing and speech development. *Journal of Research in Music Education, 28* (4), 236–242.

Soong, A. C. K., & Stuart, I. J. M. (1989). Evidence of chaotic dynamics in underlying the human alpha-rhythm electroencephalogram. *Biological Cybernetics, 62,* 55–62.

Sornson, R. (1993). Special education. In R. Russell (Ed.), *Using the whole brain: Integrating the right and left brain with Hemi-Sync sound patterns* (pp. 116–122). Norfolk, VA: Hampton Roads Publishing Co.

Soshensky, R. (2001). Music therapy and addiction. *Music Therapy Perspectives, 19* (1), 45–52.

Sperry, R. (1991). In defense of mentalism and emergent interaction. *Journal of Mind and Behavior, 12,* 221–246.

Sperry, R. (1993). Psychology's mentalist paradigm and the religion/science tension. In J. Ashbrook (Ed.), *Brain, culture, and the human spirit: Essays from an emergent evolutionary perspective.* Lanham, MD: University Press of America.

Spiegel, D., Bloom, J. R., Kraemer, H. K., & Gottheil, E. (1989). Effect of psychosocial treatment on survival of patients with metastatic breast cancer. *Lancet, 2,* 888–891.

Spintge, R., & Droh, R. (Eds.). (1992). *Music medicine.* St. Louis, MO: MMB Music, Inc.

Spintge, R. K. W. (1989). The anxiolytic effects of music. In M. H. M. Lee (Ed.), *Rehabilitation, music and human well-being* (pp. 82–97). St. Louis, MO: MMB Music, Inc.

Spurr, B. (2000). Awakening the healing power of spirit in health care. *Bridges, 11* (3), 9–14.

Squire, L. (1987). *Memory and brain.* New York: Oxford University Press.

Squire, L. (1998). Memory and brain systems. In S. Rose (Ed.), *From brains to consciousness* (pp. 53–72). Princeton, NJ: Princeton University Press.

Srinivasan, T. M. (1997). Machines with promise: Electromedicine. *Bridges, 8* (4), 1, 4–6.

Srinivasan, T. M. (2001). Personal peace to global peace: A Tibetan perspective. *Bridges, 12* (2), 4–8.

Srinivasan, T. M. (Ed.). (1988). *Energy medicine around the world.* Phoenix: Gabriel Press.

Standley, J., & Madsen, C. (1990). Comparisons of infant preferences and responses to auditory stimuli: Music, mother, and other female voices. *Journal of Music Therapy, 27* (2), 54–97.

Standley, J. M. (1986). Music research in medical/dental treatment: Meta-analysis and clinical applications. *Journal of Music Therapy, 23* (2), 56–122.

Standley, J. M. (1991). The effect of vibrotactile and auditory stimulation perception on comfort, heart rate and peripheral finger temperature. *Journal of Music Therapy, 28* (3), 120–134.

Staum, M. (1983). Music and rhythmic stimuli in the rehabilitation of gait disorders. *Journal of Music Therapy, 20* (2), 69–87.

Staum, M. (1987). Music notation to improve the speech prosody of hearing impaired children. *Journal of Music Therapy, 24* (3), 146–159.

Steele, A. L. (1968). Programmed use of music to alter uncooperative problem behavior. *Journal of Music Therapy, 5* (4), 103–107.

Steele, A. L. (1984). Music therapy for the learning disabled: Intervention and instruction. *Music Therapy Perspectives, 1* (3), 2–7.

Steele, A. L., & Jorgensen, H. (1971). Effect of contingent preferred music in reducing two stereotyped behaviors of a profoundly retarded child. *Journal of Music Therapy, 8* (4), 139–143.

Steele, K. M., Brown, J. D., & Stoecker, J. A. (1999). Failure to confirm the Rauscher and Shaw description of recovery of the Mozart effect. *Perceptual and Motor Skills, 88* (3), 945–948.

Stein, A. H. (1996). The self-organizing psyche: Nonlinear and neurobiological contributions to psychoanalysis. In W. Sulis & A. Combs (Eds.), *Nonlinear dynamics in human behavior* (pp. 256–275). Singapore: World Scientific.

Stein, A. M. (1991). Music to reduce anxiety during Cesarean births. In C. D. Maranto (Ed.), *Applications of music in medicine* (pp. 163–178). Washington, DC: National Association for Music Therapy.

Steinberg, R. (Ed.). (1995). *Music and the mind machine: The psychophysiology and psychopathology of the sense of music.* Berlin: Springer-Verlag.

Steiner, R. (1983). *The inner nature of music and the experience of tone.* New York: Anthrosophic Press.

Steinke, W. R. (1991). The use of music, relaxation, and imagery in the management of postsurgical pain for scoliosis. In C. Maranto (Ed.), *Applications of music in medicine* (pp. 141–162). Washington, DC: National Association for Music Therapy.

Sternheimer, J. (1983, January). La musque des particles elementaires. *Compte-rendi de l'Academic des Sciences.*

Stewart, R. J. (1987). *Music and the elemental psyche.* Rochester, VT: Destiny Books.

Storr, A. (1992). *Music and the mind.* New York: Ballantine Books.

Stratton, V. N., & Zalanowski, A. (1984). The relationship between music, degree of liking, and self-reported relaxation. *Journal of Music Therapy, 21* (4), 184–192.

Stravinsky, I. (1947). *Poetics of music.* New York: Vintage Books.

Subrahamanian, S., Moinuddin, M., & Kalyansundaram. (1988). Pulsed magnetic fields in therapy. In T. M. Srinivasan (Ed.), *Energy medicine around the world* (pp. 191–203). Phoenix: Gabriel Press.

Sugano, H., Uchida, S., & Kuramoto, I. (1994). A new approach to the studies of subtle energies. *Subtle Energy, 5* (2), 143–166.

Sulis, W., & Combs, A. (Eds.). (1996). *Nonlinear dynamics in human behavior.* Singapore: World Scientific.

Summer, L. (1988). *Imagery and music in the institutional setting.* St. Louis, MO: MMB Music, Inc.

Summer, L. (1996). *Music: The New Age elixir.* Amherst, NY: Prometheus Books.

Sutherland, G., Newman, B., & Rachman, S. (1982). Experimental investigations of the relations between mood and intrusive, unwanted cognitions. *British Journal of Medical Psychology, 55,* 127–138.

Swanwick, K. (1994). *Musical knowledge.* London: Routledge.

Swicord, M. L., & Davis, C.C. (1983). Acoustic oscillations of DNA. *Bioelectromagnetics, 4,* 21.

Takakura, K., Kosugi, Y., Ilebe, J., & Musha, T. (1987). 1/f controlled transcutaneous electrical stimulation for pain relief. In C. M. Van Vliest (Ed.), *Ninth International Conference on Noise in Physical Systems* (pp. 279–282). Singapore: World Scientific.

Talbot, M. (1991). *The holographic universe.* San Francisco: HarperCollins.

Tame, D. (1984). *The secret power of music.* New York: Destiny Books.

Tarnas, R. (1991). *The passion of the Western mind.* New York: Balantine Books.

Tarnas, R. (1998). The great initiation. *Noetic Sciences Review, 47,* 24–31, 57–59.

Tart, C. (1975). *States of consciousness.* New York: E. P. Dutton.

Tart, C. (1983). *Transpersonal psychologies.* El Cerrito, CA: Psychological Processes.

Taylor, A. M. (1976). Process and structure in socio-cultural systems. In E. Jantsch & C. H. Waddington (Eds.), *Evolution and consciousness: Human systems in transitions.* Reading, MA: Addison-Wesley.

Taylor, D. B. (1981). Music in general hospital treatment from 1900–1950. *Journal of Music Therapy, 18* (2), 62–73.

Taylor, D. B. (1997). *Biomedical foundations of music as therapy.* St. Louis, MO: MMB Music, Inc.

Taylor, E., Murphy, M., & Donovan, S. (1997). *The physical and psychological effects of meditation: A review of contemporary research with a comprehensive bibliography: 1931–1996.* Sausalito, CA: Institute of Noetic Sciences.

Taylor, I. A., & Paperte, F. (1958). Current theory and research in the effects of music on human behavior. *Journal of Aesthetic Art Quarterly, 17,* 251–258.

Taylor, J. A., Barry, N. H., & Walls, K. C. (1997). *Music and students at risk: Creative solutions for a national dilemma.* Reston, VA: MENC.

Teich, M. C. (1989). Fractal character of the auditory neural spike train. *IEEE Transactions Biomedical Engineering, 36,* 150–160.

Teich, M. C., Johnson, D. H., Kunan, A. R., & Turcott, R. G. (1990). Rate fluctuation and fractional power-law noise recorded from cells in the lower auditory pathway of the cat. *Hearing Research, 46,* 41–52.

Temoshok, L. (1987). Personality, coping style, emotions, and cancer: Toward an integrative model. *Cancer Surveys, 6*, 545–567.

Ten Dan, H. (1990). *Exploring reincarnation*. London: Penguin.

Terhardt, E. (1995). Music perception in the auditory hierarchy. In R. Steinberg (Ed.), *Music and the mind machine: The psychophysiology and psychopathology of the sense of music* (pp. 81–87). Berlin: Springer-Verlag.

Thaut, M. (1985). The use of auditory rhythm and rhythmic speech to aid temporal muscular control in children with gross motor dysfunction. *Journal of Music Therapy, 22* (3), 129–145.

Thaut, M. (1989). The influence of music therapy interventions on self-rated changes in relaxation, affect, and thought in psychiatric prisoner-patients. *Journal of Music Therapy, 26* (3), 155–166.

Thaut, M. (1990a). Neuropsychological processes in music perception and their relevance in music therapy. In R. Unkefer (Ed.), *Music therapy in the treatment of adults with mental disorders* (pp. 3–32). New York: Schirmer Books.

Thaut, M. (1990b). Physiological and motor responses to music stimuli. In R. Unkefer (Ed.), *Music therapy in the treatment of adults with mental disorders* (pp. 33–49). New York: Schirmer Books.

Thaut, M. (1997). Rhythmic auditory stimulation in rehabilitation of movement disorders: A review of current research. In D. J. Schneck & J. K. Schneck (Eds.), *Music in human adaptation* (pp. 223–230). Blacksburg: Virginia Polytechnic Institute and State University.

Thaut, M. (2000). *A scientific model of music in therapy and medicine*. St. Louis, MO: MMB Music, Inc.

Thaut, M. H., McIntosh, G. C., & Rice, R. R. (1997). Rhythmic facilitation of gait training in hemiparetic stroke rehabilitation. *Journal of Neurological Sciences, 151*, 207–212.

Thaut, M. H., McIntosh, G. C., Rice, R. R., Metler, R. A., Rathbun, J., & Brault, J. (1996). Rhythmic auditory stimulation in gait training with Parkinson's disease patients. *Movement Disorders, 11*, 193–200.

Thaut, M. H., McIntosh, G. C., Rice, R. R., & Prassas, S. G. (1993). Effect of rhythmic cueing on temporal stride parameters and EMG patterns in hemiparetic gait of stroke patients. *Journal of Neurologic Rehabilitation, 7*, 9–16.

Thaut, M. H., Miller, R. A., & Schauer, M. L. (1997). Rhythm in human motor control. In D. J. Schneck & J. K. Schneck (Eds.), *Music in human adaptation* (pp. 191–198). Blacksburg: Virginia Polytechnic Institute and State University.

Thaut, M. H., Schleiffers, S., & Davis, W. (1992). Changes in EMG patterns under the influence of auditory rhythm. In R. Spintge & R. Droh (Eds.), *Music medicine* (pp. 80–101). St. Louis, MO: MMB Music, Inc.

Thomas, L. (1974). *The lives of a cell: Notes of a biology watcher*. New York: Viking Press.

Thompson, W. I. (1976). *Evil and world order*. New York: Harper & Row.

Tiller, W. A. (1997). *Science and human transformation: Subtle energies, intentionality and consciousness*. Walnut Creek, CA: Pavior.

Tillich, P. (1959). *Theology of culture*. New York: Oxford University Press.

Timbergen, N. (1952). Derived activities: Their causation, biological significance, origin, and emancipation during evolution. *Quarterly Review of Biology, 27,* 127–132.

Tomaino, C. M. (Ed.). (1998). *Clinical applications of music in neurologic rehabilitation.* St. Louis, MO: MMB Music, Inc.

Tomatis, A. A. (1987). Ontogenesis of the faculty of listening. In T. R. Verny (Ed.), *Pre- and perinatal: An introduction* (pp. 23–35). New York: Van Nostrand Reinhold.

Tomatis, A. A. (1991). *The conscious ear.* Barrytown, NY: Station Hill Press.

Tombs, D. L. (1994). *Introduction to addictive behaviors.* New York: Guilford Press.

Torrance, D. J. (1980). *Encouraging creative learning for the gifted and talented: A handbook of methods and techniques.* Ventura, CA: Ventura County Superintendent of Schools.

Tortora, G. J., & Anagnostakos, N. P. (1987). *Principles of anatomy and physiology,* 5th ed. New York: Harper & Row.

Traub, R. D., Jeffreys, J. G. R., & Whittington, M. A. (1999). *Fast oscillations in cortical circuits.* Cambridge, MA: MIT Press.

Trauger-Query, B., & Haghighi, K. R. (1999). Balancing the focus: Art and music therapy for pain control and symptom management in hospice care. *Hospice Journal: Physical, Psychological and Pastoral Care of the Dying, 14* (1), 25–38.

Treffinger, D. J. (1983). Fostering creativity and problem solving. In *Documentary report of the Ann Arbor Symposium on the Applications of Psychology to the Teaching and Learning of Music: Session III* (pp. 55–59). Reston, VA: MENC.

Treitler, L. (1997). Language and the interpretation of music. In J. Robinson (Ed.), *Music and meaning* (pp. 23–56). Ithaca, NY: Cornell University Press.

Trevarthen, C. (1984). Emotions in infancy: Regulators of contact and relationships with persons. In K. Scherer & P. Ekman (Eds.), *Approaches to emotion* (pp. 129–157). Hillsdale, NJ: Erlbaum.

Tronick, E., & Adamson, L. (1980). *Babies as people: New findings on our social beginnings.* New York: Collier.

Tsao, C. C., Gordon, T. F., Maranto, C. D., Lerman, C., & Murasko, D. (1991). The effects of music and directed biological imagery on immune response (S-IgA). In C. Maranto (Ed.), *Applications of music in medicine* (pp. 85–121). Washington, DC: National Association for Music Therapy.

Turnbull, C. (1966). *Wayward servants.* Garden City, NY: Natural History.

Turnbull, D. (1992). Maps, perception, and reality. In B. Rubik (Ed.), *The interrelationship between mind and matter* (pp. 21–28). Philadelphia: Center for Frontier Sciences.

Turner, V. (1969). *The ritual process.* Ithaca, NY: Cornell University Press.

Turry, A. E. (1997). The use of clinical improvisation to alleviate procedural distress in young children. In J. V. Loewy (Ed.), *Music therapy and pediatric pain* (pp. 89–106). Cherry Hill, NJ: Jeffrey Books.

Tyler, P. E. (Ed.). (1975). Biological effects of non-ionizing radiation. Special issue, *Annals of New York Academy of Science, 24.*

Tyson, F. (1981). *Psychiatric music therapy: Origins and development.* New York: Fred Weidner & Sons Printers.

Ulfardsother, L. O., & Erwin, P. G. (1999). The influence of music on social cognitive skills. *The Arts in Psychotherapy, 26* (2), 81–84.

Underhill, D., & Harris, L. (1974). The effect of contingent music on establishing imitation in behaviorally retarded children. *Journal of Music Therapy, 11* (3), 156–166.

Underhill, R. (1938). *Singing for power: The song magic of the Papago Indians of southern Arizona.* Berkeley: University of California Press.

Unkefer, R. F. (1961). The music therapist. In E. H. Schneider (Ed.), *Music therapy 1960* (pp. 27–31). Lawrence, KS: Allen Press.

Unkefer, R. F. (Ed.). (1990). *Music therapy in the treatment of adults with mental disorders.* New York: Schirmer Books.

U.S. Special Committee on Aging. (1992). *Hearing testimony: Forever young, music and aging.* Washington, DC: U.S. Government Printing Office.

VanderArk, S., Newman, I., & Bell, S. (1983). The effects of music participation on quality of life of the elderly. *Music Therapy, 3* (1), 71–81.

VanderArk, S. D., & Ely, D. (1992). Biochemical and galvanic skin responses to music stimuli in biology and music. *Perceptual and Motor Skills, 74* (3 pt. 2), 1079–1090.

Vandervert, L. R. (1992). The emergence of brain and mind amid chaos through maximum evolution: World futures. *Journal of General Evolution, 33,* 253–273.

Vandervert, L. R. (1996). The fractal maximum-power. In E. MacCormac & M. I. Stamenov (Eds.), *Fractals of brain, fractals of mind* (pp. 235–271). Philadelphia: John Benjamins North America.

Van de Wall, W. (1936). *Music in initiations.* New York: Russell Sage Foundation.

Van Eenwyk, J. R. (1996). Chaotic dynamics. In F. MacCormac & M. I. Stamenov (Eds.), *Fractals of brain, fractals of mind* (pp. 322–346). Philadelphia: John Benjamins North America.

Vargas, A., & Koss-Chioino, D. (Eds.). (1992). *Working with culture: Psychotherapeutic interventions with ethnic minority children and adolescents.* San Francisco: Jossey-Bass.

Vaughan, F. (1980). Transpersonal psychotherapy: Context, content, and process. In R. N. Walsh & F. Vaughan (Eds.), *Beyond ego: Transpersonal dimensions in psychology* (pp. 182–189). Los Angeles: Jeremy P. Tarcher.

Vaughan, F. E. (1979). *Awaking intuition.* Garden City, NY: Anchor Press, Doubleday.

Vaughan, F. E. (1998). Multiple ways of knowing. *Noetic Sciences Review, 47,* 34–37.

Vaughan, M. (1971). An examination of music processes as related to creative thinking. *Journal of Research in Music Education, 19,* 35–37.

Verny, T. R. (Ed.). (1982). *Pre- and peri-natal psychology: An introduction.* New York: Van Nostrand Reinhold.

Verny, T. R., & Kelly, J. (1981). *The secret life of the unborn child.* New York: Delacorte.

Vescelius, E. A. (1918). Music and health. *The Musical Quarterly, 4* (3), 376–401.

Voss, R. F. (1989). Fractals in nature: From characterization to simulation. In H-O. Peitgen & D. Saupe (Eds.), *The science of fractal images* (pp. 21–70). Berlin: Springer-Verlag.

Voss, R. F., & Clark, J. (1975). 1/f noise in music and speech. *Nature, 258,* 317–318.

Voss, R. F., & Clark, J. (1978). 1/f noise in music: Music from 1/f noise. *Journal of the Acoustical Society of America, 63,* 258–263.

Wade, J. (1996). *Changes of mind: A holonomic theory of the evolution of consciousness.* Albany: State University of New York Press.

Wagner, M. J. (1975). Effects of music and biofeedback on alpha brainwaves, rhythm and attentiveness. *Journal of Research in Music Education, 23,* 3–13.

Wagner, M. J. (1994). *Introductory musical acoustics,* 3d ed. Raleigh, NC: Contemporary Publishing Co.

Wagner, M. J., & Menzel, M. B. (1977). The effect of music listening and attentiveness training on the EEGs of musicians and non-musicians. *Journal of Music Therapy, 14* (4), 151–164.

Wald, E. (1994, February 11). To the tune of an ancient therapy. *Boston Globe,* A21–A22.

Waldrop, M. M. (1992). *Complexity.* New York: Simon & Schuster.

Walker, J. (1995). Music therapy, spirituality and chemically dependent clients. *Journal of Chemical Dependency Treatment, 5* (2), 145–166.

Walker, J. B. (1972). The use of music as an aid in developing functional speech in the institutionalized mentally retarded. *Journal of Music Therapy, 9* (1), 1–12.

Wallin, N. L. (1991). *Biomusicology.* Stuyvesant, NY: Pendragon Press.

Wallin, N. L., Merker, B., & Brown, S. (Eds.). (2000). *The origins of music.* Cambridge, MA: MIT Press.

Walsh, R. (1979). Meditation research: An introduction and review. *Journal of Transpersonal Psychology, 11,* 161–174.

Walsh, R. (1983). Meditation practice and research. *Journal of Humanistic Psychology, 23* (1), 18–50.

Walsh, R. (1988). Two Asian psychologies and their implications for Western psychotherapies. *American Journal of Psychotherapy, 42* (4), 543–560.

Walsh, R. (1990). *The spirit of shamanism.* Los Angeles: Jeremy P. Tarcher.

Walsh, R. (1999). *Essential spirituality.* New York: John Wiley & Sons.

Walsh, R. (2002). The practices of essential spirituality. *Noetic Sciences Review, 58,* 9–15.

Walsh, R., & Vaughan, F. (1993). *Paths beyond ego: The transpersonal vision.* Los Angeles: Jeremy P. Tarcher.

Walsh, R. N., Elgin, D., Vaughan, F., & Wilber, K. (1980). Paradigms in collision. In R. N. Walsh & F. Vaughan (Eds.), *Beyond ego: Transpersonal dimensions in psychology* (pp. 36–53). Los Angeles: Jeremy P. Tarcher.

Walsh, R. N., & Vaughan, F. (Eds.) (1980). *Beyond ego: Transpersonal dimensions in psychology.* Los Angeles: Jeremy P. Tarcher.

Ward, D. (1993). Aesthetic education, therapy and children with special needs. In R. R. Pratt (Ed.), *Music therapy and music education for the handicapped* (pp. 112–124). St. Louis, MO: MMB Music, Inc.

Warja, M. (1994). Sounds of music through the spiraling path of individuation: A Jungian approach to music psychotherapy. *Music Therapy Perspectives, 12* (2), 75–83.

Washburn, M. (1995). *The ego and the dynamic ground,* 2d ed. Albany: State University of New York.

Watson, A., & Drury, N. (1987). *Healing music.* Bridport, England: Prism Press.

Webster, P. (1983, December). Refinement of a measure of musical imagination in young children and a comparison to aspects of musical aptitude. Paper presented at the Armington Symposium, Case Western Reserve University.

Webster, P. (2001). Creative thinking in music. *Music Educators Journal, 88,* 19–23.

Weil, A. (1972). *The natural mind.* Boston: Houghton Mifflin.

Weiler, C. (1995). Recovery from Werniche's aphasia: A positron emission topographic study. *Annals of Neurology, 37,* 723–732.

Weinberg, H., Stroink, G., & Kalila, T. (1988). *Biomagnetism: Applications and theory.* New York: Pergamon Press.

Weinberger, N. M. (1993). Music, the brain, and science. NAMM news special report. Reston, VA: National Association of Music Merchants.

Weinstock, C. (1977). Notes on "spontaneous" regression of cancer. *American Society of Psychosomatic Dentistry and Medicine, 24* (4), 106–110.

Wells, D. R. (1970). Dynamic stability of closed plasma configurations. *Journal of Plasma Physiology, 4,* 654.

Wertheim, N. (1977). Is there an anatomical localization for musical facilities? In M. Crutchley & R. Henson (Eds.), *Music and the brain* (pp. 282–297). London: Heinemann Medical Books.

Wesley, S. (1998–1999). Music, Jung and making meaning. *Journal of the Association for Music and Imagery, 6,* 3–14.

West, B. J., & Goldberger, A. L. (1987). Physiology in fractal dimensions. *American Science, 75,* 354–365.

West, M. (Ed.) (1987). *The psychology of meditation.* Oxford: Clarendon Press.

Westgate, G. E. (1996). Spiritual wellness and depression. *Journal of Counseling and Development, 75,* 26–35.

Wheeler, B. L. (1981). The relationship between music therapy and theories of psychotherapy. *Music Therapy, 1* (1), 9–16.

Wheeler, B. L. (1987). Levels of therapy: The classification of music therapy goals. *Music Therapy, 6* (2), 39–49.

Wheeler, B. L. (Ed.). (1995). *Music therapy research.* Phoenixville, PA: Barcelona Publishers.

Wheeler, C. P. (2003). Chaos theory in psychology: A practical application of music therapy as a potential treatment for PTSD. Unpublished M.A. thesis, Walden University, Minneapolis.

Whelan, J. (1999). American soul. *Noetic Sciences Review, 48,* 22–31.

Whipple, J., & Lindsey, R. S. (1999). Music for the soul: A music therapy program for battered women. *Music Therapy Perspectives, 17* (1), 61–67.

White, J. M. (1997). Effects of relaxing music on cardiac autonomic balance and anxiety following acute myocardial infarction. *Dissertation Abstracts International, 57* (11), 6856B (University Microfilms No. AAM 9711866).

White, J. M. (1999). Effects of relaxing music on cardiac autonomic balance and anxiety after acute myocardial infarction. *American Journal of Critical Care Nursing, 8* (4), 220–230.

Whitmont, E. C. (1994a). *The alchemy of healing: Psyche and soma.* Berkeley, CA: North Atlantic Books.

Whitmont, E. C. (1994b). Form and information. *Noetic Sciences Review, 31,* 11–18.

Wigram, T. (1997). The development of vibroacoustic therapy. In T. Wigram & C. Dileo (Eds.), *Music vibration* (pp. 11–26). Cherry Hill, NJ: Jeffrey Books.

Wigram, T., & Dileo, C. (Eds.). (1997). *Music vibration.* Cherry Hill, NJ: Jeffrey Books.

Wigram, T., Saperston, B., & West, R. J. (Eds.). (1995). *The art and science of music therapy: A handbook.* Chur, Switzerland: Harwood Academic Publishers.

Wilber, K. (1977). *The spectrum of consciousness.* Wheaton, IL: Theosophical Publishing House.

Wilber, K. (1982). *The holographic paradigm and other paradoxes.* Boston: Shambhala.

Wilber, K. (1986). The spectrum of development. In K. Wilber, J. Engler, & D. P. Brown (Eds.), *Transformations of consciousness* (pp. 66–105). Boston: Shambhala.

Wilber, K. (1990). *Eye to eye: The quest for the new paradigm.* Boston: Shambhala.

Wilber, K. (1996). *A brief history of everything.* Boston: Shambhala.

Wilber, K. (1998). *The marriage of sense and soul.* New York: Random House.

Wilber, K. (1999). *One taste: The journals of Ken Wilber.* Boston: Shambhala.

Wilber, K., Engler, J., & Brown, D. P. (Eds.) (1986). *Transformations of consciousness.* Boston: Shambhala.

Wilkes, J. (1993). Flow design research relating to flowforms. In W. Forward & A. Wolpert (Eds.), *Chaos, rhythm and flow in nature* (pp. 72–84). Edinburgh: Floris Books.

Williams, C. B., Frame, M. W., & Green, E. (1994). Counseling groups of African American women: A focus on spirituality. *Journal for Specialists in Group Work, 24* (3), 260–273.

Williams, G. P. (1997). *Chaos theory tamed.* Washington, DC: Joseph Henry Press.

Wilson, B. J. (Ed.). (2002). *Models of music therapy interventions in school settings.* Silver Spring, MD: American Music Therapy Association.

Wilson, C. V. (1976). The use of rock music as a reward in behavior therapy with children. *Journal of Music Therapy, 13* (1), 39–48.

Wilson, C. W., & Hopkins, B. L. (1973). The effects of contingent music on the intensity of noise in junior high school home economics classes. *Journal of Applied Behavior Analysis, 6,* 269–276.

Wilson, E. S. (1993a). A technical report. In R. Russell (Ed.), *Using the whole brain: Integrating the right and left brain with Hemi-Sync sound patterns* (pp. 227–230). Norfolk, VA: Hampton Roads Publishing Co.

Wilson, E. S. (1993b). The transits of consciousness. In R. Russell (Ed.), *Using the whole brain: Integrating the right and left brain with Hemi-Sync sound patterns* (pp. 193–203). Norfolk, VA: Hampton Roads Publishing Co.

Wilson, F. R. (1986). *Tone deaf and all thumbs?* New York: Viking Penguin.

Wilson, F. R., & Roehmann, F. L. (Eds.). (1990). *Music and child development*. St. Louis, MO: MMB Music, Inc.

Winckel, F. (1967). *Music, sound and sensation*. New York: Dover Publications.

Winkelman, M. (1991a). Physiological and therapeutic aspects of shamanic healing. *Subtle Energies, 1,* 1–18.

Winkelman, M. (1991b). Therapeutic effects of hallucinogens. *Anthropology of Consciousness, 2* (3–4), 15–19.

Winkelman, M. (1996). Psychointegrator plants: Their roles in human culture and health. In M. Winkelman & W. Andritzky (Eds.), *Yearbook of cross-cultural medicine and psychotherapy, 1995,* vol. 6 (pp. 9–52). Berlin: Verlag & Vertrieb.

Winkelman, M. (2000). *Shamanism: The neural ecology of consciousness and healing*. Westport, CT: Bergin & Garvey.

Winkelman, M. (2003). Complementary therapy for addiction: "Drumming out drugs." *American Journal of Public Health, 93* (4), 647–651.

Winkelman, M., & Andritzky, W. (Eds.). (1996). *Yearbook of cross-cultural medicine and psychotherapy, 1995,* vol. 6. Berlin: Verlag & Vertrieb.

Winner, W. (1982). *Invented worlds*. Cambridge, MA: Harvard University Press.

Winson, J. (1985). *Brain and psyche: The biology of the unconscious*. New York: Vintage Books.

Wise, A. (2002). *Awakening the mind: A guide to mastering the power of your brain waves*. New York: Jeremy P. Tarcher.

Wise, G., Hartmann, D., & Fisher, B. (1992). Exploration of the relationship between choral singing and successful aging. *Psychology Reports, 70,* 1175–1183.

Wisneski, L. A. (2000). Psychoneuroimmunology: From biochemistry to energy medicine. *Subtle Energy, 11* (1), 23–41.

Wittrock, M. C. (Ed). (1977). *The human brain*. Englewood Cliffs, NJ: Prentice Hall.

Wolf, F. A. (1986). *The body quantum*. New York: Macmillan.

Wolf, F. A. (1989). *Taking the quantum leap: The new physics for nonscientists,* 2d ed. New York: HarperCollins.

Wolf, F. A. (1999). *The spiritual universe: One physicist's vision of spirit, soul, matter, and self*. Portsmouth, NH: Moment Point Press, Inc.

Wolfe, D. E., & Horn, C. (1993). Use of melodies as structural prompts for learning and retention of sequential verbal information by pre-school students. *Journal of Music Therapy, 30* (2), 100–118.

Wolman, B. O., & Ullman, M. (1986). *Handbook of states of consciousness*. New York: Van Nostrand Rheinhold.

Woodman, M. (1993). Stepping over the threshold. *Noetic Sciences Review* (Winter), 10–15.

Woodward, S. C., Guidozzi, F., Hofmeyer, G. J., Dijong, P., Anthony, J., & Woods, D. (1992). Discoveries in fetal and neonatal worlds of music. In H. Lees (Ed.), *Music education: Sharing musics of the world* (pp. 58–66). New Zealand: University of Canterbury.

Wright, P. A. (1995). The interconnectivity of mind, brain, and behavior in altered states of consciousness: Focus on shamanism. *Alternative Therapies in Health and Medicine, 1* (3), 50–56.

Yalom, I. D. (1985). *The theory and practice of group psychotherapy.* London: Basic Books.

Yamadori, A., Osumi, Y., Masuhara, S., & Okubo, M. (1977). Preservation of singing in Broca's aphasics. *Journal of Neurology, Neurosurgery and Psychiatry, 40,* 221–224.

Yarbough, C., Charboneau, M., & Wapnich, J. (1977). Music as reinforcement for correct math and attending in ability assigned math class. *Journal of Music Therapy, 14* (2), 77–88.

Yates, R. E. (1980). Physical causality and brain theories. *American Journal of Physiology, 238,* R277.

Zatorri, R. J., Evans, A. C., & Meyer, E. (1994). Neural mechanisms underlying melodic perception and memory for pitch. *Journal of Neuroscience, 14,* 1908–1919.

Zelazny, C. M. (2001). Therapeutic instrumental music playing in hand rehabilitation for older adults with osteoarthritis: Four case studies. *Journal of Music Therapy, 38* (2), 97–113.

Zukav, G. (1979). *The dancing Wu Li masters.* New York: Bantam Books.

Zukav, G. (1989). *The seat of the soul.* New York: Simon & Schuster.

Index

1/f spectrum, xviii, 43, 64, 93–94, 219;
    brain functioning and, 124, 128–29;
    content of healing and, 184, 191;
    DNA and, 181; emotion and, 243;
    intelligence and, 156; low-frequency
    sound, 129; memory and, 151;
    perception and, 128; rhythm and, 64,
    223; sleep and, 146. See also fractal
    structure

acoustical energy, 203, 211
acoustic reflex, 58
acoustic waves, 55, 206, 211, 213
action potential, 104
activity interventions, 10–11, 13–21;
    behavior reinforcement, 20–21;
    composing music and songs, 16–17;
    movement to music/dance, 17; music
    activity therapy, 16; music-based
    discussion, 21; music combined with
    other art forms, 17–18; music
    performance/skill building, 15–16;
    neurological interventions, 20; process-
    oriented, 11–12, 18–21; product-
    oriented, 14–18. See also improvisation
acupuncture, 184, 204

Adagio for Strings (Barber), 68–69
adaptive ability, 155–56
addictions, 325–30
adolescents, 23, 248–49, 289
Aescelepius, temple of, 283–84, 318
aesthetic judgment, 353–54
aesthetic response, 77–78, 274–76, 297
affect, 140, 238, 263
affiliation, 298–99
after potential, 104
aging process, 194–95. See also older
    adults
AIDS, 331
Alcoholics Anonymous, 328–29
alertness, 110, 167, 215
altered states of consciousness (ASC),
    151, 176, 209–10; brain structures and,
    314–15; dreams and imagery, 320–23;
    human spirit and, 293; meditation,
    323–25; relaxed wakefulness, 306;
    spirit and, 308–17; transcendence,
    273–76
Alvin, Juliette, 11
Alzheimer's disease, 20, 22, 99, 125, 175
American Association for Music Therapy,
    11

~

About the Author

Barbara J. Crowe, MT-BC, has been director of music therapy at Arizona State University since 1981, having held a similar position at Indiana University–Purdue University at Fort Wayne from 1977 until 1981. She holds a bachelor's degree (1973) and master's degree (1977) in music therapy from Michigan State University, and completed her clinical internship at Ypsilanti State Hospital in Michigan. Her clinical experience in music therapy includes work with adolescents with emotional disturbances at the University of Michigan Neuropsychiatric Institute and adolescents with moderate mental retardation at the Beekman School in Lansing, Michigan, and consulting with music therapy in geriatric care in Fort Wayne, Indiana, and Phoenix, Arizona. Professor Crowe's research interests include the historical antecedents of modern music therapy and the theoretical foundations of music therapy practice. She has published numerous articles in periodicals such as the *German Journal of Music Therapy* and a chapter in *Music: Physician for Times to Come* by Don Campbell. She presents extensively at conferences and workshops for associations such as the Academy of Osteopathic Physicians and the International Society for the Study of Subtle Energy and Energy Medicine. Professor Crowe is past president of the National Association for Music Therapy and was executive director of the Rhythm for Life Project from 1992 to 1996.